Outline of Ortho...ary

for you, wherever you are

For Elsevier:

Commissioning Editor: Alison Taylor/Laurence Hunter
Development Editor: Helen Leng
Project Manager: Elouise Ball
Designer/Design Direction: Kirsteen Wright
Illustration Manager: Bruce Hogarth

Adams's
Outline of Orthopaedics

David L Hamblen
PhD DSc FRCS (Edinburgh, England, Glasgow)

Emeritus Professor of Orthopaedic Surgery,
University of Glasgow
Visiting Professor University of Strathclyde,
Glasgow, UK

A Hamish R W Simpson
DM(Oxon) FRCS(Ed & England)

Professor of Orthopaedics and Trauma,
University of Edinburgh, UK

Contributor
Nigel Raby
MRCP FRCR

Consultant Musculoskeletal Radiologist,
Western Infirmary, Glasgow

Fourteenth Edition

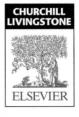

CHURCHILL
LIVINGSTONE

ELSEVIER

EDINBURGH LONDON NEW YORK OXFORD PHILADELPHIA ST LOUIS SYDNEY
TORONTO 2010

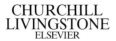

First edition 1956   Eighth edition 1976
Second edition 1958   Ninth edition 1981
Third edition 1960   Tenth edition 1986
Fourth edition 1961   Eleventh edition 1990
Fifth edition 1964   Twelfth edition 1995
Sixth edition 1967   Thirteenth edition 2001
Seventh edition 1971   Fourteenth edition 2010

ISBN 9780702030611
International ISBN 9780702030604

British Library Cataloguing in Publication Data
A catalogue record for this book is available from the British Library

Library of Congress Cataloging in Publication Data
A catalog record for this book is available from the Library of Congress

Notice
Neither the publisher nor the authors assume any responsibility for any loss or injury and/or damage to persons or property arising out of or related to any use of the material contained in this book. It is the responsibility of the treating practitioner, relying on independent expertise and knowledge of the patient, to determine the best treatment and method of application for the patient.

The Publisher

Printed in China

 your source for books,
journals and multimedia
in the health sciences
www.elsevierhealth.com

Working together to grow
libraries in developing countries

www.elsevier.com | www.bookaid.org | www.sabre.org

ELSEVIER   BOOK AID International   Sabre Foundation

The publisher's policy is to use
paper manufactured from sustainable forests

Preface

This new 14th edition of *Outline of Orthopaedics* is the first without the direct input of John Crawford Adams. It appears just over 50 years from the publication of his first edition of this book and its companion volume *Outline of Fractures*. To mark this remarkable achievement it was decided to add his name to both titles, which still contain evidence of his lucid writing style and clear illustrative line drawings. His original aim of providing a broader coverage of orthopaedic diseases and their diagnosis and treatment than that required for undergraduate examinations has been preserved. We make no apology for this, since musculoskeletal disorders now make up at least 20% of the clinical material presenting to primary care. This book should provide a valuable reference tool for general practitioners, physiotherapists, orthopaedic nurses, and basic surgical trainees, as well as instructing the undergraduate medical student.

The broad arrangement of material into three parts; clinical methods, a general survey of orthopaedic disorders, and regional orthopaedics, has been retained in the new edition. All the text has now been put into the same standard font size which should ease the task of the reader. To make space for this change without enlarging the book to a cumbersome size, we decided to eliminate the literature references previously included. It was felt that these are now more readily available in an up-to-date digital format using computer technology. We have also eliminated some of the duplication of material in the regional chapters where this has already been covered in the general survey of Part 2.

Professor Hamish Simpson, the co-author for the latest edition of *Outline of Fractures*, has now joined the editorial team for this revision of *Outline of Orthopaedics*. His input has provided valuable material on the fast-changing nature of today's orthopaedic practice. We also welcome the collaboration of Dr Nigel Raby, who has contributed a new expanded chapter on the role of imaging in orthopaedic diagnosis and treatment. This development probably represents the most important change to orthopaedic practice in the past ten years and has revolutionised clinical care. The danger is that these sophisticated investigations may also be used as a substitute for the clinical skills of history taking and physical examination of the patient. Without this, other co-morbid conditions may be missed and the opportunity to make a provisional diagnosis allowing more focused investigation may be lost. With the assistance of Dr Raby and other clinical collaborators we have been able to include a large number of new illustrations to replace and enhance some of the older redundant images. We hope that the new edition, while retaining the strength of its predecessors, will provide today's trainees, whether undergraduate or postgraduate, with a broad overview of the constantly expanding field of orthopaedic surgery.

David L Hamblen
Hamish Simpson
2010

Acknowledgements

The authors must first pay tribute to the original author, John Crawford Adams, whose inspiration and enthusiasm produced the original volume and steered it through twelve further editions. The success the book has enjoyed for over 50 years is a tribute to his writing skills which have provided us with a sound base on which to develop this new edition.

A major contribution to the latest revision has come from Dr Nigel Raby, Radiologist at the Western Infirmary, Glasgow, who has written the new chapter on 'Imaging in Orthopaedics' and co-edited the material on bone and soft tissue tumours. In addition he has supplied a large number of new and replacement radiographs and scans in many of the other chapters to reflect the advances in this field of investigation. Because of the increasing specialisation within orthopaedics we have had to seek help from other clinical colleagues to fill gaps in the illustrative material. For this we thank Dr Robin Reid, Dr Martin Sambrook, Mr Nick Geary, Mr Thanos Tsirikos, and Mr Graham Lawson. Thanks also go to Dr Helen Frost for editing and updating the material on the role of physiotherapy in treatment. We acknowledge the assistance of Morag Macleod and the staff at the National Centre for Prosthetics and Orthotics, University of Strathclyde, for supplying the pictures of patient appliances and prostheses.

Particular thanks are due to Helen Leng, our Development Editor, who has shown great patience and understanding in accommodating our frequent and confusing alterations to the text and figures. We are also grateful to all the staff at Elsevier for all their help and encouragement in the production of this new edition.

Our respective secretaries Catherine Davidson and Linda Digance have played a key role in the typing of the manuscript and their efforts are very much appreciated.

Finally we record our appreciation for the support and forbearance of our wives and families during the time devoted to the writing of the book, which might otherwise have been spent in their company.

David L Hamblen
Hamish Simpson

Note by
John Crawford Adams

Outline of Orthopaedics evolved from bedside teaching of medical students over many years. Despite inevitable flaws and omissions in the original version, the book proved popular and revised editions were called for every few years. Indeed, so many changes have been made in successive editions that the present one is hardly recognisable as the same book.

In the half century that has elapsed since the book was first published there has been spectacular progress in the practice of orthopaedic surgery – more so than in most other branches of surgery. One field in which developments have been particularly striking is that concerned with diagnostic procedures. Notable among the sophisticated refinements that now make diagnosis easier, more accurate, and substantially less traumatic for the patient include image intensification; computerised tomographic scanning; magnetic resonance imaging, contrast radiography; ultrasound scanning; radio-isotope scanning; and interventional radiology using intra-arterial cannulas. These diagnostic methods, together with techniques of direct inspection of the inside of joints or other cavities (arthroscopy, endoscopy) have nearly all been introduced or greatly refined since this book was first published.

In the field of operative surgery the development of total replacement arthroplasty – at first confined mainly to the hip – was the most spectacular landmark. For several decades surgeons had striven to create a mobile artificial hip joint, but success generally eluded them and forced them to rely mainly upon arthrodesis for relief of arthritic pain. Only when a two-part (ball and socket) prosthesis of special metal, or metal and plastic, was developed was successful arthroplasty achieved. The technique was refined very quickly and was soon extended to the knee and other joints. Today many thousands of replacement arthroplasties are undertaken every year in Britain alone.

Another major surgical landmark in the last half century was the refinement of arthroscopic examination of major joints – at first mainly the knee – which led naturally to the development of arthroscopic surgery. This proved so successful – at first in the knee – that open operations for damaged semilunar cartilages and ligaments of the knee were soon almost wholly superseded. At the same time minimal access surgery was extended to other sites – notably the spine – as well as to the separate fields of abdominal and gynaecological surgery. These major developments are still relatively new: hardly mentioned in the earliest editions of this book half a century ago.

One of the consequences of these developments has been a trend for surgeons to concentrate on a particular field of surgery – for instance hip surgery, knee surgery, spine surgery or hand surgery – while largely abandoning other fields to their colleagues. While this trend towards "super-specialisation" may be generally applauded, care must be taken to ensure that it does not go too far, to the point where a surgeon, initially trained in general orthopaedic techniques, becomes incapable of undertaking routine work.

Note by John Crawford Adams

The stage has already been reached at which it is no longer practicable for a single author to undertake the production of a book covering the whole range of orthopaedic surgery. Some degree of collaboration is clearly desirable, and it is with much pleasure that I now hand over this work to the capable hands of Professor David Hamblen, my long-term co-author, and Professor Hamish Simpson, his new collaborator.

John Crawford Adams

Note on terminology

The anatomical nomenclature used in this book conforms to that recommended by the International Anatomical Nomenclature Committee and approved at the Eighth International Congress of Anatomists at Wiesbaden in 1965. This nomenclature, which differs only in minor respects from the earlier Birmingham revision of the Basle nomenclature, has been adopted at most schools of anatomy and it is to be hoped that it will become the standard terminology acceptable to anatomists and surgeons alike.

The recommended method of recording and expressing joint movement conforms to that laid down by the American Academy of Orthopaedic Surgeons in the booklet *Joint Motion* published by the Academy in 1965 (reprinted 1966), and approved by most of the Orthopaedic Associations of the English-speaking world. (See also McRae, R. (2003): *Clinical Orthopaedic Examination*, 5th edn. Edinburgh: Churchill Livingstone.) The guiding principle of the method is that for any joint the extended 'anatomical position' is regarded as zero degrees (0°), and movement at the joint is measured from this starting position. For example, in the knee the straight position is described as 0° and the fully flexed position is expressed as (say) 145 degrees (145°) of flexion; likewise at the elbow. At the ankle the anatomical position, with the foot at a right angle to the leg, is the zero position, from which plantarflexion and dorsiflexion (extension) are measured.

The Academy booklet also gives figures for the normal range of movement at each joint. In some instances these do not accord with authors' experience and they have not always been followed in this text. Individual variations are common, so that any statement of the normal must necessarily be imprecise.

Contents

Introduction

The orthopaedic surgeon today is concerned with diseases and injuries of the trunk and limbs. His field is not confined to the bones and joints; it includes in addition the muscles, tendons, ligaments, bursae, nerves, and blood vessels. He is not concerned with injuries of the skull, which fall within the province of the neurosurgeon; or with injuries of the jaws, which are the responsibility of the facio-maxillary or dental surgeon.

The term orthopaedic is derived from the Greek words ορθοζ (straight) and παιζ (child). It was originally applied to the art of correcting deformities by Nicolas Andry, a French physician, who in 1741 published a book entitled *Orthopaedia: Or the Art of Correcting and Preventing Deformities in Children: By such Means, as may easily be put in Practice by Parents themselves, and all such as are Employed in Educating Children.*

In Andry's time orthopaedic surgery in the form known today did not exist. Surgery was still primitive. Indeed, except for sporadic attempts by ingenious individuals, it is probable that little real progress had been made since the days of Hippocrates, who lived in about 400 BC.

That is not to say that surgeons were unintelligent or that they lacked a capacity for careful study and research. Early writings prove that many of them were shrewd observers, and from the time of John Hunter (1728–1793) onwards this was increasingly true. Take, for example, the words of Sir Astley Cooper (1768–1841) in his *Treatise on Dislocations and Fractures of the Joints*: 'Nothing is known in our profession by guess; and I do not believe, that from the first dawn of medical science to the present moment, a single correct idea has ever emanated from conjecture. It is right, therefore, that those who are studying their profession should be aware that there is no short road to knowledge; that observations on the diseased living, examinations of the dead, and experiments upon living animals are the only sources of true knowledge; and that inductions from these are the sole basis of legitimate theory.'

The enthusiasm and the capacity for study were there. The real obstacle to progress was the lack of the essential facilities that we now take so much for granted – anaesthesia, asepsis, powerful microscopes, and X-rays. Any surgical operation that could not be completed within a few minutes was out of the question when the patient's consciousness could be clouded only by intoxication or exsanguination. And when every major operation was inevitably followed by suppuration which often proved fatal, it is small wonder that operations were seldom advised except in an attempt to save life.

Thus orthopaedic surgery, until relatively recent times, was confined largely to the correction of deformities by rather crude pieces of apparatus, to the reduction of fractures and dislocations by powerful traction, and to amputation of limbs (Fig. 1).

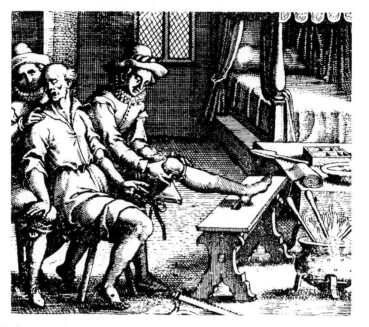

Fig.1 A seventeenth century amputation scene. (From Fabricus: *Opera*, 1646.)

LANDMARKS OF SURGERY IN THE NINETEENTH CENTURY

Fundamental advances in surgery were in fact dependent upon the development of other branches of science and of industry which provided, for instance, the high-powered microscope and the X-ray tube. It is therefore not surprising that, after centuries of stagnation, the facilities that were lacking were all made available within the span of a single life-time, at the period of the Industrial Revolution.

The first epoch-making advance was the introduction of anaesthesia. The credit for this should be given jointly to Crawford Long, of Athens, Georgia, who was the first to use ether in 1842 but delayed publication of his observations for seven years; and to W.T.G. Morton, of Boston, Massachusetts, whose use of ether anaesthesia was reported in 1846.

A few years later Louis Pasteur (1822–1895), working in Paris and equipped at last with an adequate microscope, was carrying out his fundamental research on bacteria as a cause of disease. Then in 1867 Joseph Lister (1827–1912), working in Glasgow, Scotland, on the basis of Pasteur's work introduced his antiseptic surgical technique which allowed the surgeon, for the first time in history, to look for primary healing of his operation wounds. Finally, in 1896, came Roentgen's report from Würzburg in Germany of his discovery of X-rays, which within a short time were put to practical use in surgical diagnosis.

THE EMERGENCE OF ORTHOPAEDICS AS A DISTINCT SPECIALITY

Thus at the dawn of the 20th century the stage was set for the phenomenally rapid evolution of surgery that has been witnessed by many still alive today. With the consequent widening of the scope of surgical practice orthopaedic surgery, at first encompassed by the general surgeon, began to branch off as a distinct science and art; but it was not until after the First World War that it came to be widely recognised as a separate speciality.

In Great Britain many of the fundamental principles of orthopaedics had been propounded, just before the 20th century began, by Hugh Owen Thomas[1] (1834–1891) of Liverpool. Thomas was not primarily concerned with operative surgery but rather with manipulative surgery and with conservative methods such as rest and splintage, and it was left to his nephew, Sir Robert Jones (1857–1933) to set orthopaedic surgery upon the sound foundation that it now enjoys. During and after the First World War Robert Jones trained many of the surgeons, British and American, who were among the first to devote their professional lives entirely to the practice of orthopaedics.

THE PRESENT

The second half of the 20th century saw major technological advances in biomaterials, instrumentation, and diagnostic techniques. These have had a major impact on the practice of orthopaedic surgery, particularly in the development of reliable methods for joint replacement in the treatment of arthritis. The results have been spectacular for the major joints of the hip and knee, where success rates are better than 90% after 10 years, even in the younger patient. This success has brought its own problems, with an increasing demand for complex and expensive revision surgery in the few patients who develop late failure with implant loosening and bone destruction.

Another significant advance has been the development of microsurgical techniques, allowing the anastomosis or repair of very small blood vessels and nerves, and thus facilitating the transfer of living tissue – whether skin or bone or nerve – from one site to another, and even the replacement of severed parts. Major advances have been made in the field of arthroscopy and arthroscopic surgery, allowing patients the benefits of minimally invasive surgery on most of the major joints in both upper and lower limbs. This has dramatically reduced the time patients spend in a hospital bed, and in many cases allows operations to be carried out as day case procedures with reduced morbidity and a more rapid return to normal function.

At the same time, orthopaedic surgeons – particularly in Western countries – have seen the virtual elimination of many diseases that were formerly prevalent, notably tuberculosis, poliomyelitis, tertiary syphilis, and rickets. The reduction in infective disease owes much to the advent of more powerful antibiotics, but their widespread use – particularly for prophylaxis in surgical operations – has resulted in an alarming increase in the emergence of resistant strains of bacteria. If this trend continues the risk of severe infection as a feared post-operative complication may again become a factor in limiting surgical treatment.

[1] Thomas's name is remembered in the widely used Thomas's knee splint and in Thomas's test for fixed flexion at the hip.

THE FUTURE

The limits to the development of improved technology and biomaterials for orthopaedic surgery may now have been reached. As a result there has been an increasing interest in methods for restoring normal tissues, as an alternative to replacing them. This will require new developments in the field of tissue engineering to allow composites of cultured autogenous or donor stem cells to be combined with a synthetic biodegradable matrix to repair bone and articular cartilage. Surgical skill will still be required to provide access to bones and joints for their repair, but this will need to be combined with an increased knowledge in the new disciplines of molecular biology and cell genetics. At the same time the completion of the project to map the entire human genome has enabled scientists to identify the genetic basis for many of the diseases which affect the musculoskeletal system. This new knowledge of the DNA make up of genes can be combined with the techniques of molecular biology to produce 'designer drugs', such as the recombinant bone morphogenetic proteins (BMPs) now being used to stimulate bone healing in difficult clinical situations. Other monoclonal antibodies are now widely available and used to enhance diagnostic and imaging techniques in orthopaedics.

The aim must be to consolidate the new knowledge gained and to develop an even more sound clinical judgement, so that in devising treatment for our patients we do the right thing at the right time. 'Get it right first time' should be the slogan. This is still quite a challenge; the challenge that adds to the fascination of orthopaedic surgery.

REFERENCES AND BIBLIOGRAPHY

Titles printed in italics refer to books or monographs; those in roman type refer to papers in journals.

Andry, N. (1741, reprod. 1961): *Orthopaedia*. Philadelphia: Lippincott.

Bigelow, H. J. (1846): Insensibility during surgical operations produced by inhalation. Boston Medical and Surgical Journal, **35**, 309.

Cooper, A. (1823): *Treatise on Dislocations and Fractures of the Joints*, 2nd edn. London: Longmans [etc.].

Dubos, R. J. (1951): *Louis Pasteur: Freelance of Science*. London: Gollancz.

Evans, C.H. & Rosier, R.N. (2005): Molecular biology in orthopaedics: the advent of molecular orthopaedics. Journal of Bone and Joint Surgery, **87A**, 2550.

Jones, A. Rocyn (1948): Hugh Owen Thomas. Journal of Bone and Joint Surgery, **30B**, 547.

Jones, A. Rocyn (1948): Lister. Journal of Bone and Joint Surgery, **30B**, 196.

Jones, A. Rocyn (1948): John Hunter. Journal of Bone and Joint Surgery, **30B**, 357.

Jones, A. Rocyn (1956): A review of orthopaedic surgery in Britain. Journal of Bone and Joint Surgery, **38B**, 27.

Lister, J. (1867): On the antiseptic principle in the practice of surgery. Lancet, **2**, 353.

Long, C. W. (1849): An account of the first use of sulphuric ether by inhalation as an anaesthetic in surgical operations. Southern Medical and Surgical Journal, **5**, 705.

Mayer, L. (1950): Orthopaedic surgery in the United States of America. Journal of Bone and Joint Surgery, **32B**, 461.

Morrey, B. (2003): *Joint Replacement Arthroplasty*. 3rd edn. Philadelphia: Churchill Livingstone.

Morton, W. T. G. (Quoted by Bigelow; see above).

Morton, W. T. G: Letheon [a circular]. Boston: Dutton & Wentworth.

Osmond-Clarke, H. (1950): Half a century of orthopaedic progress in Great Britain. Journal of Bone and Joint Surgery, **32B**, 620.

Platt, H. (1950): Orthopaedics in Continental Europe, 1900–50. Journal of Bone and Joint Surgery, **32B**, 570.

Röntgen, W. C. (1896): On a new kind of rays. Nature, **53**, 274, 377.

Part 1

PRINCIPLES OF DIAGNOSIS AND TREATMENT

In this part guidance is given on the correct line of approach to an orthopaedic problem, with particular reference to diagnosis and treatment.

As in all branches of medicine and surgery, proficiency in diagnosis can be acquired only from long experience. There is no short cut to a familiarity with physical signs or to skill in radiographic interpretation. Nevertheless the inexperienced surgeon who tackles the problem methodically step by step will often achieve a better result than a more experienced colleague who makes a 'snap' diagnosis after no more than a cursory investigation.

The essential clinical skills to obtain an adequate differential diagnosis remain the ability to take a careful history and perform an appropriate physical examination. The dramatic improvements in imaging techniques and other sophisticated investigations, though valuable, should not be allowed to replace these vital preliminary steps. Instead they should be used in a more efficient and cost-effective manner to complement and refine the clinical diagnostic skills. To reflect the increased importance of imaging, a new chapter has been added describing the range of methods available and their role in diagnosing and facilitating the treatment of orthopaedic disease. It is also worth noting the expansion of arthroscopy as a diagnostic tool for viewing the internal structure of most of the larger joints of the limbs, in addition to its use in treatment.

In the choice of treatment, whether conservative or surgical, the development of a sound judgement is also largely a matter of experience. Yet more than that is needed. Other essential qualities are common sense and a sympathetic appreciation of human problems. There are surgeons who never acquire a sound judgement, however long their apprenticeship. Others seem to have a natural aptitude that quickly matures under proper guidance and training.

1

Clinical methods of history taking and examination

As in other fields of medicine and surgery, diagnosis of orthopaedic disorders depends first upon an accurate determination of all the abnormal features from:

1. the history
2. clinical examination
3. radiographic examination and other methods of imaging
4. special investigations.

Secondly, it depends upon a correct interpretation of the findings.

HISTORY TAKING

In the diagnosis of orthopaedic conditions the history is often of first importance. In cases of torn meniscus in the knee, for instance, the clinical diagnosis sometimes depends upon the history alone. Except in the most obvious conditions, a detailed history is always required.

First the exact nature of the patient's complaint is determined. Then the development of the symptoms is traced step by step from their earliest beginning up to the time of the consultation. The patient's own views on the cause of the symptoms are always worth recording: often they prove to be correct. Enquiry is made into activities that have been found to improve the symptoms or to make them worse, and into the effect of any previous treatment. Facts that often have an important bearing on the condition are the age and present occupation of the patient, previous occupations, hobbies and recreational activities, and previous injuries.

When a full history of the local symptoms has been obtained, do not omit to enquire whether there have been symptoms in other parts of the body, and whether the general health is affected. Ask also about previous illnesses.

Finally, in cases that seem trivial, a tactful enquiry as to why the patient decided to seek advice, and to what extent he is worried by his disability, will often give a valuable clue to the underlying problem. It should be remembered that very often patients seek advice not because they are handicapped by a disability (which is often insignificant) but because they fear the development of some serious disease such as cancer, paralysis, or progressive crippling deformity.

CLINICAL EXAMINATION

The part complained of is examined according to a rigid routine which should become habitual. If this is done, familiarity with the routine will ensure that no step in the examination is forgotten. Accuracy of observation is essential: it can be acquired only by much practice and by diligent attention to detail.

The examination of the part complained of does not complete the clinical examination. It sometimes happens that symptoms felt in one part have their origin in another. For example, pain in the leg is often caused by a lesion in the spine, and pain in the knee may have its origin in the hip. The possibility of a distant lesion must therefore be considered and an examination made of any region under suspicion.

Finally, localised symptoms may be the first or only manifestation of a generalised or widespread disorder. A brief examination is therefore made of the rest of the body with this possibility in mind.

Thus the clinical examination may be considered under three headings:

1. examination of the part complained of
2. investigation of possible sources of referred symptoms
3. general examination of the body as a whole.

1. EXAMINATION OF THE PART COMPLAINED OF

The following description of the steps in the clinical examination is intended only as a guide. The technique of examination will naturally be varied according to individual preference. Nevertheless, it is useful to stick to a particular routine, for a familiarity with it will ensure that no step in the examination is forgotten.

Exposure for examination

It is essential that the part to be examined should be adequately exposed and in a good light. Many mistakes are made simply because the student or practitioner does not insist upon the removal of enough clothes to allow proper examination. When a limb is being examined the sound limb should always be exposed for comparison.

Inspection

Inspection should be carried out systematically, with attention to the following four points:

1. **The bones** Observe the general alignment and position of the parts to detect any deformity, shortening, or unusual posture.
2. **The soft tissues** Observe the soft-tissue contours, comparing the two sides. Note any visible evidence of general or local swelling, or of muscle wasting.
3. **Colour and texture of the skin** Look for redness, cyanosis, pigmentation, shininess, loss of hair, adventitious tufts of hair or other changes.
4. **Scars or sinuses** If a scar is present, determine from its appearance whether it was caused by operation (linear scar with suture marks), injury (irregular scar), or suppuration (broad, adherent, puckered scar).

Palpation

Again there are four points to consider:

1. **Skin temperature** By careful comparison of the two sides judge whether there is an area of increased warmth or of unusual coldness. An increase of local temperature denotes increased vascularity. The usual cause is an

inflammatory reaction; but it should be remembered that a rapidly growing tumour may also bring about marked local hyperaemia, with increase in skin warmth.

2. **The bones** The general shape and outline of the bones are investigated. Feel in particular for thickening, abnormal prominence, or disturbed relationship of the normal landmarks.

3. **The soft tissues** Direct particular attention to the muscles (are they in spasm, or wasted?), to the joint tissues (is the synovial membrane thickened, or the joint distended with fluid?), and to the detection of any local swelling (?cyst; ?tumour) or general swelling of the part.

4. **Local tenderness** The exact site of any local tenderness should be mapped out and an attempt made to relate it to a particular anatomical structure.

Determining the cause of a diffuse joint swelling. The question often arises: what is the cause of a diffuse swelling of a joint? The answer can be supplied after careful palpation. For practical purposes a *diffuse* swelling of the joint as a whole can have only three causes:

1. thickening of the bone end
2. fluid within the joint
3. thickening of the synovial membrane.

In some cases two or all three causes may be combined, but they can always be differentiated by palpation. *Bony thickening* is detected by deep palpation through the soft tissues, the bone outlines being compared on the two sides. A *fluid effusion* generally gives a clear sense of fluctuation between the two palpating hands. *Synovial thickening* gives a characteristic boggy sensation – rather as if a layer of soft sponge-rubber had been placed between the skin and the bone. It is nearly always accompanied by a well-marked increase of local warmth, for the synovium is a very vascular membrane.

Measurements

Measurement of limb length is often necessary, especially in the lower limbs, where discrepancy between the two sides is important. Measurement of the circumference of a limb segment on the two sides is also important if any asymmetry is suspected. It provides an index of muscle wasting, soft-tissue swelling or bony thickening. Details will be given in the chapters on individual regions.

Estimation of fixed deformity

Fixed deformity exists when a joint cannot be placed in the neutral (anatomical) position. Its causes are described on page 56. The degree of fixed deformity at a joint is determined by bringing the joint as near as it will come to the neutral position and then measuring the angle by which it falls short.

Valgus and varus. Explanation is needed of the commonly used terms *valgus* and *varus*, which are often confusing to students. In valgus deformity the distal part of a member is deviated laterally (outwards) in relation to the proximal part. Thus, for example, in hallux valgus the toe is deviated outwards in relation to the foot; and in genu valgum the lower leg is deviated outwards in relation to the thigh. Varus deformity is the opposite: the distal part of a member is deviated medially (inwards) in relation to the proximal part (examples – cubitus varus and genu varum).

Movements

In the examination of joint movements information must be obtained on the following points:

1. What is the range of active movement?
2. Is passive movement greater than active movement?
3. Is movement painful?
4. Is movement accompanied by crepitation?
5. Is there any spasticity (stiff resistance to free movement)?

In measuring the range of movement it is important to know what is the normal. The range is recorded as an angle usually measured from the straight position of the joint as neutral. Measurement can be facilitated by the use of a jointed protractor with long arms, termed a goniometer. With some joints the normal varies considerably from patient to patient; as, for instance, at the metacarpo-phalangeal joint of the thumb: so it is wise always to use the unaffected limb for comparison. Restriction of movement in all directions suggests some form of arthritis, whereas selective limitation of movement in some directions, with free movement in others, is more suggestive of a mechanical derangement.

Except in two sets of circumstances passive movement will usually be found equal to the active range. The passive range will exceed the active only in the following circumstances:

1. when the muscles responsible for the movement are paralysed
2. when the muscles or their tendons are torn, severed, or unduly slack.

Stability

The stability of a joint depends partly upon the integrity of its articulating surfaces, partly upon intact ligaments, and to some extent upon healthy muscles. When a joint is unstable there is abnormal mobility – for instance, lateral mobility in a hinge joint. It is important, when testing for abnormal mobility, to ensure that the muscles controlling the joint are relaxed; for a muscle in strong contraction can often conceal ligamentous instability.

Power

The power of the muscles responsible for each movement of a joint is determined by instructing the patient to move the joint against the resistance of the examiner. With careful comparison of the two sides it is possible to detect gross impairment of power. By general convention, the strength of a muscle is recorded according to the Medical Research Council grading, as follows:

0 = no contraction;
1 = a flicker of contraction;
2 = slight power, sufficient to move the joint only with gravity eliminated;
3 = power sufficient to move the joint against gravity;
4 = power to move the joint against gravity plus added resistance;
5 = normal power.

Sensation

Patients often complain of 'numbness' or tingling, and it is important to test sensibility both to light touch and to pin prick throughout the whole of the affected area. In unilateral affections the opposite side should be similarly tested for comparison. The precise area of any blunting or loss of sensibility should be carefully mapped out, and from a knowledge of the sensory dermatomes and the cutaneous distribution of the peripheral nerves the particular nerve or nerves affected may be identified and the root value established.

Reflexes

As part of the neurological examination the appropriate deep and superficial reflexes must be tested. Details will be given in the sections on individual regions of the body.

Peripheral circulation

Symptoms in a limb may be associated with impairment of the arterial circulation. Time should therefore be spent in assessing the state of the circulation by examination of the colour and temperature of the skin, the texture of the skin and nails, and the arterial pulses; and by such special investigations as may be necessary. This examination is particularly important in the case of the lower limb. Further details are given on page 420.

Tests of function

It is necessary next to test the function of the part under examination. How much does the disorder affect the part in its fulfilment of everyday activities? Methods of determining this vary according to the part affected. To take the lower limb as an example, the best test of function is to observe the patient standing, walking, running and jumping, or climbing and descending stairs. Special tests are required to investigate certain functions – for example, the Trendelenburg test for abductor efficiency at the hip (p. 340).

2. INVESTIGATION OF POSSIBLE SOURCES OF REFERRED SYMPTOMS

When the source of the symptoms is still in doubt after careful examination of the part complained of, attention must be directed to possible extrinsic disorders with referred symptoms. This will entail examination of such other regions of the body as might be responsible. For instance, in a case of pain in the shoulder it might be necessary to examine the neck for evidence of a lesion interfering with the brachial plexus, and the thorax and abdomen for evidence of diaphragmatic irritation, because either of these conditions may be a cause of shoulder pain. Again, in a case of pain in the thigh the examination will often have to include a study of the spine, abdomen, pelvis, and genito-urinary system as well as a local examination of the hip and thigh.

3. GENERAL EXAMINATION OF THE BODY AS A WHOLE

The mistake is sometimes made of confining the attention to the patient's immediate symptoms and failing to assess the patient as a whole. It should be made a rule in every case, however trivial it may seem, to form an opinion not only of the patient's general physical condition but also of his psychological outlook. In simple and straightforward cases this general survey may legitimately be brief and rapid, but it should never be omitted.

DIAGNOSTIC IMAGING

Until recent years radiography was the only method by which bone and other relatively dense tissues could be shown as a visual image contrasting with adjacent less-dense tissues. This is no longer the case, for technical developments have led to alternative methods of imaging. These include:

1. ultrasound scanning
2. radioisotope scanning
3. X-ray computerised tomography (CT scanning)
4. magnetic resonance imaging (MRI).

A more detailed consideration of these methods and their applications to the diagnosis of orthopaedic disorders will be dealt with in Chapter 2.

Clinical methods of history taking and examination

2 Imaging for orthopaedics

Nigel Raby

Imaging has now assumed a greater role in the management of patients with orthopaedic disease than ever before. For many years imaging was limited to the use of plain radiographic films which really only gave useful information on bony structures. Over the past 25 years orthopaedics has benefited greatly from newer imaging modalities which are able to give much greater information, not only on the bony structures, but also of the surrounding soft tissues. While plain films remain the mainstay of imaging in trauma, in other orthopaedic conditions they are now less important. Cross-sectional imaging, in particular the use of magnetic resonance imaging (MRI), has now become the most important imaging modality for many orthopaedic conditions. MRI allows detailed identification of the soft-tissue structures in and around joints and for this reason has assumed a very prominent position in imaging of orthopaedic patients.

PLAIN RADIOGRAPHIC FILMS AND DIGITAL RADIOGRAPHY

In a modern medical imaging department the plain radiograph taken on X-ray film is now almost obsolete. Plain radiographic images are mostly obtained with digital equipment using a much smaller X-ray dose compared to conventional film. The resulting image is displayed on a computer screen where it can be manipulated to alter the image brightness and contrast, magnify areas of interest, and measure the size of abnormalities. Whether obtained with a digital system or on 'hard copy' X-ray film, plain radiographs continue to be the commonest imaging modality used in orthopaedics. They are usually the only diagnostic images required for most cases of trauma and the great majority of degenerative disorders. Fracture diagnosis and management is satisfactorily guided by plain films, as is planning joint replacement surgery for arthritic disease in the hip and knee. The use of plain films has diminished in other areas of orthopaedic practice, where for many years they were the standard imaging investigation. An example would be patients with back pain, where it is now recognised that the plain film has little to offer in evaluation and MRI is the investigation of choice.

COMPUTERISED TOMOGRAPHY (CT)

CT is a technique that utilises X-rays, but acquires multiple thin slices axially through the area of interest. With the advances in digital technology modern CT scanners can now acquire this data very rapidly. Current models in use can obtain 16 slices simultaneously, while new machines will be able to acquire

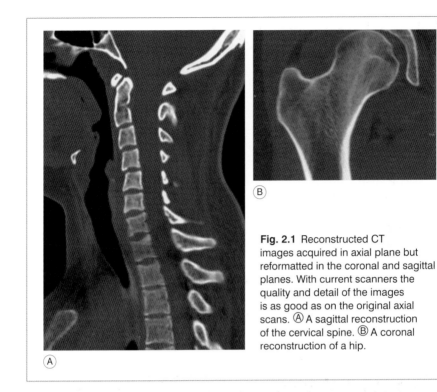

Fig. 2.1 Reconstructed CT images acquired in axial plane but reformatted in the coronal and sagittal planes. With current scanners the quality and detail of the images is as good as on the original axial scans. Ⓐ A sagittal reconstruction of the cervical spine. Ⓑ A coronal reconstruction of a hip.

64 and even 256 slices at a time. The result is a stack of very thin radiographic images, usually about 1mm in thickness. These can be manipulated by the CT computer to generate images in any plane with excellent detail. Typically these images are reformatted into coronal and sagittal planes so that images are similar to looking at AP and lateral radiographs (Fig. 2.1). These images can be acquired in only a few seconds and the reconstructions are also available within a similar short time. Modern scanners can also rapidly reconstruct a three-dimensional model of the scanned area (Fig. 2.2). The commonest role of CT in orthopaedics is assisting in the management of trauma patients with complex fractures. While the fracture is usually easily visualised on plain radiographs, the exact position, number and size of the fracture fragments may be more difficult to identify correctly. This is where CT and its multiplanar capability is of most use in orthopaedic patient management. Typical areas where CT is of most value are in the assessment of fractures in complex anatomical sites, such as the spine, pelvis, tibial plateau and calcaneus. Fracture treatment planning is greatly aided by the multiple views that can be obtained of these complex injuries and in selected cases three-dimensional reconstructions can also add useful information.

Non-traumatic conditions where CT can be useful are the evaluation of bone- and cartilage-based tumours. Although MRI is the principal method used for the anatomical staging of these tumours, CT may add further useful information regarding the extent of the ossifying or calcified portions of these tumours which an MR scan can underestimate (Fig. 2.3). Another example is osteoid osteoma, where a CT scan provides the diagnostic finding of a very

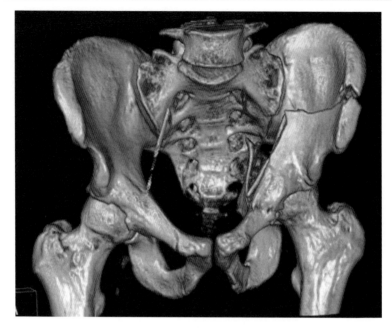

Fig. 2.2 CT scan which has been reconstructed to give a three-dimensional image. On computer screen this can be rotated on real time to allow full evaluation of the bony structures in detail.

small central sclerotic nidus (Fig. 2.4). A CT scan is also valuable for the full staging of bone and soft-tissue sarcomas, where it is used routinely to detect the presence of lung metastases (Fig. 2.5).

MAGNETIC RESONANCE IMAGING (MRI)

MRI is a new technology now commonly used in the evaluation of orthopaedic patients without the use of ionising radiation and with no known harmful effects. MR scanning can produce images in any plane and the tissue contrast can be altered to highlight particular anatomical structures and areas of pathology.

When a patient is placed into the core of a very powerful magnet the protons (hydrogen atoms) of the body align themselves to the magnetic field. If a radiofrequency pulse is then applied the protons will be tipped slightly from the line of the field and for a short time will oscillate (or resonate – hence the name). These resonating protons emit low-power radio waves which can be detected by magnetic coils within the scanner and can then be used to form a three-dimensional image. By altering how the resonance is performed and how the radio waves are captured, it is possible to formulate the images into slices in any plane. It is also possible to alter the characteristics of the image in a large variety of ways. The most common types used in orthopaedic imaging are called T1 and T2 weighted images. Images where signal from fat is suppressed, termed fat saturation, are also useful.

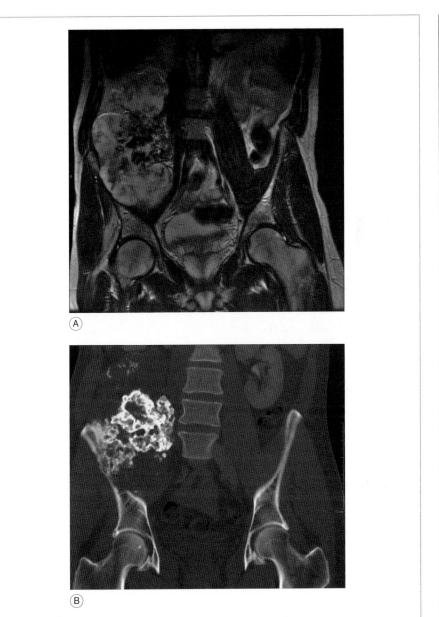

Fig. 2.3 Ⓐ MRI scan of a very large mass arising from the pelvis and occupying a large part of the abdomen. Ⓑ A coronal reformatted CT of the same lesion. This shows the bony origin and the bone content of the tumour which is not well seen on the MRI scan.

Imaging for orthopaedics

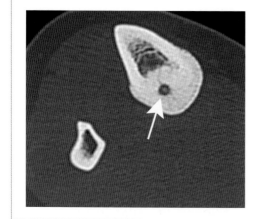

Fig. 2.4 An axial CT through an osteoid osteoma. The central sclerotic nidus is identified (arrow) and is best seen on CT.

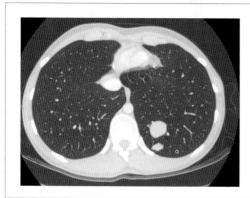

Fig. 2.5 CT of lungs in a patient with an osteosarcoma of the femur demonstrating pulmonary metastases.

The T1 images show fat as white, bone and tendons as black, with muscle and water appearing grey (Fig. 2.6A). A T2 image of the same structure is most easily recognised because water is seen as white (Fig. 2.6B). This is useful in the detection of fluid structures such as cerebrospinal fluid in the spinal canal and cystic masses in the soft tissues. If the same image then has fat saturation, the fat becomes black leaving even small amounts of fluid as the only white areas on the image. This means that subtle oedema in muscle or bone can be easily identified.

Further information can be obtained by using MR contrast agents. These substances are injected intravenously and are most commonly compounds derived from gadolinium, a heavy metal which alters the signal characteristics of various structures, particularly those with a large blood supply. Further scans obtained after injection of this contrast medium may give helpful additional information in selected cases. Typically this is used for the assessment of tumours, infection and post operative patients following spinal surgery (Fig. 2.7).

MRI is particularly helpful where the abnormality is confined to soft-tissue structures and is most commonly used for evaluation of disease and injury in the spine and knee. In the spine, MRI can identify the intervertebral discs and individual nerve roots, making it the investigation of choice for patients with suspected disc herniation causing nerve root compression (Fig. 2.8). It can also be used to identify spinal stenosis, disc space infection and spinal tumours.

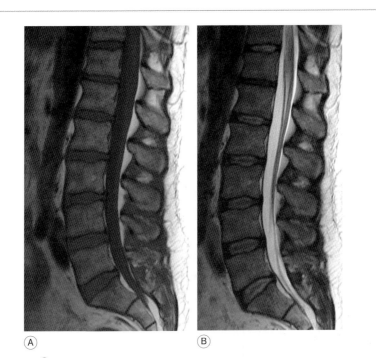

Fig. 2.6 Ⓐ A sagittal T1 weighted image of the lumbar spine. Note that the CSF in the spinal canal is dark grey. Ⓑ Sagittal T2 weighted image of same patient. Here the CSF is now white. Fluid appears white on T2 weighted images. The intervertebral discs are healthy as they can be seen to contain high signal fluid within the nucleus pulposus.

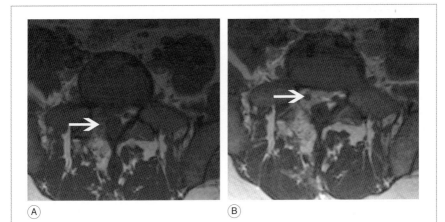

Fig. 2.7 Ⓐ Axial T1 weighted scan. This is a patient who had a microdiscectomy at L5/S1 on the right and now has recurrent symptoms. There is a mass of abnormal tissue (arrow) along the right side of the thecal sac. It is not possible to see the right S1 nerve root. A recurrent disc herniation could be the cause of this. Ⓑ Following administration of intravenous gadolinium there is enhancement of all the abnormal tissue indicating that this is post-operative granulation tissue and not disc material which would not enhance. The S1 root is now clearly visible (arrow) surrounded by the granulation tissue.

Imaging for orthopaedics

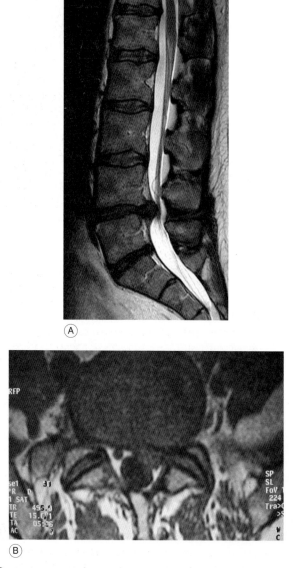

(A)

(B)

Fig. 2.8 (A) Sagittal T2 weighted image of lumbar spine. There is a large herniation of the L4/5 disc. (B) Axial scan through the disc space showing disc material has herniated into the left side of the spinal canal and compressed the left L5 nerve (compare with normal nerve on the right). By convention axial images are viewed as if looking from the patient's feet. Thus, the patient's right is on the left of the image and vice versa.

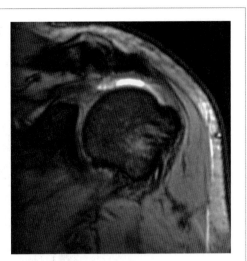

Fig. 2.9 Coronal MRI scan of shoulder. There is fluid seen as an area of bright signal within the supraspinatus tendon indicating a tear of the rotator cuff.

In patients with knee pain, MRI is highly accurate in diagnosing patients with meniscal tears and can distinguish between degenerate oblique tears and the less common bucket handle tears. It is also valuable in detecting injuries of the cruciate and collateral ligaments following trauma to the knee joint.

In the shoulder MR scans are increasingly used to identify degenerative tendinopathy of the rotator cuff muscles and tears of the individual tendons (Fig. 2.9). Around the ankle it has proved useful in the diagnosis of tears and degeneration of the Achilles tendon, as well as for osteochondral fractures of the talar dome, and injuries to the collateral ligaments of the ankle and subtalar joints.

MRI is particularly sensitive for imaging the bone marrow because of its high fat content, so that any disease associated with abnormal bone marrow will be identified. These include malignant primary bone tumours, as well as metastases and myeloma, all of which are marrow-based disorders (Fig. 2.10). Infection of bone, avascular necrosis and stress fractures, only cause changes visible on plain radiographs late in the disease process, but MR scans will identify all of these conditions at an early stage.

ULTRASOUND

Ultrasound has a useful role in orthopaedic imaging. Ultrasound machines are readily available in almost every hospital. The scan only takes a short time, but its value and reliability is very operator dependent. Like MRI, there are no known dangerous side effects associated with the use of ultrasound. While little or no information is obtained from bony structures, ultrasound can visualise the soft tissues in many areas. Particular structures which are well seen on ultrasound are tendon and muscles. Thus suspected abnormalities of the patellar tendon, Achilles tendon and rotator cuff of the shoulder can all be diagnosed by this technique (Fig. 2.11). Muscle tears are easily identified as are their associated haematomas. In skilled hands evaluation of tendon lesions around the hand and wrist can be assessed and some operators are also able to identify ligamentous

Imaging for orthopaedics

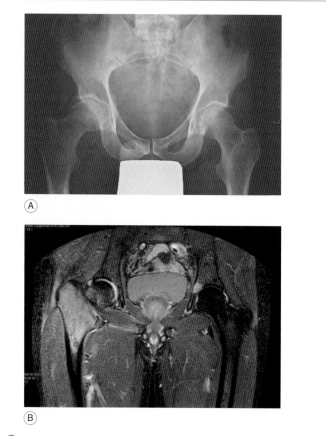

Fig. 2.10 Ⓐ Plain film of pelvis does not show any abnormality. Ⓑ MRI shows extensive abnormal signal in right proximal femur. This is due to marrow replacement by tumour. Patient subsequently shown to have metastatic disease.

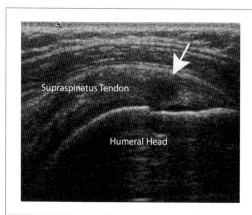

Fig. 2.11 Ultrasound of shoulder. The humeral head and overlying supraspinatus muscle and tendon are labelled. The arrow points to an area of altered reflectivity within the tendon. This indicates a tear at this site.

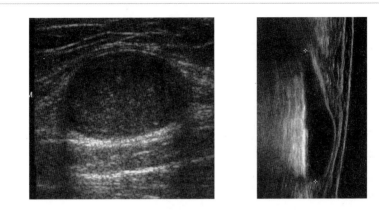

Fig. 2.12 (left) Ultrasound of a small soft-tissue lump in the mid thigh. It contains multiple echoes seen as white speckles. This indicated a solid mass rather than a fluid lesion and is clearly delineated from surrounding muscle. The appearances suggest a nerve sheath tumour and a schwannoma was confirmed at surgery.

Fig. 2.13 (right) Ultrasound of a clinical mass in the popliteal fossa. On this occasion there is an oblong structure which does not have any echoes within it. This indicated the presence of fluid (compare with Fig. 2.12) and is a popliteal or Baker's cyst.

injuries around the elbow and ankle. Ultrasound is also of use in the evaluation of soft-tissue masses (Fig. 2.12), and fluid-filled structures such as Baker's cyst of the knee (Fig. 2.13), which can be diagnosed reliably by this technique alone.

Because of the lack of ossification in the femoral head at birth, ultrasound has been advocated as a method for screening the neonatal hip joint for developmental dysplasia (DDH). Its value has not been proven for universal population screening, though it is used extensively in many European countries. However, in Britain and North America, the technique is only used for selective screening in babies showing clinical evidence of hip instability or dislocation.

ISOTOPE SCANNING

Isotope bone scanning requires the intravenous injection of a radioactive tracer, usually technetium (^{99m}Tc), linked to a molecule such as disphosphonate which will become incorporated into areas of high bone turnover where there is increased osteoblastic and osteoclastic activity. The bone-seeking radioisotope is injected intravenously and the emitted rays are charted with a gamma camera. After injection of the isotope there is an immediate diffusion of isotope into the bone matrix from the blood: thus an increased uptake of isotope locally in the skeleton denotes hyperaemia of the bone. This is seen on a scan obtained a few minutes after injection (early phase). It will only be seen in conditions with markedly increased blood flow to the area, typically in acute infection. Within 2–4 hours (late phase) the isotope is taken up by active bone-forming cells, increased uptake thus denoting increased osteogenic activity. However, this is non specific as osteoclastic activity is increased by many

Imaging for orthopaedics

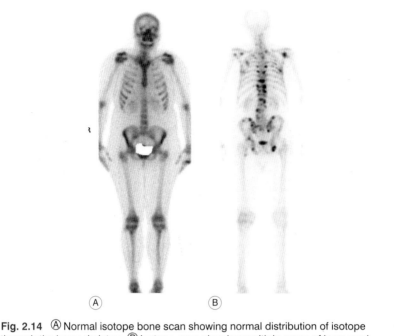

Ⓐ   Ⓑ

Fig. 2.14 Ⓐ Normal isotope bone scan showing normal distribution of isotope through the bony skeleton. Ⓑ Isotope scan showing multiple areas of increased isotope uptake. This pattern is seen in patients with multiple bone metastases.

disease processes, including the site of healing fractures as well as tumours and bone infection. Nevertheless, taken in conjunction with the history and clinical findings, areas of increased uptake can be identified and the likeliest cause suggested. The commonest use for isotope scanning is in identifying the site of bony metastases (Fig. 2.14). Bone scanning will provide images of the complete bony skeleton and this is its major advantage. It is often necessary to supplement the scan with plain radiographs of the areas showing abnormal increased isotope uptake. An example where this is required is when the plain films may be able to identify benign causes of increased isotope uptake and distinguish these from tumour (Fig. 2.15). Isotope bone scanning may also have a role in the diagnosis of infections of bone or joint, primary bone tumours, osteoid osteoma, and stress fractures.

A less common application of radioisotope imaging is for the detection of focal bone or joint infection where this is not demonstrable clinically. The technique takes 24–48 hours, uses the patient's own white cells, which are labelled with indium-111 and then reinjected intravenously to localise in areas of focal inflammation.

POSITRON EMISSION TOMOGRAPHY (PET CT)

Positron emission tomography is the newest addition to imaging, now usually combined with a CT scan. In essence it is an isotope imaging technique, but one which uses a more complex isotope which emits positrons. The isotope can be linked to various molecules but the one most commonly used is

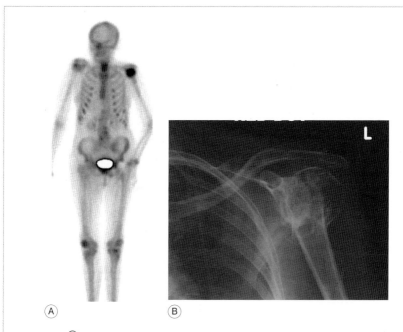

Fig. 2.15 Ⓐ Isotope scan in a patient with known breast carcinoma and left shoulder pain. There is marked increased uptake in the region of the left humeral head. In view of the history a metastatic deposit was thought likely. Ⓑ Plain radiograph of the shoulder shows that there is an old humeral neck fracture which accounts for the isotope uptake.

fluorodeoxyglucose (FDG), which accumulates in areas of altered glucose metabolism. The localisation of the site of this uptake is improved by fusing the isotope image with that of a CT scan acquired at the same time. The most common application is in the identification of active tumours and although its role in orthopaedics is currently limited, it may have a future role in the evaluation of bone and soft-tissue tumours. The technique may also be useful in the evaluation of infection around joint replacements but as yet this is not well defined. The technology for PET CT is currently limited to a few specialist centres and is not generally available.

ARTHROGRAPHY

Arthrography is a technique where an X-ray contrast is injected directly into a joint to enable visualisation of the joint surfaces and structures within the joint which would otherwise not be visible on an X-ray. This is being used much less frequently than in the past, as MRI and ultrasound can now often visualise the structures of interest without the need for any contrast. Where it is still used, it is usually in conjunction with MRI and occasionally CT. The resultant MR arthrogram can give even greater detail about intra-articular structures than plain MRI. The commonest indications are; in the shoulder to demonstrate disruption of the glenoid labrum in patients with recurrent dislocation or instability (Fig. 2.16), and in the hip when looking for evidence of impingement and labral tears.

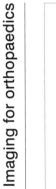

Imaging for orthopaedics

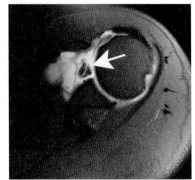

Fig. 2.16 MR arthrogram of the shoulder of a patient with recurrent dislocation. The scan demonstrates that the anterior cartilaginous glenoid labrum (arrow) is detached from the underlying bony rim. This is the so-called Bankart lesion.

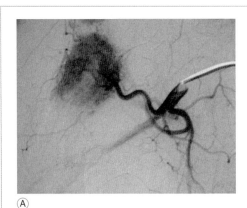

(A)

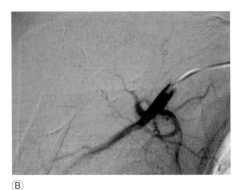

(B)

Fig. 2.17 Ⓐ Angiogram showing a large tumour blush with vessels feeding a metastasis from renal carcinoma. Ⓑ Following embolisation the blood flow to the lesion has been occluded allowing surgery to take place with much less blood loss and an easier operative field.

ANGIOGRAPHY (ARTERIOGRAPHY)

This is a specialised technique which is now used only infrequently in orthopaedics. The two major indications are trauma and tumour. Following trauma with a severely displaced bone fracture, angiography may be indicated to evaluate associated vascular injury, such as may occur in the pelvis and humerus. Note that angiography can now be carried out using CT and MRI, as well as by conventional intra-arterial catheterisation. In the evaluation of tumours, arteriography may be useful to delineate the extent of the vascular supply, or the relationship of vascular structures to the tumour, to enable safe surgical planning. In both circumstances the use of conventional catheterisation for angiography has the advantage of being able to carry out therapeutic procedures. In life-threatening haemorrhage, embolisation or stenting can be undertaken at the site of vascular damage. In cases of highly vascular tumours, preoperative embolisation of the tumour may reduce intraoperative haemorrhage. This is most commonly used in patients with metastasic renal tumour as these are generally highly vascular and prone to bleed profusely at surgery without prior embolisation (Fig. 2.17).

3 | Other investigation techniques

More often than not the diagnosis can be established from the clinical assessment and imaging studies without the aid of other special investigations. In any case the possibilities should be narrowed down to as few as possible before such investigations are ordered. If doubt then exists, appropriate tests are ordered to support or weaken each possible diagnosis.

Tests commonly employed in orthopaedic diagnosis include haematological studies; biochemical tests upon urine, faeces, plasma, and cerebrospinal fluid; serological and bacteriological tests; electrical tests; arthroscopy; and histological examination of specimens excised at biopsy or at definitive operation.

BLOOD TESTS

Haematology

Full blood count. Assessment of the haemoglobin is of great value after trauma and post-operatively, as it gives an indication as to how much blood has been lost. The white cell count is usually, but not always, raised when an infection is present. The ESR (erythrocyte sedimentation rate) and CRP (C-reactive protein) are more sensitive tests for revealing systemic inflammation. The CRP is particularly useful, as it rises rapidly when there is an infective process. The ESR and CRP are also helpful in distinguishing septic and aseptic loosening of total joint replacements. If these tests are normal on two occasions, it is unlikely that the loosening is as a result of an infection.

Biochemistry

If there are concerns about organ dysfunction, liver function tests and renal function tests are of value and part of the pre-operative work-up. Similarly, routine electrolytes can also be of value, particularly if the patient is on drugs such as diuretics.

The biochemical tests that are of particular value for assessing bone function are the plasma levels of calcium, phosphate and alkaline phosphatase. Derangements in the calcium and phosphate balance can confirm the diagnosis of rickets and osteomalacia.

MICROBIOLOGICAL TESTS

The diagnosis of musculoskeletal infection is often challenging for a number of reasons.

1. Bacteria such as the normal skin flora are grown as contaminants from specimens such as sputum. However, in orthopaedics these same organisms can be pathogens and the cause of musculoskeletal infections. To distinguish between a growth of, for example, *Staphylococcus epidermidis*, which is a contaminant as opposed to one which is a pathogen, it is vital to obtain multiple samples. At operation of a patient with suspected musculoskeletal infection, at least five samples should be obtained under sterile conditions. If two or more of these multiple specimens grow the same bacteria, it is likely that this is a true pathogen rather than a contaminant.
2. The swabs from sinus tracts are often misleading and do not accurately reflect the true deep organisms that are causing the infection. However, aspiration of fluid from the depth of a sinus is worthwhile and often will give a more accurate picture of the true range of causative organisms.
3. In 10–20% of cases with established musculoskeletal infection, despite optimum culture techniques, it may not be possible to grow an organism. Thus, it is vital to obtain material for histological analysis as well as for microbiological culture where infection is suspected (see below).

ELECTRICAL TESTS (ELECTRODIAGNOSIS)

The two most common electrodiagnostic techniques used in orthopaedic practice are nerve conduction studies and electromyography.

Nerve conduction studies are used to determine whether or not a nerve is able to transmit an electrical impulse. The principle is to apply a stimulating electrode over a point on the nerve trunk distal to the lesion, and to observe whether or not the muscles supplied by the nerve will contract in response to the stimulus. The nerves in the sound limb are examined first, to determine the threshold of current required to cause a muscle contraction. If in the affected limb a current at least twice as great as the threshold fails to produce a muscle contraction, nerve conduction is absent. A nerve conduction test provides a simple method of determining whether or not a clinical paralysis is due to a complete lesion of the nerve, which has resulted in degeneration of its myelin sheath. If nerve conduction is present the lesion cannot be complete and myelin degeneration has not occurred.

Nerve conduction tests may also be used to measure motor conduction velocity in the peripheral nerve, and the principle can also be applied to afferent sensory testing. A slowing in the velocity of conduction may indicate the site of an incomplete lesion in the nerve trunk, such as may occur in compression neuropathy. Using stimulating electrodes, applied both proximal and distal to the suspected lesion, the latent period before the appearance of the muscle action potentials is measured. The difference in conduction time and the distance between the electrodes provides a measurement of velocity, which can be compared with the normal side, or with normal values (40–70 m/s).

The measurement of sensory nerve conduction is technically more difficult, but has a useful clinical application in spinal cord monitoring. Surface electrodes are used to provide repetitive peripheral stimulations during spinal surgery, so that recordings of central cortical responses can be used to detect any interference with spinal cord function.

Electromyography. In this technique the electrical changes occurring in a muscle are picked up by a needle or surface electrode, suitably amplified and studied in the form of sound through a loudspeaker, or as a tracing on an oscillograph. Normal muscle is electrically 'silent' at rest, but on voluntary contraction shows increasing electrical discharges in the form of triphasic action potentials, as more motor units are recruited into activity. Partly denervated or totally denervated muscle shows only spontaneous contractions of individual fibres (fibrillation potentials). Repeated testing at intervals can be used to detect evidence of re-innervation, as small polyphasic motor unit action potentials reappear and spontaneous fibrillation disappears. The motor unit action potentials gradually increase in duration and amplitude, but do not return to a normal pattern until remyelination of the nerve is complete. Electromyography may show diagnostic changes in some types of myopathy, as well as in anterior horn cell disease such as poliomyelitis and motor neurone disease.

GAIT ANALYSIS

Gait analysis is the study of locomotion. In its most rudimentary form, it can be the observation of a patient during walking. Simple measures of walking speed and step length can be obtained with a stopwatch and a walkway of known length covered in powder. However, modern gait laboratories use multiple video cameras, which record simultaneously, and floor load transducers (force plates), which measure the ground reaction force in magnitude and direction. In addition, passive reflective marker balls are placed along the length of the limbs to aid in imaging the movement, and surface electrodes are placed over major muscle groups such as the quadriceps, so that electromyograms can be recorded simultaneously. Gait analysis can be used in sports medicine, Parkinson's disease and other neuromuscular diseases. In orthopaedics, it has been used to help plan surgery in children with cerebral palsy.

ARTHROGRAMS

Arthrograms consist of injecting contrast medium into a joint and then obtaining serial plain X-rays, CT/MR images. Arthrograms are commonly used with plain X-rays, for assessing children's dysplastic hip joints, and in adults for determining whether the components of an artificial joint replacement are loose. In this latter situation, the arthrogram is often combined with an aspiration of the joint (under sterile conditions), which allows fluid to be sent for microbiological assessment. CT and MRI arthrograms are frequently used in the assessment of rotator cuff injuries of the shoulder.

ARTHROSCOPY

In recent years the technique of direct inspection of the interior of a joint through a fine telescope introduced through a cannula has become highly developed. Indeed it is relied upon almost routinely in the diagnosis of mechanical derangements within the knee, and also in the study of many non-traumatic affections of doubtful nature. The use of arthroscopy has now been extended to joints other than the knee, and is increasingly used for the diagnosis and treatment of intra-articular disorders of the shoulder, hip, wrist, and ankle.

BIOPSY

Biopsy is the operation of taking a specimen of living tissue for histological, electron-microscopic or other examination in order to elucidate the nature of a disease. Very often it is done as a final step in the diagnosis and staging of a tumour. Two techniques of biopsy are available:

1. needle biopsy, in which a core of tissue is extracted by a special hollow needle
2. open biopsy.

Except in certain situations open biopsy is usually to be preferred despite a theoretically greater risk of tumour dissemination, because it is more likely to yield a representative specimen. Nevertheless needle biopsy has an important place, and with improvements in technique its application has been widened, though diagnostic accuracy may not be as good as with open biopsy, except in very specialised centres.

The main essentials in a biopsy operation are:

1. that an adequate and representative piece of tissue be obtained
2. that the incision be so placed that it does not prejudice the success of a subsequent operation for total eradication of the tumour – especially in malignant disease.

The scar must be so placed that it is conveniently included in the block of tissue to be excised at the time of definitive surgical excision.

INTERPRETATION OF THE FINDINGS

When the study of the patient is complete the abnormal findings elicited from the history, clinical examination, diagnostic imaging, and appropriate special investigations should be assembled together to form a composite clinical picture. This can then be matched against the recognised disorders of the region under consideration. It is comforting to remember that the number of disorders that commonly affect a particular region is limited. Often the number is not large. Theoretically, therefore, if all the possibilities are listed and thereafter confirmed or eliminated one by one the correct diagnosis must always be revealed.

This is, of course, an over-simplification. In practice diagnosis is not as simple as that. But it is nevertheless true that if the problem is tackled logically, step by step, in the manner described, a correct conclusion can be formed in the great majority of cases. The only essentials are a capacity for painstaking enquiry, with strict attention to detail, accurate observation, and a working knowledge of the salient features of the common disorders.

PSYCHOGENIC OR STRESS DISORDERS

This heading is included to issue a word of warning. When the cause of a patient's symptoms remains obscure despite a thorough investigation there is a prevalent tendency to discount the genuineness of the symptoms and to ascribe them to 'functional' or 'psychogenic' factors, or simply to stress. This must be deplored as a dangerous policy that has led on many occasions to the overlooking of a serious organic disease.

Just because we fail to discover the cause of a particular symptom it by no means follows that the symptom is imaginary or psychogenic; it usually means only that we are not sufficiently skilled in diagnosis. Admittedly, true hysterical

Other investigation techniques

disorders are encountered from time to time in orthopaedic practice, but they are few and far between. Much more often a long-continued organic pain leads to a distracted state of mind that is wrongly interpreted as a hysterical manifestation. It is widely accepted that physical symptoms may be prolonged or may seem to be worse if there is an associated psychological disorder. Such aggravation is often termed 'psychological overlay' or 'illness behaviour', especially in legal practice. It is far safer to err on the side of disregarding possible psychogenic factors than to overlook an organic lesion on the supposition that the symptoms are imaginary.

4 | Treatment of orthopaedic disorders

Orthopaedic treatment falls into three categories:

1. no treatment – simply reassurance or advice
2. non-operative treatment
3. operative treatment.

In every case these three possibilities of treatment should be considered one by one in the order given. At least half of the patients attending orthopaedic out-patient clinics (excluding cases of fracture) do not require treatment: all that they need is reassurance and advice. In many cases the sole reason for the patient's attendance is a fear that there may be cancer, tuberculosis, impending paralysis, crippling arthritis, or other serious disease. If reassurance can be given that there is no evidence of serious disease the patient goes away satisfied, and the symptoms immediately become less disturbing.

If active treatment seems to be required it is a good general principle that whenever practicable a trial should be given first to non-operative measures; though obviously there are occasions when early or indeed immediate operation must be advised. Most orthopaedic operations fall into the category of 'luxury' rather than life-saving procedures. Consequently the patient should seldom be persuaded to submit to operation: rather the surgeon should have to be persuaded to undertake it. When one is undecided whether to advise conservative treatment or operation it is wise always to err on the side of non-intervention.

METHODS OF NON-OPERATIVE TREATMENT

REST

Since the days of H. O. Thomas (p. 3), who, more than a century ago, emphasised its value in diseases of the spine and limbs, rest has been one of the mainstays of orthopaedic treatment. Complete rest demands recumbency in bed – which, for the most part, is deprecated today – or immobilisation of the diseased part in plaster. But by 'rest' the modern orthopaedic surgeon does not usually mean complete inactivity or immobility. Often he means no more than 'relative rest', implying simply a reduction of accustomed activity and avoidance of strain. Indeed complete rest is enjoined much less often now than it was in the past, because diseases for which rest was previously important, such as poliomyelitis or tuberculosis, can now be prevented or are more readily amenable to specific remedies such as antibacterial agents. Complete rest after operations, formerly favoured, has given place in most cases to the earliest possible resumption of activity.

SUPPORT

Rest and support often go together; but there are occasions when support is needed but not rest – for example, to stabilise a joint rendered insecure by muscle paralysis, or to prevent the development of deformity. When support is to be temporary it can be provided by a cast or splint made from plaster of Paris or from one of the newer splinting materials. When it is to be prolonged or permanent an individually made surgical appliance, or orthosis, is required. Examples in common use are spinal braces, cervical collars, wrist supports, walking calipers, knee and ankle orthoses, and devices to control drop foot (Figs 11.3–11.5, pp. 177–8).

PHYSIOTHERAPY

Physiotherapy in its various forms occupies an important place in the non-operative and post-operative treatments of orthopaedic disabilities. Emphasis on evidence-based practice has helped to produce an awareness among physiotherapists of the hazards as well as the merits of treatment. This has led to a correct emphasis being placed upon the value in many conditions of active rather than of passive treatment: in other words, of helping the patient to help him/herself. This approach is particularly rewarding in the rehabilitation of patients after injury or after operations, and in diseases such as poliomyelitis, cerebral palsy, hemiplegia, peripheral nerve palsies and mechanical low back pain. When it is used, physiotherapy should be pursued thoroughly. A number of different physiotherapy interventions have evolved over the years. These may be active, passive or a combination of the two. Passive approaches involve a range of different techniques carried out on the patient by the therapist. Active approaches require active involvement by the patient, either by exercising or changing behaviour.

Active intervention

Physiotherapists use the term physical activity, exercise and physical fitness to describe active interventions, but they are often used loosely and interchangeably. The term 'exercise' is used to include a range of methods from isometric stabilising exercise through to intensive aerobic fitness programmes. Exercise programmes aim to (1) strengthen specific muscles, (2) stretch soft tissues, (3) mobilise joints and (4) improve coordination of muscles. Exercise to improve coordination is of particular importance in cerebral palsy, multiple sclerosis, ankle and knee injuries.

Physical fitness is a multi-dimensional concept that has been defined as a set of attributes that people possess or achieve that relates to the ability to perform physical activity, and is comprised of skill-related, health-related and physiological components. Physical fitness programmes vary in intensity, design and delivery and are generally supervised in a group, but can be offered to patients on an individual basis. They usually include aerobic exercise with an aim to improve overall cardiovascular fitness, as well as specific exercises.

Hydrotherapy

Hydrotherapy is a valuable way of allowing active pain-free movements of all joints in warm water. The warmth and buoyancy of the water relieve the muscle spasm and can help to reduce pain and increase the range of movement. Hydrotherapy is often particularly useful in the treatment of rheumatoid arthritis.

Passive interventions

These techniques are carried out by the therapist and do not require any active participation by the patient. The chief use of passive movements, or 'mobilisation' is to preserve full mobility when the patient is unable to move the joint actively – i.e. when the muscles are paralysed or severed. They are important after nerve injuries, especially to preserve mobility in the hand, and in poliomyelitis in countries where it still occurs. Recently, the use of machines to provide continuous passive motion of joints after operation or injury has become popular to minimise complications and encourage healing of articular cartilage.

Manual therapy
Manual therapy includes a wide range of joint mobilisation and manipulation techniques used by osteopaths and chiropractors, as well as physiotherapists. It also includes mobilisation of soft tissue. The manipulation can be high-velocity thrust applied at the end of joint range (such as to spinal joints) or a more gentle passive low-velocity mobilisation applied in various parts of the available joint range.

Soft-tissue techniques
Soft-tissue techniques include interventions that aim to mobilise soft tissue, either by massage or passive stretching techniques. Massage techniques range from Swedish massage to deep connective tissue massage and stretching of neural tissue.

Traction
Traction for the spine is carried out both manually or using a motorised traction couch. The duration and magnitude of force can be varied, and if motorised traction is applied it can be carried out continuously or intermittently. The rationale for the use of traction therapy is based on the mechanical effects of traction on the spine, mainly stretching structures. These mechanisms are thought to cause separation of the vertebrae, widening of the intervertebral foramina, movement of the facet joints and stretching of spinal muscles and ligaments. The proposed mechanisms are not supported by research findings.

Electrotherapy
The theoretical basis for the use of these modalities is weak and they are not recommended in national or international guidelines. However, they continue to be used in clinical practice. Transcutaneous electrical nerve stimulation (TENS) and interferential therapy, short wave diathermy, laser therapy are all used by physiotherapists with the aim of providing pain relief. The interference effect uses two different medium-frequency alternating currents applied simultaneously through two electrodes to induce a current at the site of their interaction in the deep tissues. Transcutaneous nerve stimulation uses direct current pulses of adjustable frequency to stimulate the larger sensory nerve fibres selectively, and thereby to set up a gate control mechanism blocking the activity of the small fibres which conduct pain signals.

Treatment of orthopaedic disorders

Ultrasound

Ultrasound waves at approximately 10^6 Hz can be projected as a beam from a transducer to induce a heating effect in deep tissues. They may also produce benefit from their mechanical and chemical effects on collagen and proteoglycans. Ultrasound is frequently used to reduce post-traumatic haematoma, oedema and adhesions of joints and their associated soft tissues.

ALTERNATIVE THERAPIES

There has been an increasing trend for patients to seek alternative therapy (i.e. chiropractic therapy, osteopathy, acupuncture, massage and homeopathy) to relieve musculoskeletal symptoms. However, no strong evidence has emerged over the last decade that suggests that alternative therapy is any more beneficial than physiotherapy.

LOCAL INJECTIONS

The indications for local injections fall into two groups:

1. osteoarthritis or rheumatoid arthritis, in which the substance (usually hydrocortisone with or without a local anaesthetic solution) is injected directly into the affected joint with rigid aseptic precautions
2. extra-articular lesions of the type often ascribed (for want of more precise knowledge) to chronic strain, as exemplified by tennis elbow, tendonitis about the shoulder, and certain types of back pain.

The response depends upon the nature of the basic lesion: permanent relief is often gained in extra-articular lesions such as tennis elbow, but in arthritis the benefit is often no more than temporary, and repeated injections are seldom to be recommended.

DRUGS

Drugs have rather a small place in orthopaedic practice. Those used may be placed in eight categories:

1. antibacterial agents and antibiotics
2. analgesics
3. sedatives
4. anti-inflammatory drugs
5. hormone-like drugs
6. anti-osteoporosis drugs
7. specific drugs
8. cytotoxic drugs.

Antibacterial agents are of immense importance in infective lesions, especially in acute osteomyelitis and acute pyogenic arthritis. To be successful treatment must be begun very early. These drugs are also of definite value in certain chronic infections, notably in tuberculosis.

Analgesics should be used as little as possible. Many orthopaedic disorders are prolonged for many weeks or months, and it is undesirable to prescribe any but the mildest analgesics continuously over long periods, except for incurable malignant disease.

Sedatives may be given if needed to promote sleep, but as with analgesics the rule should be to prescribe no more than is really necessary.

Anti-inflammatory drugs are those that damp down the excessive inflammatory response that may occur especially in rheumatoid arthritis and related disorders, by inhibiting the cyclo-oxygenase enzymes responsible for prostaglandin formation. Non-steroidal anti-inflammatory drugs are generally to be preferred – especially in the first instance – and they are a mainstay in the treatment of rheumatoid arthritis. Many of these drugs also have an analgesic action. The powerful steroids cortisone, prednisolone, and their analogues should be used with extreme caution and indeed should be avoided altogether whenever possible, because through their side effects they may sometimes do more harm than good. Nevertheless there are times when their use may be justified – as for instance in acute exacerbations of rheumatoid arthritis, and especially in polymyalgia rheumatica and giant-cell arteritis (see p. 166).

Hormone-like drugs include the corticosteroids noted above, and sex hormones or analogues used for the prevention of osteoporosis in post-menopausal women and for the control of certain metastatic tumours such as hormone-dependent breast and prostatic tumours. These are being increasingly replaced by the bisphosphonates, a family of drugs which block the resorption of bone mineral.

Anti-osteoporosis drugs. Hormone replacement therapy and the SERMS (selective oestrogen receptor modulators) have largely been replaced by the bisphosphonates which block bone resorption and by anabolic agents such as parathyroid hormone and strontium.

Specific drugs work well in certain special diseases. Examples are vitamin C for scurvy, vitamin D for rickets and salicylates for the arthritis of rheumatic fever.

Cytotoxic drugs form the basis of chemotherapy for malignant tumours. These anti-cancer drugs include cyclophosphamide, melphalan, vincristine, doxorubicin, and methotrexate. They have serious side effects and are used only under expert supervision.

MANIPULATION

Treatment by manipulation is practised widely by orthopaedic surgeons and by others in allied professions. Strictly, the term might legitimately be used to include the passive movements, or 'mobilisations', that form part of the daily activities of a physiotherapy department and which have already been referred to above: but it is used here in a more restricted sense, to describe passive movements of joints, bones, or soft tissues carried out by the surgeon – with or without an anaesthetic, and often forcefully – as a deliberate step in treatment.

The subject will be considered under three general headings:

1. manipulation for correction of deformity
2. manipulation to improve the range of movements at a stiff joint
3. manipulation for relief of chronic pain in or about a joint, especially in the neck or spine.

Manipulation for correction of deformity

In this category manipulation has its most obvious application in the reduction of fractures and dislocations. It is also used to overcome deformity from contracted or short soft tissues – as, for example, in congenital club foot. Yet another simple example is the forcible subcutaneous rupture and dispersal of a ganglion over the dorsum of the wrist.

Technique. An anaesthetic may or may not be required, according to the nature of the condition that is being treated. In many instances – as in manipulation for a fracture or dislocation – the aim is to secure full reduction at the one sitting; but in resistant deformities such as club foot repeated manipulation may be required at intervals of a week or so, a little further improvement being gained each time.

Subsequent management. After manipulation for a deformity that is liable to recur – as in most cases of displaced fracture and in chronic deformities of joints – the limb is usually immobilised on a splint or in plaster to maintain the correction. In cases of resistant deformity gradual yielding of the soft tissue allows re-application of the splint in a more favourable position each time it is changed.

Manipulation for joint stiffness

The type of case mainly concerned with here is that in which a joint shows serious limitation of movement after an acute injury – usually a fracture of a limb bone. 'Frozen' shoulder (periarthritis) in its non-active stage may also be included in this category. In such cases the stiffness is caused by adhesions either within the joint itself or, more often, in the soft tissues about or near the joint. Forcible manipulation by the surgeon is not required very often for stiffness of this type, because it will usually respond gradually to treatment by active exercises under the care of a physiotherapist, combined with increasing use of the limb.

The joint that is most amenable to manipulation is the knee. The shoulder and the joints of the foot may also respond. Manipulation of the elbow and of the joints of the hand may increase the stiffness and should not be attempted.

Technique. Muscular relaxation should be secured by anaesthesia, supplemented if necessary by a relaxant drug. Great force should not be used: it is better to gain slight improvement by moderate force and then to repeat the manipulation after an interval. Excessive force may fracture a bone; or it may cause fresh bleeding within the joint, thereby aggravating the stiffness.

Subsequent management. Manipulation for joint stiffness should always be followed by intensive active exercises designed to retain the increased range of movement.

Manipulation for relief of chronic pain

In this third category of case treatment by manipulation is somewhat empirical, because in many instances it is impossible to determine precisely the nature of the underlying pathology, and consequently the way in which manipulation acts is a matter of conjecture and – it must be said – of misconception.[1] Manipulation is used in such cases simply because previous experience has proved that it is often successful.

[1]Non-medical practitioners – especially chiropracters and osteopaths – often postulate 'displacements' (for instance, of vertebrae) which clearly do not exist.

The painful conditions that respond best to manipulation are chronic strains, especially of the tarsal joints, the joints of the spinal column, and the sacro-iliac joints. A chronic strain may be the consequence of an acute injury that has not been followed by complete resolution, or it may be caused by long-continued mechanical overstrain. It is generally surmised that adhesions are present that prevent the extremes of joint movement (even though a restriction of movement may not be obvious clinically), that these adhesions are painful when stretched, and that the effect of manipulation is to rupture them. An alternative explanation that is advanced in certain cases is that there is a minor displacement of the joint surfaces or of an intra-articular structure (even though this can seldom be demonstrated radiologically), and that the effect of manipulation is to restore normal apposition.

Technique. Manipulation for relief of pain from chronic strain consists in putting the affected joint or joints forcibly through a full range of movement, usually while the patient is fully relaxed under an anaesthetic but sometimes without an anaesthetic. Steady longitudinal distraction of the joint is often a useful preliminary to the forcing of the extreme range.

Subsequent management. The manipulation should usually be followed by physiotherapy to maintain the function of the joint. It may be repeated after an interval if initial improvement does not progress to complete cure.

Dangers and safeguards in treatment by manipulation. Manipulation may do harm if it is undertaken for the stiffness of inflammatory arthritis in an active stage, or if a tumour or other destructive disease exists close to the joint. It is also inadvisable in cases of acute back pain due to prolapsed intervertebral disc, because it may cause further extrusion of disc material. This emphasises the importance of careful clinical and radiological examination – supplemented when necessary by other investigations such as determination of the erythrocyte sedimentation rate, radioisotope scanning, radiculography or magnetic resonance imaging – before treatment is begun. It must be emphasised again that manipulation is of no value for stiffness of the metacarpo-phalangeal joints and interphalangeal joints of the hand.

During the manipulation itself care must be taken to avoid disasters such as the fracture of a bone or massive displacement of an intervertebral disc. It is well known that a fracture – especially of the patella or humerus, or even of the femur – may be caused easily by injudicious manipulations. This risk is greatly increased if the bone is already weak from the osteoporosis of disuse or from other rarefying disease.

RADIOTHERAPY

Radiotherapy – by X-rays or by the gamma rays of radio-active substances – may be used for certain benign conditions or for malignant disease. Because of its possible ill effects – particularly the risk of inducing malignant change – it should be advised only with caution for benign lesions, but its use may rarely be justified in the treatment of some cases of giant-cell tumour of bone that are unsuitable for local excision because of their anatomical site. In malignant disease radiotherapy is occasionally curative but more often palliative. In conditions such as malignant bone tumours, for which a tumour dose in the range of 5000–6000 centiGray may be required, only the penetrating rays produced by a super-voltage linear accelerator or by a radio-active cobalt unit should be used. With such apparatus a high dose can be delivered to the tumour with the least possible damage to the skin.

OPERATIVE TREATMENT

The chief essential of any operation is that it should not make the patient worse. This is so obvious that the statement may sound almost absurd. Yet it is unfortunately true that a disturbing number of operations carried out for orthopaedic conditions do in fact cause more harm than good for one reason or another. Hence the selection of cases for operation, the choice of the most appropriate operation in given circumstances, the technical performance of the operation, and the post-operative management are matters of the highest importance, and they call for a high degree of judgement and skill. Herein lies much of the fascination of orthopaedic surgery.

A detailed account of operative techniques is unnecessary here. All that is required is a brief mention of the more important operations.

SYNOVECTOMY

Synovectomy is the operation for removal of the inflamed lining of a joint, while leaving the capsule intact. It may be of value in some types of chronic infective arthritis as well as occasionally in early rheumatoid arthritis. Because of the difficulty in gaining anatomical access, it is necessarily a subtotal procedure; but it may nevertheless afford worthwhile relief by reducing local pain and swelling. There is no clear evidence that it protects the articular cartilage from further damage; but the removal of a large part of this invasive granulation tissue or pannus may be of benefit by reducing the production of proteolytic enzymes.

OSTEOTOMY

Osteotomy is the operation of cutting a bone or creating a surgical fracture.
Indications. The general indications for osteotomy are as follows:

1. to correct excessive angulation, bowing or rotation of a long bone
2. to permit angulation of a bone in order to compensate for mal-alignment at a joint
3. to permit elongation or shortening of a bone in the lower limb in order to correct a discrepancy of length between the two sides.

In addition, there are certain special indications for osteotomy at the upper end of the femur, as follows:

4. to improve stability at the hip by altering the line of weight transmission (abduction osteotomy)
5. to improve containment in transient avascular necrosis of the epiphysis of a long bone
6. to relieve the pain of an osteoarthritic hip (displacement osteotomy, Fig. 17.28A, p. 363).

Technique. If the bone is relatively soft (as in children) it may be divided simply with an osteotome or, in the case of a thin bone, by bone-cutting forceps. The strong cortex of the major long bones in an adult is not easily divided in that way because it tends to splinter; so most surgeons weaken the bone by making multiple drill holes before applying the osteotome, or, alternatively, they use a powered saw or a high-speed dental burr. When the bone has been divided and the necessary correction made it is often convenient to fix the fragments with a plate, nail-plate, or medullary nail: this may allow external splintage to be dispensed with. If internal fixation is not used the fragments may be immobilised by an external fixator; or they may be held in position by a suitable splint or plaster until union has occurred.

ARTHRODESIS

The operation of arthrodesis, or joint fusion, is used less commonly since the advent of reliable techniques of joint reconstruction, or arthroplasty, for the major limb joints. It has the advantage of providing a painless stable joint and the disability from a single stiff joint is usually slight, and patients readily adapt themselves to it. Even when two or three joints are fused function may be surprisingly good, depending upon the particular joints affected. This gives arthrodesis its most common application for treatment of arthritis in the small joints of the hands and feet but it is now rarely used for the hip, knee, or shoulder except as a salvage procedure.

Indications. Arthrodesis is indicated mainly in the following conditions:

1. advanced osteoarthritis or rheumatoid arthritis with disabling pain, especially when confined to a single joint
2. quiescent tuberculous arthritis with destruction of the joint surfaces, to eliminate risk of recrudescence and to prevent deformity
3. instability from muscle paralysis, as after poliomyelitis
4. for permanent correction of deformity, as in hammer toe.

Methods of arthrodesis. Arthrodesis may be intra-articular or extra-articular, or the two may be combined. In *intra-articular* arthrodesis the joint is opened and the bone ends are displayed. The articular cartilage (or what remains of it) is removed so that raw bone is exposed. The joint is placed in the desired position and immobilised, usually by metallic internal fixation as well as by a plaster-of-Paris splint, until clinical tests and radiographs show sound bony fusion. In some cases an external fixation device can be used with the addition of compression across the opposed bone surfaces which seems to speed union.

In *extra-articular* arthrodesis the joint itself is left undisturbed (though it may be immobilised by a nail or screw), but it is 'by-passed' by securing bone-to-bone fusion outside the joint, usually through the medium of a bone graft. The method is applicable mainly to the spine, shoulder, and hip. It has a theoretical advantage in cases of infective joint disease, because any risk of reactivating or disseminating the infection by opening the joint is avoided.

Examples of methods for arthrodesing the spine and a metatarso-phalangeal joint of the toe are illustrated in Fig. 4.1.

Position for arthrodesis. The best position for arthrodesis should not be regarded as rigidly established for each joint: variations may be appropriate and desirable in individual cases – for instance, to conform to the requirements of the patient's work. The following is only a general guide. *Shoulder:* 30° of abduction and flexion, with 40° of medial rotation. *Elbow:* If only one elbow is affected, 75° of flexion from the fully extended position (or according to the requirements of the patient's work). If both elbows are affected, one should be in flexion 10° above the right angle and the other about 20° below the right angle. If forearm rotation is lost the most useful position of the forearm is in 10° of pronation. *Wrist:* Extended 20°. *Metacarpo-phalangeal joints:* Flexed 35°. *Interphalangeal joints:* Semiflexed. *Hip:* About 15° of flexion; no abduction or

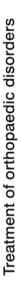

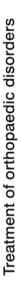

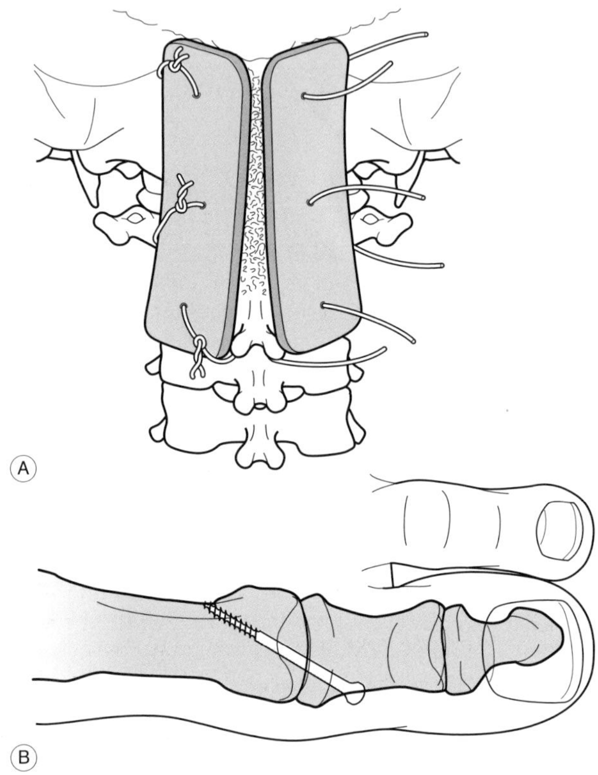

Fig 4.1 Two methods of arthrodesis (joint fusion). Ⓐ Extra-articular arthrodesis of the cervical spine using a posterior cortico-cancellous bone graft with wire fixation, proximal and distal to the intervertebral joint to be fused. Ⓑ Intra-articular arthrodesis of the metatarso-phalangeal joint of the great toe using internal fixation with a single screw to fix the raw cancellous bone surfaces in the desired position.

adduction. *Knee:* About 20° of flexion. *Ankle:* In men, right angle; in women, 15–25° of plantarflexion, according to accustomed height of heel. *Metatarso-phalangeal joint of big toe:* Slight extension, depending upon the accustomed height of shoe heel.

ARTHROPLASTY

Arthroplasty is the operation for construction of a new movable joint. Its successful development in the last 30 years has resulted from the introduction of new biomaterials to replace articular surfaces and the surgical techniques to attach these to bone. Arthroplasty of the hip has revolutionised the treatment of arthritis in that joint and its use has now been extended to the knee, as well as the ankle, the shoulder, the elbow, certain joints in the hand, and the first metatarso-phalangeal joint in the foot.

Indications. The indications for arthroplasty vary with the particular joint affected and the degree of disability. Broadly, it has a use in the following conditions:

1. advanced osteoarthritis or rheumatoid arthritis with disabling pain, especially in the hip, knee, ankle, shoulder, elbow, hand and metatarso-phalangeal joints
2. quiescent destructive tuberculous arthritis especially of the elbow or hip
3. for the correction of certain types of deformity (especially hallux valgus)
4. certain ununited fractures of the neck of the femur.

It will be realised that in several of these conditions arthroplasty is an alternative to arthrodesis. By far the commonest applications for arthroplasty are disabling osteoarthritis of the hip and the knee.

Methods of arthroplasty

Three methods are available:

1. excision arthroplasty
2. hemiarthroplasty or half-joint replacement
3. total replacement arthroplasty.

Each method has its merits, disadvantages and special applications.

Excision arthroplasty. In this method one or both of the articular ends of the bones are simply excised, so that a gap is created between them (Fig. 4.2) effectively creating a false joint or pseudarthrosis. The gap fills with fibrous tissue, or a pad of muscle or other soft tissue may be sewn in between the bones. By virtue of its flexibility the interposed tissue allows a reasonable range of movement, but the joint often lacks stability making it less suitable for the large weight-bearing joints of the lower limb. Excision arthroplasty is used most commonly at the metatarso-phalangeal joint of the big toe, in the treatment of hallux valgus and hallux rigidus (Keller's operation). It is also occasionally used at the hip, usually as a salvage operation after failed replacement arthroplasty. It is used occasionally at the elbow, the shoulder, and certain of the small joints of the hands and feet.

Hemi-arthroplasty (half-joint replacement arthroplasty). In a hemiarthroplasty only one of the articulating surfaces is removed and replaced by a prosthesis of similar shape (Fig. 4.3A). The prosthesis is usually made from

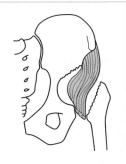

Fig. 4.2 Excision arthroplasty (pseudarthrosis) of the hip. Note the interposed soft tissue between the bony surfaces.

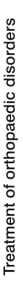

Treatment of orthopaedic disorders

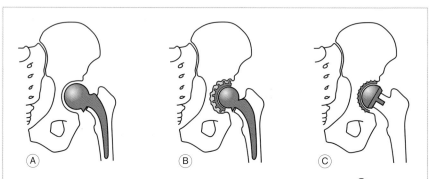

Fig. 4.3 Three methods of arthroplasty (joint replacement) used at the hip. Ⓐ Half-joint replacement arthroplasty: the femoral head is replaced by a metal prosthesis. Ⓑ Total replacement arthroplasty. The femoral head is replaced by a metal prosthesis and the acetabulum by a plastic socket. Both components may be held in place by acrylic filling compound or 'cement'. Ⓒ Resurfacing (double cup) arthroplasty. Matching metal shells are used to resurface the femoral head and acetabular socket with cemented or cementless fixation.

metal. When appropriate, it may be fixed into the recipient bone with acrylic filling compound or 'bone cement'. The opposing, normal articulating surface is left undisturbed. The technique has its main application at the hip, where prosthetic replacement of the head and neck of the femur is commonly practised for femoral neck fracture in the elderly. The disadvantage is that any degeneration in the unreplaced articular surface will accelerate with recurrence of pain and loss of movement making it unsuitable for younger patients. It has rather a limited use elsewhere, examples being the replacement of the head of the radius after certain types of fracture, and replacement of the lunate bone in Kienböck's disease.

Total replacement arthroplasty. In this technique both of the opposed articulating surfaces are excised and replaced by prosthetic components (Fig. 4.3B). In the larger joints one of the components is usually of metal and the other of high-density polyethylene, and it is usual for both components to be held in place by acrylic 'bone cement'. In small joints such as the metacarpo-phalangeal joints a flexible one-piece prosthesis made from silicone rubber may be used.

Total replacement arthroplasty has proved very successful at the hip, and at the knee. It has been extended, so far with only moderate success, to many other joints including the shoulder, elbow, ankle, metacarpo-phalangeal joints, and metatarso-phalangeal joints. A disadvantage – which applies also to half-joint replacement arthroplasty – is that there is a tendency for the prosthesis to work loose after 10–15 years. This results from bone resorption around the implant due to an aseptic inflammatory reaction triggered by the production of microscopic wear particles from the artificial materials used for the articulating surfaces. In turn this has led to a search for harder materials and improved prosthetic designs to minimise the production of wear particles.

Another approach to preserve bone in younger patients, who might require later revision surgery, is to resurface rather than replace the joint. Attempts have been made to achieve this biologically with autogenous chondrocytes in the knee, or with artificial materials as in the double cup arthroplasty of the hip (Fig. 4.3C). The longer-term results from these new techniques remain uncertain and it should be noted that a conventional well-fitted replacement joint may give good service for as long as 15–20 years, especially in the case of the hip or knee.

BONE GRAFTING OPERATIONS

Bone grafts are usually obtained from another part of the patient's body (autogenous grafts or autografts). If it is impracticable or undesirable to take bone from the patient's own body, grafts from another human subject may be used (allografts, homogenous grafts or homografts). These must be stored frozen under aseptic conditions until they have been proved to be free from transmissible infection, including HIV and other dangerous viral infections. For bone from living donors (mainly femoral heads removed during hip replacement operations) this necessitates retesting after 9 months to ensure that the donor was not incubating infectious disease at the time of removal of the bone. Cadaveric bone sterilised by irradiation is sometimes used and is increasingly available from large tissue banks. Grafts obtained from animals (xenografts, heterogenous grafts or heterografts) may be applicable if they are specially treated to reduce their antigenic properties. At some centres limited use is still made of such bone (chiefly bovine) prepared commercially in sterile packs, but it has been shown to be far inferior to the patient's own bone and cannot be relied upon to become incorporated with the host bone.

Bone transferred as a free autograft from one site to another does not survive wholly in a living state. For the most part the bone cells die, although a proportion may possibly survive, especially in cancellous bone. The purpose of the graft – as of allografts and heterografts – is mainly to serve as a scaffolding or temporary bridge upon which new bone is laid down. It also provides an osteogenic stimulus to the host cells from the bone morphogenic proteins released from the non-cellular bone matrix. Thus the whole of a graft is eventually replaced by new living bone. This process of replacement is dependent upon adequate revascularisation of the graft; so a graft that lies in a highly vascular bed is more likely to succeed than one that is surrounded by relatively ischaemic tissue.

With refinements in the technique of microvascular surgery it is now possible to transfer bone with its soft-tissue coverings on a vascular pedicle to a distant recipient site, with immediate anastomosis of its nutrient vessels to those in the new bed. Such living grafts are found to become incorporated rapidly. Vascularised grafts are especially valuable in major reconstructive procedures after extensive loss of bone and soft tissue.

Indications. Bone grafts are used mainly in three types of case:

1. in cases of ununited fracture, to promote union
2. in arthrodesis of joints, either to supplement an intra-articular arthrodesis or to promote extra-articular fusion (see p. 39)
3. to fill a defect or cavity in a bone.

Technique. Autogenous bone for grafting may be obtained as a solid slab, or it may be used in the form of multiple slivers or strips, or of small chips.

Strut grafts. A strut graft is usually obtained from strong cortical bone: the subcutaneous part of the tibia is a common site. The graft is fixed to the recipient bone either by internal fixation or by inlaying. Such a graft serves as an internal splint as well as providing a framework for the growth of new bone (Fig. 4.4A).

Treatment of orthopaedic disorders

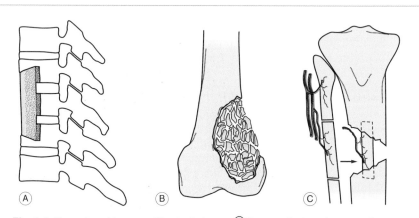

Fig. 4.4 Examples of bone grafting techniques. Ⓐ Strut graft of cortico-cancellous bone used to provide inlay fixation for anterior cervical spine fusion. Ⓑ Cancellous grafts used to fill a cavity in a bone. Ⓒ Vascularised fibula bone graft.

Strip grafts. Sliver or strip grafts are generally obtained from spongy cancellous bone – especially from the crest of the ilium. They are used commonly for ununited fractures. They are laid about the fracture, deep to the periosteum, and are held in place by suture of the soft tissues over them.

Chip grafts. These also are preferably obtained from cancellous bone. They serve the same purposes as sliver grafts but are smaller pieces of bone. The chips are packed firmly into, or around, the recipient bone and are held in place simply by suture of the soft tissues over them (Fig. 4.4B).

Vascularised grafts. These require a suitable donor site, such as the fibula, rib, or iliac crest, together with a meticulous microscopic technique to secure the necessary re-anastomosis of the nutrient vessels at the new site (Fig. 4.4C). The method is only suitable for use in specialised centres with the necessary equipment and expertise.

TENDON TRANSFER OPERATIONS

In the operation of tendon transfer, or tendon transplant, the insertion of a healthy functioning muscle is moved to a new site, so that the muscle henceforth has a different action. In this way the lost function of a paralysed or severed muscle can be taken over by one that is intact. In properly selected cases there need be no noticeable loss of power in the former sphere of action of the transferred muscle, because there is often considerable duplication or overlap in the function of individual muscles. Thus a tendon of flexor digitorum superficialis may be transferred to a new site without appreciably impairing the power of finger flexion, which can be adequately controlled by the flexor profundus. Similarly the extensor indicis can be spared for a new function without seriously interfering with the power of extension of the index finger (Fig. 4.5).

Indications. Tendon transfers have their main application in three groups of conditions:

1. in cases of muscle paralysis, to restore or improve active control of a joint by re-routing a healthy muscle to act in place of a paralysed one

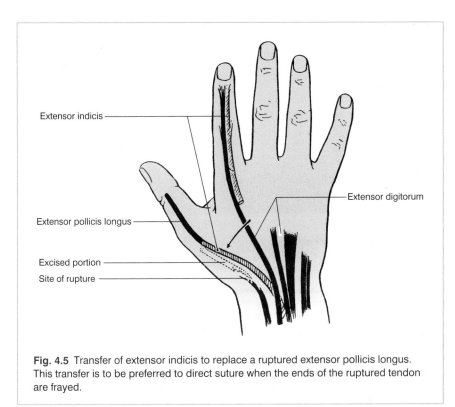

Extensor indicis

Extensor digitorum

Extensor pollicis longus

Excised portion

Site of rupture

Fig. 4.5 Transfer of extensor indicis to replace a ruptured extensor pollicis longus. This transfer is to be preferred to direct suture when the ends of the ruptured tendon are frayed.

2. in cases of deformity from muscle imbalance, to maintain correction by switching healthy muscles to restore proper balance
3. in cases of ruptured or cut tendon, when direct suture of the ends is impracticable.

Technique. The tendon to be transferred is divided at an appropriate point, re-routed in the direction of its new action, and secured to its new insertion. If it is to be inserted into bone it is passed through a drill hole and held by suturing back on itself or by suturing to the periosteum or soft tissues on the deep aspect of the bone. If it is to be united to a tendon stump the junction may be secured by end-to-end suture or, preferably, by interlacing the tendons one through the other and transfixing them with mattress sutures.

Examples. 1. In a case of paralysis of the radial nerve, with loss of active extension of the wrist, fingers, and thumb, function may be restored by the following tendon transfers: pronator teres is transferred to extensor carpi radialis brevis; flexor carpi ulnaris is transferred to extensor digitorum and extensor pollicis longus; and palmaris longus is transferred to abductor pollicis longus. 2. In a case of congenital talipes equino-varus (p. 434) transfer of the tendon of the tibialis anterior or tibialis posterior to the outer side of the foot will help to prevent recurrence of the deformity. 3. In a case of rupture of the extensor pollicis longus, with extensive fraying of the tendon, direct repair may be impracticable. Function may be restored by transfer of the extensor indicis to the extensor pollicis longus (Fig. 4.5).

Treatment of orthopaedic disorders

TENDON GRAFTING OPERATIONS

In tendon grafting a length of free tendon is used to bridge a gap between the severed ends of the recipient tendon.

Indications. The chief use of free tendon grafts is in the reconstruction of flexor tendons severed and adherent in the fibrous digital sheaths of the hand (p. 324).

Technique. The free tendon graft is usually obtained from the palmaris longus or from one of the toe extensors at the dorsum of the foot. The original, adherent tendon is removed. Proximally, the graft is joined to the recipient tendon by sutures of stainless steel wire. Distally, it may be secured to the distal stump of the recipient tendon or it may be attached directly to bone through a drill hole.

EQUALISATION OF LEG LENGTH

If a patient's legs are of markedly unequal length, as in certain cases of congenital anomaly, previous poliomyelitis, or damage to a growth epiphysis, the discrepancy may be reduced or eliminated by operation. The methods available are:

1. leg lengthening
2. leg shortening
3. arrest of epiphysial growth.

Leg lengthening is suitable mainly for children. It is achieved by dividing the appropriate bone (usually the tibia, sometimes the femur) and then gradually elongating the limb in a special screw-distraction apparatus at the rate of about 2 mm a day. A maximum of about 5 cm may be gained. The procedure is time-consuming and trying for the patient, and should be reserved for carefully selected cases in which the discrepancy in length is marked. A more recent innovation is the technique of *bone transport*, in which a length of the diaphysis is moved slowly downwards to fill a gap, while new bone forms to fill in the space created by its advancement (Fig. 4.6). These techniques have been facilitated by the introduction of the ring frame distraction apparatus of Ilizarov[1], which allows correction of angulation as well as lengthening (Fig. 4.7).

Leg shortening, by removing an appropriate length from the shaft of the longer femur or tibia, is less hazardous but not to be undertaken lightly because it disturbs a limb that was previously normal. In a patient who is fairly tall, and especially in adults, it is often preferable to leg lengthening.

Arrest of epiphysial growth (on the longer side) is applicable only to children with considerable growth still to come. It entails either destruction, or bridging by bone grafts or by metal staples, of the lower femoral epiphysis or of the upper tibial epiphysis, or both. The correction to be expected depends upon the amount of growth still to come from the corresponding epiphysis of the opposite (shorter) leg, which depends in turn upon the patient's age at the time of operation, and upon the nature of the abnormality that is responsible for the shortening.

[1]Gauril Abramovich Ilizarov (1921–1992) Russian surgeon with little formal research training who developed practical application of tension stress to tissues. Became Professor at Kurgen Institute in Siberia and was elected to the Soviet Academy of Medicine.

Bone transport
= Movement of segment of bone in its soft
  tissue sleeve with the formation of new bone
  in its path

Length of limb maintained throughout treatment

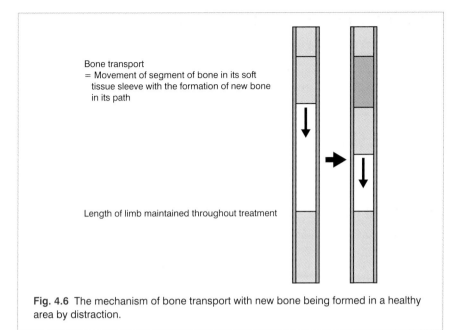

Fig. 4.6 The mechanism of bone transport with new bone being formed in a healthy area by distraction.

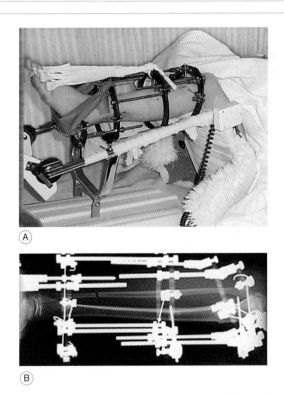

Ⓐ

Ⓑ

Fig. 4.7 Ⓐ Ilizarov frame applied to tibia for leg lengthening. Ⓑ Radiograph of leg in frame to show position of fixator pins in relation to osteotomy of tibia.

Tissue distraction techniques

Relatively recently, the principle of tissue distraction was described by Ilizarov. This states that if a tissue is very gradually pulled apart it responds by creating new tissue. The principle was initially described for bone, where it was shown that if a bone was divided and following a delay period of 3–10 days, was pulled apart at approximately 1 mm/day, the body responded by creating a column of callus, which eventually would consolidate into healthy new bone.

This process is now used extensively in limb lengthening, bone transport and the correction of deformity. In the latter case, the bone is gradually straightened and rotated to the desired position. In bone transport, the same process is used to fill a bone defect (which may have arisen as a result of trauma or from the treatment of bone infection or tumours), the bone is divided through a healthy area and a segment of bone is pulled through the defect in order to create a column of new bone which fills the defect (Fig. 4.6).

The same principle can be used to create soft tissues such as muscle, nerve, tendon and skin during the gradual correction of contractures of joints.

BONE FIXATION TECHNIQUES

The same modalities of bone stabilisation that are used during fracture treatment are used for reconstructive surgery. Osteotomies are often stabilised with casts in children, but in adults are more commonly stabilised with plates, intramedullary nails, or external fixation. During the arthrodesis of joints, both internal and external fixation methods are used. Limb lengthening is usually carried out with specific external fixators, but more recently internal lengthening nails have been developed which are applicable for some patients.

External fixation frames consist of a frame that lies external to the skin, which is connected to the bone via 'half pins' or fine wires that pass from the frame through the skin and into the bone. The half pins are relatively broad (4–6 mm) and pass from the external frame through the soft tissues on one side of the limb and finally through both cortices of the bone. Fine wires (1.5–2 mm) are used with circular external fixators and completely transfix the limb, going through both cortices of the bone and the soft tissues on each side of the limb. The fine wires are placed under tension and then clamped to the circular external frame. During lengthening and the correction of deformity, fine adjustments are made to the connecting struts on the external frame which bring about the desired amount of lengthening or deformity correction.

AMPUTATION

Amputation can be a useful treatment option. It may be necessary for malignant tumours for which it is not possible to perform a limb salvage procedure. In certain patients with congenital conditions, such as pseudarthrosis, a below-knee amputation may be the best treatment. Most commonly, amputations are carried out for peripheral vascular disease, infection or trauma.

With improvements in the design and manufacture of modern prosthetic limbs, the function after below-knee amputation is usually extremely good

Treatment of orthopaedic disorders

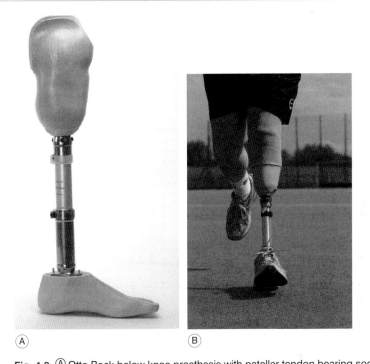

(A)　　　　　　　　(B)

Fig. 4.8 Ⓐ Otto Bock below knee prosthesis with patellar tendon bearing socket and a SACH foot. Ⓑ Amputee wearing the below knee prosthesis, without its cosmetic covering, to demonstrate the level of functional activity that can be achieved.

(Fig. 4.8). However after above-knee amputation, walking is more difficult and requires approximately a third more energy than normal. Function after upper limb amputation is also far less good, and upper limb amputation should be avoided if at all possible. As many as 80% of patients may experience 'phantom limb' sensation after amputation, that is they feel a limb that is no longer there and this may be accompanied by persistent pain.

Common levels for amputation are through the mid-foot (Chopart, Lisfranc), distal tibia (Syme's, Pyrogroff), proximal tibia (below-knee amputation), distal femur (above-knee amputation). The aim is to provide a soundly healed end bearing stump with good muscle control and this should not be compromised in order to maintain length.

Part 2

This part, comprising seven chapters, is devoted to a broad preliminary review of the field of orthopaedics. The main groups of disorders will be described without a detailed consideration of their local manifestations. Against this general background the features of the common disorders as they affect each particular region will be discussed in the subsequent chapters.

Recent injuries of the limbs and spine form a subject of separate study, and are dealt with in the companion volume to this work, *Outline of Fractures*.

CLASSIFICATION OF ORTHOPAEDIC DISORDERS

Most orthopaedic disorders fall within the following groups:

Deformities Congenital deformities Acquired deformities	**Soft tissue tumours and other diseases** Tumours of soft tissue Inflammatory lesions of soft tissue
General affections of the skeleton Bone dysplasias Inborn errors of metabolism Metabolic bone disease Endocrine disorders	**Arthritis and other joint disorders** Arthritis Dislocation and subluxation Internal derangements
Infections of bone and joints Infections of bone Joint infections	**Neurological disorders** Cerebral palsy Spina bifida Poliomyelitis Peripheral nerve lesions
Bone tumours and other local conditions Tumours of bone Osteochondritis Cystic change	

5 | Deformities and congenital disorders

Deformities may be congenital or acquired, and they may reflect an underlying abnormality of bone, joint, or soft tissue.

CONGENITAL DEFORMITIES

Congenital deformities or malformations, by definition, are attributable to faulty development and are present at birth, though they may not be recognised until later. They vary from severe malformations that are incompatible with life and may be found in still-born infants, to minor abnormalities of structure that have no practical significance. Incidence varies in different countries and among different races: in Britain probably 2 or 3% of infants are born with some significant developmental abnormality, but only about half of these affect the musculo-skeletal system. Some of the better-known anomalies are summarised in Table 5.1 (p. 53).

Causes

An abnormality of development may be caused by:

1. genetic abnormality
2. environmental abnormality
3. combined genetic and environmental abnormalities.

Studies of families and twins have helped geneticists to determine the influence of genetic and environmental factors, alone or combined, in the causation of many of the recognised malformations.

Genetic causes include mutation of a whole chromosome, as in Down's syndrome (mongolism), and mutation of a small part of a chromosome or of a single gene, as in achondroplasia. The defect is not necessarily always inherited from an affected parent: it may arise from a fresh mutation in the germ cell.

Environmental causes are not well understood. Experiments in animals have shown that many different types of environmental influence – dietetic, hormonal, chemical, physical, or infective – may cause abnormalities of development, and the system of the body that is mainly affected depends upon the timing of the environmental 'insult'. But except for a few specific agents acting early in pregnancy there is no conclusive evidence that similar influences are important causes of malformations in man. The specific agents whose influence in man is well attested include radiation, the virus of rubella, and certain drugs (notably aminopterin and thalidomide).

Combined genetic and environmental factors seem to be the usual cause of the more common congenital malformations in man, on the evidence of twin and family studies. It is thought probable that developing embryos react

Table 5.1 Some of the better-known congenital deformities or anomalies of orthopaedic interest, with their salient clinical features. (When a fuller description appears elsewhere in this book the relevant page number is given. Conditions not thus designated are either so rare or of such little importance to the student that further description is unnecessary.)

Name of deformity or anomaly	Clinical or pathological features
Generalised	
Osteogenesis imperfecta (fragilitas ossium) (p. 62)	Fragile soft bones, easily broken or deformed. Often blue sclerotics. Joint laxity. Otosclerosis
Diaphysial aclasis (multiple exostoses) (p. 63)	Cartilage-capped bony outgrowths from metaphyses. Deficient remodelling. Stunted growth
Dyschondroplasia (multiple chondromatosis; Ollier's disease) (p. 65)	Masses of cartilage in metaphyses of long bones. Impaired growth. Deformity. Often unilateral
Achondroplasia (chondro-dystrophy) (p. 61)	Short-limb dwarfing from defective growth of long bones. Trident hand. Large head
Osteopetrosis (Albers–Schönberg disease; 'marble bones')	Hard dense bones, but with increased liability to fracture. Anaemia from obliteration of medulla
Gargoylism (Hurler's syndrome)	Dwarfing. Kyphosis from deformed vertebrae. Corneal opacity. Large liver and spleen. Mental deficiency
Cranio-cleido dysostosis (p. 71)	Impaired ossification of skull. Deficient clavicles. Often deficient symphysis pubis
Arthrogryposis multiplex congenita (amyoplasia congenita)	Stiff deformed limb joints from defective development of muscles, usually secondary to nerve cell deficiency though a type due to primary dysplasia of muscle is also recognised. Hips often dislocated. Club feet
Pseudohypertrophic muscular dystrophy	Genetic transmission to boys through female carriers. Progressive muscle weakness evident at age 3–6 years. Raised urinary creatine phosphokinase: carriers may thus be identified. The defect may be diagnosed in early pregnancy, when abortion may be advised
Fibrodysplasia ossificans progressiva (p. 71)	Ectopic ossification, often beginning in trunk but extending to limbs. Short great toe
Familial hypophosphataemia (p. 76)	Rachitic bone changes corrected only by massive doses of vitamin D. Hypophosphataemia not responsive to vitamin D
Cystinosis (renal tubular rickets) (p. 78)	Rachitic rarefied bones with consequent deformity. Hypophosphataemia. Glycosuria; amino-aciduria
Neurofibromatosis (von Recklinghausen's disease) (p. 70)	*Café au lait* areas or spots. Cutaneous fibromata. Neurofibromata on cranial or peripheral nerves. Often scoliosis. Occasionally, overgrowth of bone
Haemophilia (p. 145)	Prolonged blood clotting time from deficiency of Factor VIII. Bleeding into joints or soft tissue
Gaucher's disease (p. 72)	Deposition of kerasin in reticulum cells, causing cyst-like appearance in bones, and large liver and spleen
Down's syndrome (mongolism)	Mental and physical impairment from trisomy of chromosome 21, giving 47 instead of 46 chromosomes

Continued

Table 5.1 *Cont'd.*

Name of deformity or anomaly	Clinical or pathological features
Trunk and spine	
Congenital short neck (Klippel–Feil syndrome) (p. 188)	Short stiff neck with low hair-line. Fused or deformed cervical vertebrae
Congenital high scapula (Sprengel's shoulder) (p. 189)	Scapula tethered high up, usually only on one side. Scapular movement impaired
Cervical rib (p. 202)	Often symptomless. Vascular symptoms (partial ischaemia) or nerve symptoms (paraesthesiae, lower trunk paresis)
Hemivertebra (congenital scoliosis) (pp. 213, 218)	Defective development of vertebra (and often of adjacent structures) on one side. Scoliosis
Spina bifida (spinal dysraphism) (p. 171)	Spina bifida occulta, meningocele or myelocele. Often leg deformities from paralysis or muscle imbalance. Often incontinence. Often associated hydrocephalus. Diagnosable in early pregnancy from excess of alpha-fetoprotein in urine and amniotic fluid
Limbs	
Congenital arterio-venous fistula	Hypertrophy and lengthening of limb. Bruit
Congenital amputation	Part or whole of one or more limbs absent
Phocomelia	Aplasia of proximal part of limb, the distal part being present ('seal-limb'). Diagnosable in pregnancy by ultrasonography
Constriction rings	Limb or digit constricted as if by a tight string. May be associated with syndactyly
Absence of radius (radial club hand)	Hand deviated laterally from lack of normal support by radius. Thumb often absent
Absence of thumb	Thumb alone may be absent, but other deformities may co-exist
Absence of proximal arm muscles	Trapezius, deltoid, sternomastoid, or pectoralis major absent
Radio-ulnar synostosis	Forearm bones fused at proximal ends, preventing rotation
Madelung's deformity (dyschondrosteosis) (p. 303)	Head of ulna dislocated dorsally from lower end of radius. Radius bowed
Syndactyly	Webbing of two or more digits
Polydactyly	More than five digits
Ectrodactyly	Lobster-claw appearance of hand, with pincer grip
Congenital dislocation of hip (p. 343)	Neonatal: diagnostic click obtainable. Later infancy: shortening; limited abduction. Radiographs diagnostic
Congenital coxa vara (p. 376)	Defective ossification of femoral neck, with reduced neck–shaft angle
Congenital short femur	Proximal end of femur deficient or rudimentary. Thigh short
Congenital tibial pseudarthrosis	Resembles ununited fracture in tibial shaft. Aetiology unknown, may be neurofibromatosis

Table 5.1 *Cont'd.*

Name of deformity or anomaly	Clinical or pathological features
Absence of fibula	Leg under-developed on outer side. Foot small and everted; lateral two or three digital rays may be absent
Congenital club foot (p. 434)	Foot inverted and plantarflexed (equino-varus), or everted and dorsiflexed (calcaneo-valgus)
Congenital curled toe (p. 458)	Lateral angulation of one or more toes. Toe may lie over or under adjacent toe

differently to environmental influences: some have a natural resistance whereas others are susceptible. A malformation is therefore likely to arise when an environmental 'insult' is inflicted upon cells that have a genetically determined lack of resistance to it.

CONGENITAL PSEUDARTHROSIS

Pseudarthrosis (false joint) occurs when a fractured bone fails to unite and remains mobile. Congenital pseudarthrosis can be present at birth, or the bone can bend (resulting in anterolateral bowing), and then fracture in the first few years of life. Congenital pseudarthrosis is a rare condition. It occurs most often in the tibia (1 in 200 000) births, but also is seen in other long bones such as the fibula, femur, radius, and ulna.

The aetiology of congenital pseudarthrosis is unknown, but the periosteum for several centimetres either side of the pseudarthrosis is abnormally thickened.

Approximately 50% of cases of congenital pseudarthrosis of the tibia have neurofibromatosis type I (but only 3% of neurofibromatosis patients have pseudarthrosis). Congenital pseudarthrosis is also associated with fibrous dysplasia and amniotic constriction bands.

The affected limb usually grows more slowly, and shortening of the limb ensues. Treatment options include bone grafting, Ilizarov procedures, intramedullary nailing, and below-knee amputation.

Practical significance

Many of the recognised congenital abnormalities of the musculo-skeletal system have little practical importance, either because they are very rare or because there is little that can be done for them: these will not all be considered further in this book. There are others, however, that present major problems to the orthopaedic surgeon and may demand energetic treatment. These include developmental or congenital dislocation of the hip (p. 343), congenital club foot (p. 434), spina bifida (p. 171), congenital scoliosis (p. 218), osteogenesis imperfecta (p. 62), and cervical rib (p. 202).

Inborn predisposition to disease in adults

It is well recognised that, quite apart from the overt congenital anomalies discussed above, there exists in some patients a genetically determined predisposition to abnormalities developing in later life. Examples of orthopaedic conditions to which a susceptibility may exist include certain types of osteo-arthritis (especially of the hips), ankylosing spondylitis, gouty arthritis, rheumatic fever, idiopathic scoliosis, osteochondritis dissecans, and Dupuytren's contracture.

ACQUIRED DEFORMITIES

Acquired deformities may be classified in two groups: those in which deformity arises at a joint, and those in which it arises in a bone.

DEFORMITY ARISING AT A JOINT

Deformity may be said to exist at a joint when the joint cannot be placed voluntarily in the neutral anatomical position.

Causes

The causes of deformity arising at a joint may be summarised under the following headings (Fig. 5.1):

1. dislocation or subluxation
2. muscle imbalance
3. tethering or contracture of muscles or tendons
4. contracture of soft tissues
5. arthritis
6. prolonged abnormal posture
7. unknown causes.

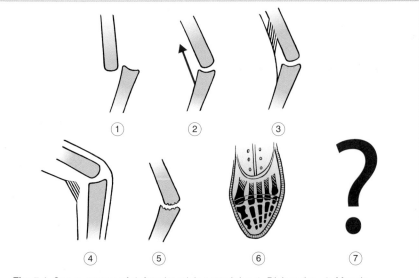

Fig. 5.1 Seven causes of deformity arising at a joint. 1. Dislocation. 2. Muscle imbalance. 3. Tethering of muscle or tendon. 4. Soft-tissue contracture. 5. Arthritis. 6. Posture 7. Idiopathic (cause unknown).

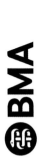

BMA

1

BMA Library

Freepost RTKJ-RKSZ-JGHG
British Medical Association
PO Box 291
LONDON
WC1H 9TG

Dislocation or subluxation

This is usually caused by injury, but it may occur as a congenital deformity, or it may follow disease of the joint (pathological dislocation).

Muscle imbalance

Unbalanced action of muscles upon a joint may hold it continuously in a particular arc of its range. In time, secondary contractures occur in the dominant muscles or in the soft tissues, preventing the joint from returning to the neutral position (Fig. 5.1 (2)). The two fundamental causes of muscle imbalance are:

1. weakness or paralysis of muscles
2. spasticity of muscles.

Thus equinus deformity at the ankle may follow paralysis of the dorsiflexor muscles (for instance, from damage to the lateral popliteal nerve) because the action of the plantarflexors and of gravity is unopposed. Or a similar deformity may be caused by spasticity of the calf muscles, which overpower their antagonists. This occurs commonly in cerebral palsy (p. 168).

Tethering or contracture of muscles or tendons

If something happens to muscles or tendons that prevents their normal to-and-fro gliding, or their elongation and retraction, the joint may be held in a position of deformity. Thus a muscle or tendon may be tethered to the surrounding tissues in consequence of local infection or injury (Fig. 5.1 (3)). An example is the anchoring of a flexor tendon of a finger within its fibrous sheath as a result of suppurative tenosynovitis, with consequent flexion deformity at the interphalangeal joints. Or a muscle may lose its elasticity and contractile power from impairment of its blood supply. An important example is Volkmann's ischaemic contracture of the forearm flexor muscles (p. 299) from occlusion of the brachial artery or from increased intra-compartmental pressure, with consequent flexion deformity of the wrist and fingers.

Contracture of soft tissues

Apart from any disturbance of the muscles, contracture of other soft tissues alone can account for joint deformity. An example is the common condition of Dupuytren's contracture (p. 321), in which the thickened and contracted palmar aponeurosis pulls the metacarpophalangeal and proximal interphalangeal joints of one or more fingers into flexion. Similarly, a flexion deformity of the knee or elbow, or indeed of any joint, may occur from contracture of the scarred skin after burns of the flexor surface of the limb (Fig. 5.1 (4)).

Arthritis

The various types of arthritis will be discussed in a later chapter. Any type of arthritis may lead to joint deformity. In some cases the joint is firmly fixed in a deformed position by bony or fibrous ankylosis. In other instances the joint retains some movement but is prevented from reaching the neutral position. Thus flexion and adduction deformity is common in osteoarthritis of the hip, flexion deformity is common in arthritis of the knee, and the deformity of ulnar deviation of the fingers (Fig. 16.11A, p. 305) is a well-known feature of rheumatoid arthritis of the metacarpo-phalangeal joints.

Posture

The habitual adoption of a deformed position of a joint often leads in time to permanent deformity. A common example is the lateral deviation of the great toe at the metatarso-phalangeal joint – hallux valgus – so common in women who cramp their feet into narrow pointed shoes (Fig. 5.1 (6)). Another postural deformity that is still seen occasionally – though it should never be allowed to occur – is fixed flexion of the knees in a patient confined to bed for a long time with the knees bent over a pillow.

Unknown causes

In some cases deformity occurs at a joint for no apparent reason. Thus many children develop knock-knee deformity between the ages of 3 and 5 years without demonstrable cause. It is usually unimportant because it tends to correct itself spontaneously. Another common and more serious example is the inversion deformity of the foot known as talipes equino-varus or congenital club foot. A more sinister deformity that is equally ill explained is the idiopathic scoliosis of adolescents (p. 215).

DEFORMITY ARISING IN A BONE

Deformity exists in a bone when it is out of its normal anatomical alignment.

Causes

There are three causes of deformity arising in bone:

1. fracture
2. bending
3. uneven epiphysial growth (Fig. 5.2).

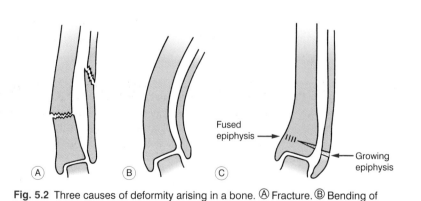

Fig. 5.2 Three causes of deformity arising in a bone. Ⓐ Fracture. Ⓑ Bending of softened bone. Ⓒ Uneven epiphysial growth.

Fracture

This is by far the most common cause. Unless a fracture is reduced so that the fragments are perfectly aligned, deformity will result. Examples are the genu valgum (knock knee) that is often the consequence of compression fractures of the lateral condyle of the tibia, the cubitus valgus that may follow displaced fractures of the lateral condyle of the humerus, and the common 'dinner-fork' deformity of an unreduced fracture of the lower end of the radius.

Congenital tibial pseudarthrosis may mimic an ununited fracture, but is often present at birth and may be linked to neurofibromatosis (see p. 70).

Bending of softened bone

Many unrelated conditions can cause softening of bone, with liability to bending and consequent deformity. They are mostly generalised disorders in which several or all of the bones are affected. The following are examples. *Metabolic disorders*: rickets, osteomalacia. *Endocrine disturbances*: parathyroid osteodystrophy, Cushing's syndrome. *Affections of unknown cause*: Paget's disease (osteitis deformans), fibrous dysplasia of bone, idiopathic osteoporosis. The main features of these disorders will be described in a later chapter.

Uneven growth of bone

In children any disturbance of the growing epiphysial cartilage (growth plate) may lead to uneven growth and consequent deformity. The usual effect of interference with a growing epiphysial cartilage is that its growth is retarded; occasionally it is accelerated. Deformity will follow only if the growing cartilage is affected more in one part than another, or if the interference with growth affects only one bone of a pair, as in the forearm or leg (Fig. 5.2C). The most frequent causes of retarded epiphysial growth are:

1. crushing fracture involving the epiphysial growth plate
2. infection of the cartilage, usually from adjacent osteomyelitis or joint infection
3. enchondroma (a benign tumour) adjacent to the cartilage, as in Ollier's disease (multiple enchondromatosis (p. 65)).

In the relatively uncommon cases in which epiphysial growth is accelerated the usual cause is local hyperaemia induced by an adjacent focus of infection or by a vascular tumour such as a haemangioma.

TREATMENT OF DEFORMITIES

Each deformity must be considered as an individual problem. Many do not require treatment, or are not amenable to it. In other cases an attempt may be made to correct or improve the deformity. One or more of the following methods may be used in appropriate cases:

1. manipulative correction and retention in a plaster or splint (example – for displaced fracture)
2. gradual correction by prolonged traction (example – for deformity in certain types of arthritis)

3. Alternatively, the gradual exertion force may be applied by an external frame such as the Ilizarov external fixator.
4. division or excision of contracted or tethered soft tissues (examples – for Dupuytren's contracture or scarring from burns)
5. osteotomy or osteoclasis (examples – for deformity from rickets or malunited fracture)
6. arthrodesis (example – for scoliosis)
7. selective retardation of epiphysial growth (in children) (example – for deformity from uneven epiphysial growth).

6 General affections of the skeleton

A large number of general affections of the skeleton have been described. Even an incomplete description could occupy a large volume. Fortunately many of these affections are so rare that it is unnecessary for the student to concern himself with them. Most of the others require only brief consideration. Clearly, many of the affections to be described have a congenital basis and many of them cause deformity; so there is inevitably some overlap between this chapter and Chapter 5.

CLASSIFICATION

The following classification is based on that of Wynne-Davies and Fairbank (1976).

Bone dysplasias and malformations	Metabolic bone disease
Achondroplasia	Hyperparathyroidism
Osteogenesis imperfecta	Nutritional rickets
Hereditary multiple exostosis (diaphysial aclasis)	Other forms of rickets
	Nutritional osteomalacia
Dyschondroplasia (Ollier's disease)	Other forms of osteomalacia
Paget's disease (osteitis deformans)	Vitamin C deficiency
Polyostotic fibrous dysplasia	
Neurofibromatosis	**Endocrine disorders**
Fibrodysplasia ossificans progressiva (myositis ossificans)	Osteoporosis
Cranio-cleido dysostosis	Hypopituitarism
Inborn errors of metabolism	Gigantism
	Acromegaly
Gaucher's disease	Hypothyroidism
Histiocytosis X	Glucocorticoid excess

BONE DYSPLASIAS

ACHONDROPLASIA

Achondroplasia is a congenital affection in which there is marked shortness of the limbs, with consequent dwarfing. It is of autosomal dominant inheritance but many cases arise from a fresh gene mutation.

Pathology. There is a failure of normal ossification in the long bones, which may be only half their normal length. Growth of the trunk is only slightly impaired.

General affections of the skeleton

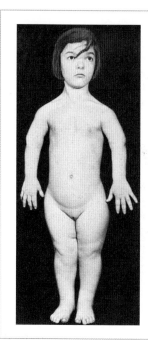

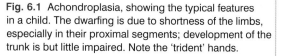

Fig. 6.1 Achondroplasia, showing the typical features in a child. The dwarfing is due to shortness of the limbs, especially in their proximal segments; development of the trunk is but little impaired. Note the 'trident' hands.

Clinical features. Achondroplasia is apparent at birth, the child being strikingly dwarfed, with very short limbs that are out of proportion to the trunk: shortness is especially marked in the proximal segments of the limbs (Fig. 6.1). Adult achondroplasts are seldom more than 130 cm (4 feet 3 inches) in height. The hands are short and broad, the central three digits being divergent and of almost equal length ('trident' hand). The head is slightly larger than normal, with a bulging forehead and depressed nasal bridge. There is marked lumbar lordosis, often with thoracic kyphosis, which may occasionally lead to compression of the spinal cord. There is no mental impairment and life expectancy is usually normal.

Radiographic features. Apart from striking shortness of the limbs, there are characteristic changes in the pelvis, the inlet being widened from side to side but narrowed in the antero-posterior diameter, with notably small greater sciatic notches. The spinal canal is also narrowed in the antero-posterior diameter, which predisposes to spinal stenosis. The calvarium of the skull is large, but the base short.

Treatment. With improved techniques of leg lengthening, there may be increasing scope in the future for worthwhile gain in stature.

OSTEOGENESIS IMPERFECTA (Fragilitas ossium)

Osteogenesis imperfecta is a congenital and inheritable disorder – or more probably a heterogeneous group of disorders – in which the bones are abnormally soft and brittle, on account of defective collagen formation. In addition to the bones, other collagen-containing tissues such as teeth, skin, tendons, and

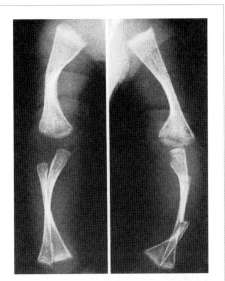

Fig. 6.2 Recent and old fractures of the bones of the upper limbs in an infant with osteogenesis imperfecta (fragilitas ossium).

ligaments may be abnormal. It is usually transmitted as an autosomal dominant, but in a severe variant of the disease the parents are normal and a fresh gene mutation or autosomal recessive inheritance is postulated.

Clinical features. In the worst cases, which occur sporadically rather than from inheritance and probably represent a distinct entity, the child is born with multiple fractures and does not survive. In the less severe examples fractures occur after birth, often from trivial violence. As many as fifty or more may be sustained in the first few years of life. The fractures unite readily, but in the more severe cases marked deformity often develops, either from malunion or from bending of the soft bones (Fig. 6.2), and such patients may be badly crippled. In the milder cases there is a tendency for fractures to occur less frequently in later life.

Additional features, not always present, are a deep blue colouration of the sclerotics of the eyes, deafness from otosclerosis (which becomes worse in later life), and ligamentous laxity.

Treatment. Fractures are generally treated in the ordinary way, but in a severe case intramedullary nailing of affected long bones should be considered as a means of preventing crippling deformity and permitting earlier resumption of activity. Newer techniques have been developed with telescoping rods, to obviate the need for multiple operations. Protective appliances, such as walking calipers, may be required in older children and adults.

MULTIPLE HEREDITARY EXOSTOSES
(Diaphyseal aclasis)

This is a congenital affection characterised by the formation of multiple exostoses (osteochondromata) at the metaphysial regions of the long bones. It is transmitted by an autosomal dominant mutant gene without any gender predisposition.

Pathology. The fault is in the epiphysial cartilage plate. Nests of cartilage cells become displaced and give rise to bony outgrowths, which are capped by proliferating cartilage. Growth of the exostoses may cease at skeletal maturity. These exostoses, or osteochondromata, constitute one type of benign bone tumour (p. 109). The number of outgrowths varies; often there are between ten and twenty, of varying size. In severe cases the process of remodelling by which a bone attains its normal adult shape is impaired, and there may be marked deformity, with reduction of longitudinal growth and consequent shortness of stature. Malignant change in the cartilaginous cap of one of the tumours can lead to the development of a chondrosarcoma (the lifetime risk is approximately 5%).

Clinical features. Usually the only symptoms and signs are those caused by the local swellings, or by their pressure effects. The patient is often of short stature, and there may be marked deformity of the limbs. Malignant change – often lethal – is suggested by rapid enlargement of one of the swellings in a patient, often at the age of skeletal maturity.

Radiographs show the bony outgrowths. In severe cases the bones are broad and ill modelled (Fig. 6.3).

Treatment. An outgrowth that is causing symptoms should be excised at its base and sent for routine histological examination to exclude any malignant change. Some deformities, particularly when they interfere with function, may require corrective osteotomies. Leg length discrepencies may also require correction, by either epiphyseal arrest or lengthening procedures.

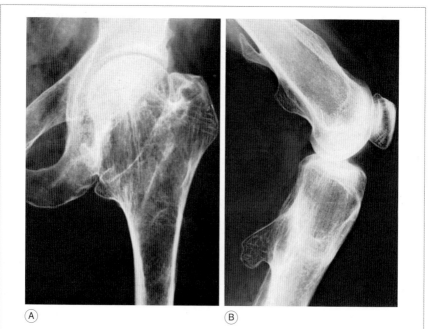

Ⓐ Ⓑ

Fig. 6.3 Diaphysial aclasis (multiple exostoses). Ⓐ shows stunting of the upper end of the femur due to failure of the remodelling process that accompanies normal growth. Defective remodelling is a characteristic feature of the disease in its more severe forms. Ⓑ shows typical exostoses (osteochondromata) projecting from femur and tibia. Such outgrowths are always directed away from the end of the bone.

General affections of the skeleton

MULTIPLE ENCHONDROMATOSIS (Dyschondroplasia; Ollier's disease[1])

In dyschondroplasia masses of unossified cartilage persist within the metaphyses of certain long bones, and the growth of the bone is retarded. The condition becomes evident in childhood, but the cause is unknown. In contrast with multiple hereditary exostoses, just described, heredity plays no part.

Pathology. The fault is in the epiphysial cartilage plate. In this respect dyschondroplasia resembles multiple exostoses, but this is the only resemblance between them: in other respects they are entirely distinct. Nests of cartilage cells are displaced from the epiphysial plate into the metaphysis, where they persist as enchondromata.

Any bone formed in cartilage may be affected. The more rapidly growing ends of the femur and tibia (that is, the ends near the knee) and the small long bones of the hands and feet are particularly common sites. There is a tendency for the disorder to affect one side of the body predominantly, or even exclusively. When a major long bone is affected interference with growth at the epiphysial cartilage adjacent to the lesion may lead to serious shortening and distortion of the bone (Fig. 6.4A). When skeletal growth ceases the masses of cartilage may ossify. Rarely one of the tumours undergoes malignant change, to become a chondrosarcoma (p. 117).

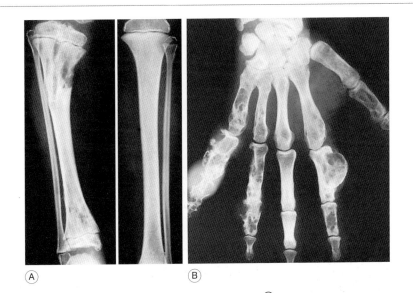

Fig. 6.4 Multiple enchondromatosis (Ollier's disease). Ⓐ Masses of proliferating cartilage occupy the metaphyses of one tibia. Growth is retarded and uneven. The normal tibia is shown for comparison. Ⓑ Multiple enchondromata in the metacarpals and phalanges.

[1]Louis Ollier (1830–1900) French surgeon who was senior surgeon at Lyons and described the clinical and radiological features of the condition in 1899. He was also an army surgeon and was decorated by the French President for his service.

Clinical and radiographic features. A limb affected by dyschondroplasia is usually short and may be markedly deformed. The hands may be grotesquely enlarged by multiple cartilaginous swellings or outgrowths. *Radiographs* show multiple areas of transradiance in the affected bones (Fig. 6.4).

Treatment. Osteotomy may be required to correct deformities resulting from uneven growth of bone. If there is marked discrepancy in the length of the lower limbs a leg equalisation procedure (p. 46) may be advisable. Lesions in the hand may be curetted and packed with bone chips.

PAGET'S DISEASE[1] (Osteitis deformans)

Paget's disease of bone is a slowly progressive disorder of one or several bones. Affected bones are thickened and spongy, and show a tendency to bend. The disease is one of the commonest general affections of the skeleton. The cause is unknown. It has been suggested that infection with a slow virus of the paramyxovirus family may be responsible, on the evidence of inclusion bodies that have been found consistently in the osteoclasts of affected bones.

Pathology. The basic abnormality is thought to be defective function of osteoclasts, with consequent irregular bone resorption and increase of bone turnover. The bones most commonly affected are the pelvis, vertebrae, femur, tibia, and skull. The disease may be confined to a single bone at first, but it often spreads to involve other bones later. The cortex of the bone loses its normal compact density and becomes spongy. At the same time the cortex is widened by the formation of new bone on both its outer and inner surfaces. The whole bone is thus thickened, but the usual sharp distinction between cortex and medulla is blurred. The marrow spaces are filled with fibrous tissue. Whereas the bone is soft and vascular at first, in the later stages there is a tendency for it to become denser and very hard.

In the spongy state the softened bones are liable to bend. Pathological fracture may occur. In rare instances osteosarcoma develops in the diseased bone.

Clinical features. The affection seldom begins before the age of 40, but a childhood form is recognised. Often there are no symptoms, the condition being discovered incidentally during routine radiographic examination. When long bones are affected pain is sometimes complained of, but it is by no means an invariable feature. Bending of the softened long bones leads to deformity, usually in the form of anterior and lateral bowing of the femur or tibia (Fig. 6.5). Thickening may be obvious clinically, especially in the case of the tibia or the skull. Thus if the patient wears a hat he may notice that he requires progressively larger sizes. More importantly, bone thickening may also cause constriction of foramina in the skull, with risk of damage to a nerve – for instance the optic nerve or the auditory nerve.

Imaging. The main *radiographic* features (Figs 6.6 and 6.7) are:

1. thickening of the bone, mainly from widening of the cortex
2. diminished density of the cortex, which loses its compact appearance and assumes a spongy or honeycombed texture
3. marked coarsening of the bone trabeculae
4. in the later stages a general increase of density of the affected bones.

[1] Sir James Paget (1814–1899) English surgeon who worked at St Bartholomew's Hospital, London and described the disease in great detail in 1877.

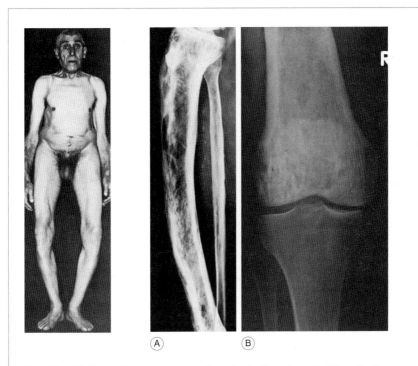

Fig. 6.5 (left) The typical appearance of a patient with widespread Paget's disease. Note the bowing of the legs and shortening of the trunk from collapse of softened vertebrae. The head was also enlarged.

Fig. 6.6 (right) Paget's disease. Ⓐ Tibia, showing bending, coarsening of trabeculae, and thickened cortex which, however, is not sharply demarcated from the medulla. Ⓑ Femur, showing broadening of the bone with loss of the normal demarcation of cortex and medulla.

The long bones are often shown to be bowed, the pelvis may be deformed, the vertebrae may be compressed and the vault of the skull thickened. *Radioisotope scanning* with ^{99m}technetium shows markedly increased uptake in the affected bones.

Investigations. The alkaline phosphatase content of the plasma is increased, often to a high level if several bones are affected. Urinary hydroxyproline is increased, reflecting the increased resorption of bone matrix.

Complications. The important complications are pathological fracture, compression of cranial nerves, and occasionally – but most importantly – osteosarcoma.

Treatment. Very often treatment is not required because the disability is negligible. Treatment is needed mainly for bone pain and for complications. Two drugs are known to affect the outcome – calcitonin and bisphosphonates.

Both drugs inhibit bone resorption. They reduce bone turnover, with lowering of plasma alkaline phosphatase, and both are effective in relieving bone pain in a high proportion of cases. Treatment must, however, be prolonged. Unlike calcitonin, which must be injected (though nasal spray and suppository forms are being tried), a bisphosphonate compound may be taken by mouth. Moreover its benefit

General affections of the skeleton

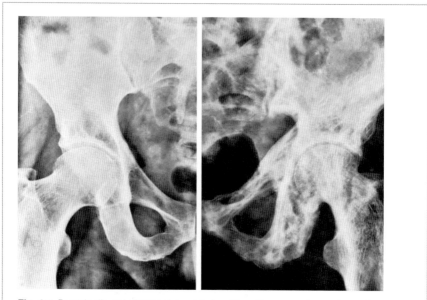

Fig. 6.7 Paget's disease. Half pelvis, side by side with a normal one shown for comparison. Note the coarse trabeculae and slight distortion of the softened pelvic ring, with deepening of the acetabulum.

often persists for up to six months after the drug has been discontinued; so it is the preferred drug in the first instance, on the basis of cost and ease of administration.

POLYOSTOTIC FIBROUS DYSPLASIA

Replacement of bone by fibrous tissue forms a conspicuous part of several unrelated bone diseases. In two conditions in particular, fibrous replacement is the predominant change. In one of these – parathyroid osteodystrophy – the changes are associated with hyperparathyroidism (p. 73). In the other, now to be described, there is fibrous replacement without any evidence of excessive parathyroid secretion.

Polyostotic fibrous dysplasia, then, is a condition in which parts of several bones are replaced by masses of fibrous tissue, but in which there is no evidence of hyperparathyroidism. The condition is rare and the cause is unknown. There is no evidence to suggest a genetic basis.

Pathology. The number of bones involved varies from two or three to twelve or more. The major long bones are those mainly affected – especially the femur. The skull and mandible are also commonly involved. Affected bones are liable to bend or break.

Clinical features. The onset is in childhood but the condition is often not recognised until adult life. The main features are deformity, from bending or local enlargement of bone, and pathological fracture. The disease progresses for years and may eventually lead to severe crippling.

Radiographs of the affected bones show well-defined transradiant areas which often have a characteristic homogeneous or 'ground-glass' appearance: these changes may be localised and patchy rather than uniform. The lesions are in the shaft and metaphyses rather than the epiphyses. When the lesion is extensive the cortex is expanded and thin, and the bone is bent when weight-bearing, producing deformities such as the 'shepherd's crook' in the proximal femur (Fig. 6.8). Sometimes the lesion has a honeycombed appearance.

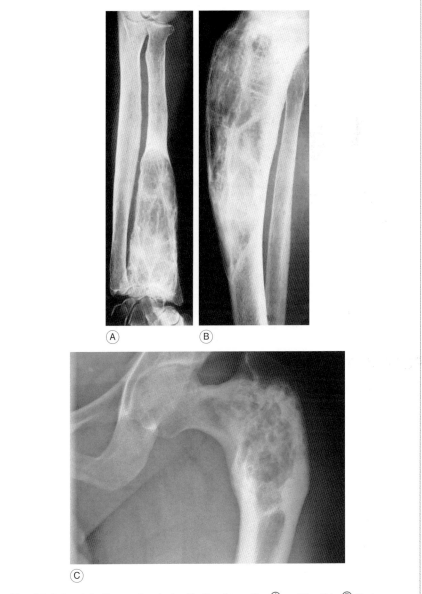

Fig. 6.8 Polyostotic fibrous dysplasia affecting the radius Ⓐ and the tibia Ⓑ. Parts of the skeleton are replaced by fibrous tissue, giving in places a 'ground-glass' appearance. Unlike hyperparathyroidism, this disorder is not associated with any known endocrine dysfunction.Ⓒ Extensive fibrous dysplasia affecting the proximal femur with softening of the bone resulting in a typical 'shepherd's crook' deformity.

Investigations. There is no consistent biochemical abnormality of the blood. In a few cases the plasma alkaline phosphatase has been raised.

Albright's syndrome

The bone lesions of polyostotic fibrous dysplasia sometimes occur in association with patchy pigmentation of the skin and, in females, sexual precocity. This combination of clinical features is known as Albright's syndrome.

NEUROFIBROMATOSIS (von Recklinghausen's disease[1])

This is a congenital inheritable affection characterised by pigmented areas on the skin, cutaneous fibromata, and multiple neurofibromata in the course of the cranial or peripheral nerves. It is ascribed to an autosomal dominant mutant gene.

Pathology. The neurofibromata consist of connective tissue arranged in whorls, with a few nerve fibres.

Clinical features. Skin lesions are seldom present at birth but often develop in early childhood. They consist of multiple *café au lait* areas, axillary or perineal freckling and of small fibromata which may be flat or raised. Neurofibromata may occur on any of the cranial or peripheral nerves, and important pressure effects may occur, including compression of the spinal cord.

The orthopaedic significance of neurofibromatosis lies mainly in the liability to scoliosis and to neurological disturbances in the limbs. There may also be pathological fracture – usually of the tibia in infants, due to fibrous infiltration of the bone (congenital pseudarthrosis).

Scoliosis. Why scoliosis should occur is unknown: but it is a common complication and it sometimes progresses to an angulation so severe that the function of the spinal cord is impaired.

Neurological disturbances. There may be impairment of function of cranial or peripheral nerves in consequence of neurofibromata lying in the course of nerve trunks. Various manifestations are observed, depending upon the site of the tumour. For instance, a tumour of a nerve root within the spinal canal may compress the spinal cord and give the typical picture of a spinal cord tumour. Or it may compress the cauda equina or an individual nerve trunk, with consequent radiating pain and impairment of function of the involved nerve. Thus neurofibromatosis enters into the differential diagnosis of brachial pain and sciatica.

Imaging. *Plain radiographs* may show erosion of a bone where a neurofibroma lies in contact with it. *CT or MR scanning* may be helpful in outlining the extent of a bulky neurofibroma.

Diagnosis. The pigmented spots or areas, and cutaneous fibromata, afford important clues to the diagnosis. A positive family history is important corroborative evidence.

[1]Frederich von Recklinghausen (1833–1910) Distinguished German pathologist working in Strasbourg who described this and several other diseases that bear his name.

Complications. Occasionally a neurofibroma may undergo malignant change, to become a neurofibrosarcoma.

Treatment. A neurofibroma that is causing symptoms should be excised.

MYOSITIS OSSIFICANS PROGRESSIVA (Fibrodysplasia ossificans)

Myositis ossificans progressiva is a congenital affection characterised by the formation of masses of bone in the soft tissues, with consequent progressive impairment of movement of the underlying joint or joints. It is often associated with shortness of the great toe or of other digits (microdactyly). Most cases are sporadic. It is caused by a defect in a gene for the receptor of the BMP family of proteins.

Pathology.[1] The ectopic bone is formed by metaplasia of connective-tissue cells, not from displaced osteoblasts.

Clinical features. Changes usually appear first in early childhood. Swellings develop in the region of the neck and trunk. At first soft and perhaps transient, they later give place to hard plates of bone which lie in the course of muscles, ligaments and fasciae. Movements of the spine and ribs, and later of the limb joints, are reduced progressively until in the worst cases there may be total immobility. In most cases the great toe is congenitally short; the thumbs or other digits may also be short.

Radiographs show the plates of bone in the soft tissues.

Progress. After many years increasing rigidity renders the patients bedridden. No curative treatment is known. Systemic treatment by bisphosphonates after excision of bony bars may retard their regeneration, but the eventual fatal outcome seems unlikely to be influenced significantly.

CRANIO-CLEIDO DYSOSTOSIS

In this dysplasia the most striking features are enlargement of the frontal and parietal regions of the head with delayed ossification and delayed fusion of the skull bones, and absence or partial absence of the clavicles. Other bones may also show less striking anomalies. The disorder is of autosomal dominant inheritance. It is caused by a mutation in the gene for osteoblast specific transcription factor 2 (osf 2) also known as (bfa-1) on chromosome 6.

Clinical features. The disorder usually becomes apparent in early childhood. The head is somewhat larger than normal, with bulging frontal and parietal regions. The clavicles are either absent or rudimentary, in consequence of which the two shoulders can be approximated anteriorly – a characteristic feature. Life expectancy is normal.

Radiographs in childhood show delayed fusion of the skull bones, with Wormian bones in the suture lines; absence of the clavicles either in whole or in the lateral parts; and delayed ossification of the pelvic bones with wide symphysis pubis.

[1]This disease, formerly known as myositis ossificans progressiva, must not be confused with post-traumatic myositis ossificans. The two conditions are entirely distinct. Post-traumatic 'myositis ossificans' is misnamed: it is nothing more than ossification within a subperiosteal haematoma.

General affections of the skeleton

INBORN ERRORS OF METABOLISM

GAUCHER'S DISEASE

Gaucher's disease is one of the group of lysosomal storage diseases included under the generic title *mucopolysaccharidoses* or *sphingolipidoses*. It is a rare lipoid storage disease of autosomal recessive inheritance, in which the enzyme beta-glucosidase is deficient and gluco-cerebroside accumulates in reticulo-endothelial cells of the spleen, liver, bone marrow, and other tissues.

Clinical features. Symptoms usually appear first in adult life. There is enlargement of the spleen and liver. There may be a feeling of weakness due to anaemia, but often the general health is good. Skeletal involvement, which takes the form of infiltration and replacement of bone by masses of lipoid-laden reticulo-endothelial cells (Gaucher cells) brings a risk of pathological fracture. Bone pain or joint pain is a common feature.

Radiographs show irregular cyst-like spaces in some of the bones, sometimes with expansion of the cortex, especially of the femur, the lower end of which may appear flask-shaped. Osteonecrosis (avascular necrosis) of the head of the femur or the head of the humerus, with consequent disorganisation of the corresponding joint, is also common.

Investigations. Bone marrow biopsy usually yields typical Gaucher cells.

Treatment. Replacement therapy with the enzyme (glucocerebrosidase) is effective but very expensive. Splenectomy relieves local discomfort and may help the anaemia but it does not influence the chronic course of the disease.

HISTIOCYTOSIS X (Skeletal granulomatosis)

The title histiocytosis X comprises a group of diseases characterised by proliferation of histiocytes and storage within them of cholesterol. The three clinical entities to be briefly described are:

1. eosinophilic granuloma
2. Hand–Schüller–Christian disease
3. Letterer–Siwe disease.

All occur mostly in children or young adults.

Eosinophilic granuloma

In eosinophilic granuloma the bone lesion is usually solitary. It consists of brownish granulation tissue containing abundant histiocytes and eosinophils, with leucocytes and giant cells. Often there are no symptoms, but there may be local pain, or occasionally a pathological fracture.

Radiologically the lesion is seen as a clear-cut hole in the bone – usually a rib, skull bone, vertebra, pelvic bone, femur, or humerus. An affected vertebral body may collapse, becoming compressed into a thin wafer (see Calvé's vertebral compression, p. 235). Examination of the blood usually fails to show any abnormality.

Eosinophilic granuloma may simulate a bone cyst, a primary or metastatic bone tumour, or tuberculosis. If multiple, it resembles Hand–Schüller–Christian disease.

Treatment. The lesion often heals spontaneously. Surgical curettage may accelerate healing. Radiotherapy has sometimes been given but it is now widely regarded as unnecessary.

Hand–Schüller–Christian disease

In this condition there is proliferation of reticulo-endothelial cells to form multiple lesions, often in the skull but also in other bones. The yellowish deposits consist of granulation tissue with abundant histiocytes, many of which contain cholesterol esters and from their vacuolated appearance are known as foam cells.

Radiologically the lesions appear as punched-out areas, without any surrounding reaction. The areas of destruction are often large. The occasional occurrence of diabetes insipidus and exophthalmos is explained by the presence of lesions in the base of the skull, involving the hypophysis and orbits. There may be other manifestations of pituitary dysfunction, such as retarded growth. The disease progresses very slowly but is often fatal eventually.

Treatment. Radiotherapy may cause the lesions to regress, but the long-term prognosis is poor.

Letterer–Siwe disease

This is the most serious form of non-lipoid granulomatosis or histiocytosis X. It begins in early childhood and progresses rapidly, usually with fatal outcome. Granulomatous deposits occur not only in bone but also in lymph glands, spleen, and liver, which may show enlargement clinically. Radiologically the skeletal lesions resemble those of Hand–Schüller–Christian disease.

METABOLIC BONE DISEASE

The majority of these disorders are associated with diffuse rarefaction of the skeleton and their causes are listed in Table 6.1.

HYPERPARATHYROIDISM (Parathyroid osteodystrophy; generalised osteitis fibrosa cystica; von Recklinghausen's disease)

The characteristic features of hyperparathyroidism are lassitude, dyspepsia, generalised osteoporosis, and cystic changes in some of the bones.

Cause. It is caused by excessive parathyroid secretion, usually from an adenoma of one of the parathyroid glands.

Pathology. The excessive secretion of parathormone causes generalised absorption of bone, the calcium from which is liberated into the blood, whence it is excreted in excessive quantities in the urine. The bone becomes spongy and the cortices are increasingly thin. Cystic changes often develop in one or more of the long bones: from their macroscopic appearance these are commonly referred to as brown cysts. A consequence of the increased excretion of calcium is that the kidneys frequently contain calculi.

Table 6.1 Ten causes of diffuse rarefaction of bone

Cause	Diagnostic features
Osteoporosis	
Prolonged recumbency	History of confinement to bed for months or years
Idiopathic	Post-menopausal. Spine predominantly affected. No biochemical change in blood
Hyperparathyroidism	Diagnostic biochemical changes in blood: plasma calcium increased; plasma phosphate decreased
Glucocorticoid excess (Cushing's syndrome)	Characteristic clinical features: obesity, hypertrichosis, hypertension, amenorrhoea in women
Osteomalacia	
Rickets (all types)	Rachitic changes at growing epiphyses. Biochemical changes depend on type of rickets (Table 6.2, p. 77)
Nutritional osteomalacia	Dietary deficiency apparent. Characteristic biochemical changes in blood: plasma calcium normal (or decreased); plasma phosphate decreased (Table 6.2, p. 77)
Idiopathic steatorrhoea	Excess of fat in faeces. Blood changes: plasma calcium decreased; plasma phosphate normal (Table 6.2, p. 77)
Tumour	
Multiple myeloma	Usually multiple circumscribed lesions, but may be diffuse. Bence Jones proteose often present in urine. Marrow biopsy shows excess of plasma cells
Diffuse carcinomatosis	Primary tumour demonstrable
Leukaemia	Blood examination and marrow biopsy show excess of immature white cells

Clinical features. The patient is adult. There are pains in the bones, indigestion, and weakness. There may also be deformity from bending of softened bone, or a pathological fracture.

Radiographic features. Radiographs show rarefaction of the whole skeleton. The loss of density may be marked, and the cortices very thin. An early sign is irregular subperiosteal cortical erosion in the phalanges of the fingers. Scattered cystic changes may be present in the long bones (Fig. 6.9A, B). The skull shows a uniform fine granular mottling, sometimes with small translucent cyst-like areas (Fig. 6.9C). Radiographs of the renal tracts often show nephrolithiasis.

Investigations. The plasma calcium is increased but the plasma inorganic phosphate is diminished. Excretion of calcium and phosphate in the urine is increased.

Diagnosis. This is from other causes of diffuse or generalised rarefaction of bone. These are summarised in Table 6.1.

Treatment. The causative parathyroid tumour should be located and removed.

NUTRITIONAL RICKETS

In rickets there is defective calcification of *growing* bone[1] in consequence of a disturbed calcium–phosphate metabolism. With the general improvement in economic conditions infantile rickets has become rare in Western countries.

---

[1]When similar influences act on mature adult bone the condition is known as osteomalacia.

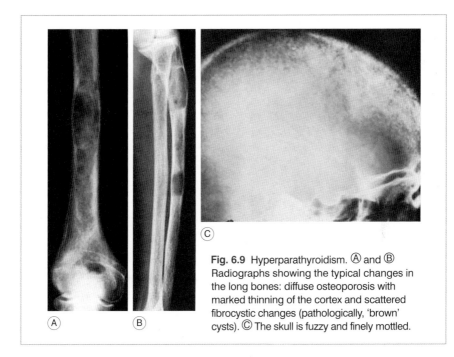

Fig. 6.9 Hyperparathyroidism. Ⓐ and Ⓑ Radiographs showing the typical changes in the long bones: diffuse osteoporosis with marked thinning of the cortex and scattered fibrocystic changes (pathologically, 'brown' cysts). Ⓒ The skull is fuzzy and finely mottled.

There is, however, a relatively higher incidence among immigrants from the West Indies and from Asia.

Cause. Nutritional rickets is caused by a deficiency of vitamin D in the diet and by inadequate exposure to sunlight, which promotes the synthesis of vitamin D in the body.

Pathology. Vitamin D promotes the absorption of calcium and phosphorus from the intestine. Its deficiency therefore leads to inadequate absorption of calcium and phosphorus. The level of calcium in the blood can then be maintained only at the expense of the skeletal calcium. Proliferating osteoid tissue in the growing epiphyses remains uncalcified, and there is a general softening of the bones already formed (Fig. 6.10).

Clinical features. The ordinary nutritional rickets usually occurs in children about one year old. The general health is impaired. The predominant signs are a large head, retarded skeletal growth, enlarged epiphyses, curvature of long bones, and deformity of the chest, which may show a transverse sulcus. In a typical case these signs produce an easily recognised clinical picture.

Radiographic features. There is a general loss of density of the skeleton with thinning of the cortices. The most striking changes, however, are in the growing epiphyses. The vertical depth of the epiphysial lines is increased, the epiphyses are widened laterally, and the ends of the shafts are hollowed out or 'cupped' (Fig. 6.10). Bending of the bones may be obvious.

Investigations. The plasma phosphate level is usually decreased. The plasma calcium is normal. The alkaline phosphatase is increased, often markedly: its level gives some indication of the severity of the disease and of the response to treatment. Measurement of the serum levels of 25-hydroxyvitamin D is a useful guide to diagnosis and treatment.

General affections of the skeleton

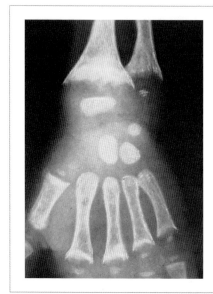

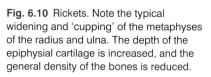

Fig. 6.10 Rickets. Note the typical widening and 'cupping' of the metaphyses of the radius and ulna. The depth of the epiphysial cartilage is increased, and the general density of the bones is reduced.

Diagnosis. If rickets is suspected an antero-posterior radiograph of a wrist should be obtained. The radiographic features are diagnostic of rickets, but biochemical examinations are required to indicate its type (Table 6.2, p. 77).

Treatment. Nutritional rickets responds well to vitamin D in ordinary doses. Severe bony deformity persisting after vitamin therapy should be corrected by osteotomy or osteoclasis.

OTHER FORMS OF RICKETS

The characteristic epiphysial changes seen in nutritional rickets occur in a number of other diseases, the primary factor responsible for the disordered calcium–phosphate metabolism being different in each type. Four types will be described: familial hypophosphataemia, cystinosis, uraemic osteodystrophy, and coeliac (gluten-induced) rickets.

Familial hypophosphataemia (chronic phosphate diabetes; vitamin-resistant rickets)

Familial hypophosphataemia is a hereditary disorder transmitted by an X-linked dominant gene. The nature of the primary defect is uncertain: it may be a failure of normal reabsorption of phosphate by the renal tubules, or it may be a fault in the absorption of calcium from the intestine. Bone changes, which are like those of nutritional rickets, may become manifest soon after the first year of life. The characteristic biochemical features are: normal plasma calcium, low plasma phosphate level *not corrected by vitamin D*, increased alkaline phosphatase, and excess of phosphate in the urine (Table 6.2, p. 77). Relatives who are clinically unaffected may nevertheless show hypophosphataemia.

Table 6.2 Summary of the biochemical changes in the various forms of rickets and osteomalacia

	Primary fault and mechanism	Plasma calcium	Plasma inorganic phosphate	Urine	Stools
Nutritional rickets (children); nutritional osteomalacia (adults)	Deficiency of vitamin D in diet → impaired absorption of calcium and phosphorus	Normal	Low	Normal	Normal
Familial hypophosphataemia	Inherited fault: impaired reabsorption of phosphates by renal tubules → excessive excretion of phosphates in urine	Normal	Low	Excess of phosphate	Normal
Cystinosis (Fanconi syndrome)	Impaired reabsorption of phosphates, glucose, and some amino acids by renal tubules→ excessive excretion of phosphates, etc. in urine	Normal	Low	Glucose, amino acids, excess of phosphate	Normal
Uraemic osteodystrophy	Mechanism uncertain. Possibly impaired glomerular function → retention of phosphorus → excretion in bowl → combination with calcium preventing its normal absorption	Low	High	Albumin	Normal
Coeliac rickets (children); idiopathic steatorrhoea (adults)	Digestive deficiency → impaired absorption of vitamin D and calcium	Low	Normal	Normal	Excess of fat

Note: The plasma alkaline phosphatase is increased in all types of rickets in the active stage. It is an index of activity rather than of type.

Treatment. Vitamin D in high doses should be combined with the administration of phosphates. Treatment on these lines corrects the bone changes but does not restore the plasma phosphate to a normal level. Improved results have been achieved by the use of a synthetic vitamin D analogue, 1α-hydroxyvitamin D3. Surgical correction of residual deformities may be required.

Cystinosis (Fanconi syndrome; renal tubular rickets with glycosuria and amino-aciduria)

In cystinosis (Fanconi syndrome) rachitic changes in the bones are associated with renal glycosuria and amino-aciduria. The primary defect, a congenital fault transmitted by a recessive mutant gene, is a failure of the proximal renal tubules to reabsorb phosphate, glucose, and certain amino acids in the normal way. The excessive loss of phosphates in the urine leads to depletion of the bone phosphate. Onset may be later in childhood than that of nutritional rickets, but the bone changes are the same. The characteristic biochemical features are: normal plasma calcium; low plasma phosphate; increased alkaline phosphatase; and excess of phosphate in the urine, which also contains glucose and certain amino acids (Table 6.2, p. 77).

Treatment. The intake of calcium, phosphate, and vitamin D should be increased. Alkalis (sodium citrate) should be given to combat the associated acidosis.

Related disorders

A number of similar disorders from renal tubular defects are recognised. In all of them there is deficient reabsorption of phosphate, but they differ in the extent to which other functions of the tubules are impaired.

Uraemic osteodystrophy (renal osteodystrophy; renal (glomerular) rickets; renal dwarfism)

In uraemic osteodystrophy general skeletal changes are associated with chronic renal impairment. The skeletal changes often become manifest between the ages of 5 and 10 years.

Pathology. The renal impairment may be due to congenital cystic changes, to ureteric obstruction with hydronephrosis, or to chronic nephritis. The mechanism by which the renal deficiency leads to rachitic changes in the skeleton is uncertain, and probably complex. One factor may be that impaired excretion of phosphorus by the kidneys leads to retention of phosphorus in the blood, and its excretion in the intestine. There it forms an insoluble compound with calcium, which in consequence is not absorbed in proper amounts.

The skeletal changes consist in deficient epiphysial growth and multiple deformities from bone softening. The parathyroid glands are hypertrophied, probably as a secondary effect.

Clinical features. The child is dwarfed and deformed. There are symptoms of renal impairment, such as excessive thirst and sallow complexion. The common skeletal deformities are coxa vara, genu valgum, and severe valgus deformity of the feet.

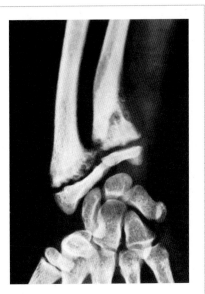

Fig. 6.11 Rachitic changes in the epiphyses of a renal dwarf aged 14 years. There was diffuse rarefaction of the skeleton, with multiple deformities from bending of softened bones.

Radiographs show epiphysial changes that are generally similar to those of nutritional rickets (Fig. 6.11).

Investigations. The biochemical changes are characteristic (Table 6.2). The plasma phosphate is markedly increased. The plasma calcium is low. The blood urea is raised, often to a high figure. Albumin is usually present in the urine.

Prognosis. Unless the renal lesion is remediable gradual progression is likely, with poor prognosis.

Treatment. This should be directed primarily against the underlying renal condition. The diet should be supplemented with calcium and vitamin D.

Coeliac (gluten-induced) rickets

Coeliac disease (gluten-induced enteropathy) is a digestive disorder character-ised by malabsorption and consequently by an excess of fat in the stools. Before a knowledge was gained of how to control the disease it was often compli-cated by rachitic changes in the bones. Such changes will now be seen only in neglected cases.

The primary fault is a susceptibility of the villi of the small intestine to atrophy under the influence of gluten, the protein fraction of flour. This villous atrophy leads to deficient absorption of fats and of fat-soluble vitamin D.

The disease begins in infancy or early childhood. The general features are wasting, impaired growth, failure to gain weight, muscular hypotonia, dis-tended abdomen, and loose offensive stools containing 40–80% fat after drying (normal = 25%). The skeletal changes, which do not develop for several years, are like those of nutritional rickets.

Investigations. The biochemical changes in the blood differ from those of nutritional rickets. The plasma calcium is low. The plasma phosphate is normal or low (Table 6.2, p. 77). Diagnosis should be confirmed by jejunal biopsy effected by a swallowed capsule with a special cutting device.

Treatment. There is steady improvement in the calcification of the skeleton as the primary disorder is brought under control. The diet should be free from gluten and should contain an abundant supply of calcium and vitamin D.

NUTRITIONAL OSTEOMALACIA

Nutritional osteomalacia is the adult counterpart of infantile (nutritional) rickets. It is regarded as rare except in certain Asiatic countries. Nevertheless it may be more common than is generally realised, especially in elderly women.

Cause and pathology. As in infantile rickets, there is a deficiency of vitamin D (and often of calcium) in the diet. In consequence the intestinal absorption of calcium and phosphorus is inadequate, and calcium is withdrawn from the bones to maintain a reasonable level in the blood. The bone trabeculae are not abnormally thin, but they are largely composed of poorly calcified osteoid tissue. There is an abundance of fibrous tissue in the marrow.

Clinical features. The main features are pain in the bones, and deformity. Because of the porosity of the bones fractures are common.

Radiographic features. There is rarefaction of the whole skeleton. The bone cortices are abnormally thin. The long bones may be curved and the pelvis triradiate. Multiple spontaneous fractures (Looser's zones), seemingly ununited though possibly bridged by unmineralised osteoid tissue, may be shown in ribs, pelvic rami, or elsewhere. These are characteristic of osteomalacia and are not seen in osteoporosis.

Investigations. The plasma calcium is normal or low. Plasma phosphate is low. Alkaline phosphatase is increased. The calcium balance is negative (Table 6.2, p. 77). Serum levels of 25-hydroxyvitamin D are low.

Diagnosis. Nutritional osteomalacia must be distinguished from other causes of diffuse rarefaction of bone (Table 6.1, p. 74). In the elderly it may be mistaken for idiopathic osteoporosis.

Treatment. Recalcification of the skeleton is induced by adequate diet and administration of vitamin D and calcium. Osteotomy may be required to correct deformity.

OTHER FORMS OF OSTEOMALACIA

Just as in children rachitic changes in the bones may occur from a number of different metabolic faults, so in adults osteomalacia may arise from causes other than purely nutritional. Such causes include advanced renal disease, and malabsorption syndromes such as chronic obstruction of the bile ducts, chronic pancreatic disease, and adult coeliac disease.

VITAMIN C DEFICIENCY (Infantile scurvy)

Scurvy is a haemorrhagic disease caused by a deficiency of vitamin C (ascorbic acid) in the diet. It is rare in Western countries, especially in adults.

Pathology. The most striking changes are in the long bones. There is a lack of osteoblastic activity in the epiphysial growth cartilage (growth plate). Haemorrhage, beginning at the epiphysial cartilage, extends beneath the periosteum, which may be raised from the bone throughout its whole length.

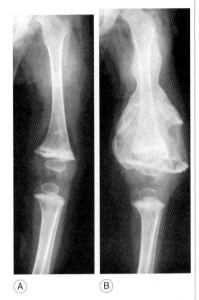

Fig. 6.12 Infantile scurvy. Ⓐ Early active stage. Note the clear zone in the metaphysis, indicating arrest of osteoblastic activity, and the dense zone adjacent to the epiphysial cartilage. Ⓑ Later stage, showing well-marked ossification in the subperiosteal haematoma.

Haemorrhages also occur from other sites, especially from the gums or within the orbit.

Clinical features. Scurvy affects infants during the second six months of life if the diet is deficient in fresh milk or other sources of vitamin C. The onset is rapid, with loss of use of a limb or limbs because of pain (pseudoparalysis). An affected limb is swollen and exquisitely tender over the affected bone or bones. The gums are often spongy and bleed, and there may be a 'black' eye.

Radiographic features. Plain radiographs show a dense line at the junction between metaphysis and epiphysial cartilage, with a clear band of rarefaction on the diaphysial side (Fig. 6.12A). Later there is ossification in the subperiosteal hae-matoma, as a result of which the bone is often markedly thickened (Fig. 6.12B).

Investigations. Ascorbic acid is deficient in the plasma.

Diagnosis. The skeletal features of scurvy in infants resemble those of syphi-litic metaphysitis, which, however, occurs at an earlier age – namely during the first 6 months of life. Other distinctive features are the positive Wassermann reaction in syphilis and bleeding from the gums in scurvy. Scurvy may also be confused clinically with acute osteomyelitis. Deficiency of plasma ascorbic acid is diagnostic.

Treatment. The disease responds readily to the administration of vitamin C.

ENDOCRINE DISORDERS

OSTEOPOROSIS (Idiopathic osteoporosis; post-menopausal osteoporosis)

This condition is characterised by diffuse osteoporosis of unknown cause. It affects the elderly, especially post-menopausal women, but it may be seen also in patients of middle age. It may possibly have an endocrine basis.

Pathology. The whole skeleton is affected, but the changes in the spine are more obvious than those elsewhere. The cortices of the vertebrae are thinner than normal, and the bone is rarefied throughout from thinning of the individual trabeculae and widening of the vascular canals. In other words there is a reduction of total bone mass. Compression fracture of one or more of the vertebral bodies is liable to occur from only trivial violence. Even without fracture the thoracic vertebrae tend gradually to become wedge-shaped so that the spine bends forward to produce a rounded kyphosis. The long bones – particularly the upper end of the femur and the lower end of the radius – are also prone to fracture easily.

Clinical features. The patient is often a woman of over 60. The osteoporosis may be symptomless and may be found only by chance. In other cases there is pain in the back. The pain occurs in two forms – a mild generalised ache, and a sharper pain of sudden onset, denoting a compression fracture. Examination reveals a rounded kyphosis in the thoracic region. If a vertebral body has collapsed there may be a more angular kyphosis with prominence of a spinous process in the thoracic or thoraco-lumbar region. The trunk is shortened, with consequent loss of height, and there is a transverse furrow across the abdomen (Fig. 6.13A).

Radiographic features. The striking feature is the reduced density of the vertebral bodies, which become concave at their upper and lower surfaces from pressure of the intervertebral discs. Often there is wedging of one or more of the vertebral bodies from compression fracture (Fig. 6.13B). Other parts of the skeleton are also rarefied, but less obviously.

Investigations. The biochemistry of the blood is normal. Metabolic balance studies may show a negative calcium balance. Bone density is best measured by dual X-ray absorptiometry.

Diagnosis. Osteoporosis may be confused with other forms of diffuse rarefaction of bone, especially that caused by parathyroid osteodystrophy, glucocorticoid excess (Cushing's syndrome), osteomalacia of various types, carcinomatosis, myelomatosis, or leukaemia (Table 6.1, p. 74). Diagnosis rests largely on the exclusion of these specific disorders.

Prevention. Hormone replacement therapy (HRT) with oestrogens, supplemented by progesterone for 10 days of the month unless the patient has had a hysterectomy, is an important option in post-menopausal women.

Treatment. Once osteoporosis is established, treatment is rather unsatisfactory. It may be possible to restore the patient to positive calcium balance by high-dosage calcium supplements to the diet, combined with calcitriol if malabsorption is present; but the gain is slow because of the slow turnover rate of bone tissue. Thus a dramatic improvement in the radiographic appearance cannot be expected.

A number of drugs have been used in trials to treat established osteoporosis in the older patient, particularly after vertebral or femoral neck fractures. These are selected for their ability to decrease osteoclastic bone resorption or to stimulate the formation of new bone by osteoblasts. The most widely used inhibitors of bone resorption are bisphosphonates, while strontium and the peptide of parathyroid hormone may promote new bone formation.

HYPOPITUITARISM

Deficient secretion of the anterior lobe of the pituitary gland leads to various types of disturbance of skeletal growth, often with impairment of sexual development and sometimes with learning disabilities. The patient may be dwarfed, or on the other hand there may be good stature with marked obesity. The orthopaedic importance of this latter condition is that it may predispose to slipping

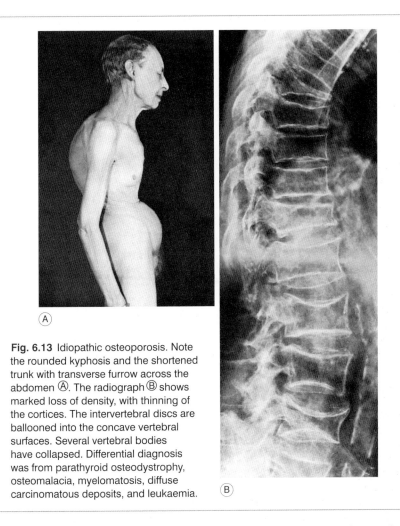

Fig. 6.13 Idiopathic osteoporosis. Note the rounded kyphosis and the shortened trunk with transverse furrow across the abdomen Ⓐ. The radiograph Ⓑ shows marked loss of density, with thinning of the cortices. The intervertebral discs are ballooned into the concave vertebral surfaces. Several vertebral bodies have collapsed. Differential diagnosis was from parathyroid osteodystrophy, osteomalacia, myelomatosis, diffuse carcinomatous deposits, and leukaemia.

of the upper femoral epiphyses in adolescents (p. 371) – as indeed may obesity from any cause.

GIGANTISM

In gigantism (one form of hyperpituitarism) skeletal overgrowth is caused by an excess of anterior pituitary hormone occurring before the growth epiphyses have fused.

Pathology. There is an eosinophilic adenoma of the anterior lobe of the pituitary. Excessive growth occurs at the epiphysial cartilages. Despite this overactivity, epiphysial fusion occurs at about the normal time.

Clinical features. The patient, usually a boy, may grow to a height of 7 feet or more, the main increase being in the limbs. Sexual development is often impaired and the mentality may be subnormal. Signs of acromegaly often develop later. Most of the giants, whose skeletons are preserved in medical museums, some more than 9 feet tall, are examples of this condition.

Diagnosis and treatment are as for acromegaly (see below).

ACROMEGALY

The primary fault is the same as in gigantism – namely, an excessive secretion of pituitary growth hormone – but it occurs after the epiphyses have fused. It is characterised by enlargement of the bones, especially of the hands, feet, skull, and mandible.

Pathology. As in gigantism, there is usually an eosinophilic adenoma of the anterior lobe of the pituitary. The enlargement of the bones is caused by deposition of new bone upon the surface of the original cortex.

Clinical features. The disease often begins in early adult life. The physical features become coarse and heavy, the skin is thickened, and the hands and feet slowly enlarge. At first strong, the patient often becomes weak and sluggish later. *Radiographs* show marked enlargement of the bones of the hands and feet, and especially of the mandible. The vertebral bodies are also enlarged, especially in the antero-posterior diameter. The sella turcica of the skull may be expanded and eroded.

Diagnosis. This is made from the clinical appearance and by demonstration of excessive growth hormone excretion by radio-immunoassay.

Treatment. Early treatment – often by removal of the pituitary adenoma or sometimes by irradiation or by drug therapy – is important in preventing deterioration.

INFANTILE HYPOTHYROIDISM (Cretinism)

Infantile hypothyroidism (cretinism) is characterised by dwarfism, with sexual and mental retardation. It is caused by congenital deficiency of thyroid secretion. From the orthopaedic viewpoint the important features are retarded growth of the limb bones, kyphosis, and distortion of the joint surfaces. Early diagnosis is important because marked improvement follows treatment with thyroxine.

GLUCOCORTICOID EXCESS (Cushing's syndrome)

This endocrine disorder is characterised by obesity, hypertrichosis, hypertension and, in women, amenorrhoea. It is induced by excessive secretion of adrenocortical hormones, caused either by a tumour of the adrenal cortex or by hyperplasia of the gland which may be secondary to a basophil adenoma of the pituitary. A similar condition may also be caused by prolonged administration of cortisone, prednisone, or related steroid drugs.

The orthopaedic significance of Cushing's syndrome lies in the fact that it is accompanied by generalised rarefaction of the skeleton, with liability to pathological fracture of porotic bone (Table 6.1, p. 74).

7 | Infections of bone and joints

Infection of bone by pyogenic organisms is termed osteomyelitis.[1] It occurs in acute and chronic forms. The only other infections of bone with which the student in Western countries need concern himself are tuberculous infections, although syphilitic infections and fungal infections may still occur occasionally in other parts of the world.

ACUTE OSTEOMYELITIS (Acute pyogenic infection of bone; acute osteitis)

Two distinct types of acute osteomyelitis must be considered:

1. haematogenous osteomyelitis, a disease mainly of childhood in which organisms reach the bone through the blood stream
2. osteomyelitis complicating open fracture or surgical operation, in which organisms gain entry directly through the wound.

The two types are sufficiently distinct to require separate descriptions.

ACUTE HAEMATOGENOUS OSTEOMYELITIS

Acute haematogenous osteomyelitis is one of the important diseases of childhood. Only about 5% of cases occur in adults. Early diagnosis is especially important because a satisfactory outcome depends upon prompt and efficient treatment.

Cause. It is caused by infection of the bone with pyogenic organisms – usually *Staphylococcus aureus*, though a variety of other organisms are occasionally responsible, including *Salmonella*. A minor injury to a bone may render it vulnerable to infection by organisms circulating in the blood.

Pathology. Organisms reach the bone through the blood stream from a septic focus elsewhere in the body – for instance from a boil in the skin. In a rare atypical form in adults infection reaches the vertebral column through the spinal venous plexus from an infected intrapelvic lesion.

In the usual childhood manifestation, the infection begins in the metaphysis of a long bone, which must be presumed to form a productive medium for bacterial growth (Fig. 7.1A); thence it may spread to involve a large part of the bone. The organisms induce an acute inflammatory reaction, but the marshalling

---

[1]There is nothing to be gained by distinguishing between *osteitis* (inflammation of bone) and *osteomyelitis* (inflammation of bone and bone marrow). For practical purposes the two terms may be regarded as synonymous.

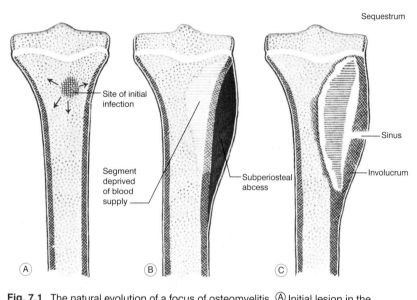

Fig. 7.1 The natural evolution of a focus of osteomyelitis. Ⓐ Initial lesion in the metaphysis. Ⓑ Pus has escaped to the surface of the bone and formed a subperiosteal abscess. Part of the bone has lost its blood supply from septic thrombosis of vessels. Ⓒ The devitalised area eventually separates as a sequestrum. Meanwhile new bone (involucrum) is formed beneath the stripped-up periosteum; it is perforated by sinuses through which pus escapes. This is the stage of chronic osteomyelitis. With prompt treatment the disease can often be arrested at the stage shown in Ⓐ.

of the body's defensive forces is greatly handicapped in bone because its rigid structure does not allow swelling. Pus is formed and soon finds its way to the surface of the bone where it forms a subperiosteal abscess (Fig. 7.1B); later the abscess may burst into the soft tissues and may eventually reach the surface to form a sinus.

Often the blood supply to a part of the bone is cut off by septic thrombosis of the vessels (Fig. 7.1B). The ischaemic bone dies and eventually separates from the surrounding living bone as a sequestrum (Fig. 7.1C). Meanwhile new bone is laid down beneath the stripped-up periosteum, forming an investing layer known as the involucrum (Fig. 7.1C).

The epiphysial cartilage plate is a barrier to the spread of infection, but if the affected metaphysis lies partly within a joint cavity the joint is liable to become infected (acute pyogenic arthritis). Metaphyses that lie wholly or partly within a joint cavity include the upper metaphysis of the humerus, all the metaphyses at the elbow, and the upper and lower metaphyses of the femur (Fig. 7.2). Even when the joint is not infected it may swell from an effusion of clear fluid (sympathetic effusion).

With efficient treatment, the infection may be aborted in its earliest phase. But when it has progressed to the stage of septic thrombosis and death of bone it almost inevitably passes into a state of chronic osteomyelitis.

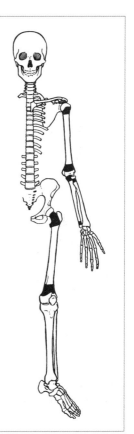

Fig. 7.2 The metaphyses shown in black are wholly or partly intracapsular. Infection at one of these sites is liable to involve the adjacent joint, with consequent pyogenic arthritis.

Clinical features. Except for rare exceptions acute haematogenous osteo-myelitis is confined to children, especially boys. The bones most commonly affected are the tibia, the femur and the humerus. The onset is rapid. The child complains of feeling ill, and of severe pain over the affected bone. There may be a history of recent boils or of a minor injury.

On examination there is obvious constitutional illness with pyrexia. Locally there is exquisite tenderness over the affected bone. The area of tenderness is clearly circumscribed; it is usually near the end of the bone in the metaphysial region. The overlying skin is warmer than normal, and often the soft tissues are indurated; later a fluctuant abscess may be present. The neighbouring joint is sometimes distended with clear fluid, but a good range of movement is retained unless the infection has spread to the joint (septic arthritis): in that event movement would be greatly restricted.

Imaging. *Radiographic examination* in the early stage does not show any alteration from the normal (Fig. 7.3A). Only after two or three weeks do visible changes appear, and they may never do so if efficient treatment is started very early. The important changes are diffuse rarefaction of the metaphysial area and new bone outlining the raised periosteum (Figs 7.3B and 7.4).

Radioisotope scanning with ^{99m}technetium is reserved for the diagnosis of bone infection in the less clinically accessible sites such as the hip, pelvis and spine.

Infections of bone and joints

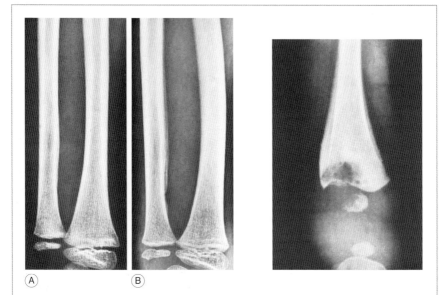

(A)   (B)

Fig. 7.3 (left) Acute osteomyelitis of the ulna in a child. Ⓐ The initial film taken 2 days after the onset does not show any abnormality. Ⓑ Two weeks later a faint shadow along the radial side of the ulna denotes new bone formation beneath the raised periosteum.

Fig. 7.4 (right) Osteomyelitis of the femur in an infant, three weeks after onset. Note new bone outlining the raised periosteum, and area of rarefaction in metaphysis and epiphysis. The infection spread to the knee joint.

Accumulation of isotope depends upon the rate of bone turnover and its vascularity, so that in the early stages of disease inadequate blood supply may result in a 'cold' lesion. More commonly, within a few hours or days of the onset of symptoms there is an increased uptake of isotope, giving a 'hot' scan at the site of the bone lesion. In the more obscure low-grade infections associated with prostheses and other surgical implants in bone, scanning with re-injected leucocytes labelled with [111m]indium may provide improved diagnostic accuracy.

MRI. In many centres this has now superseded isotope scanning as it provides more anatomical information on the infection.

Investigations. Blood culture may be positive in the incipient stage but this is not an invariable feature. Later there is a marked polymorphonuclear leucocytosis. The C-reactive protein and erythrocyte sedimentation rate is increased.

Diagnosis. Acute osteomyelitis is to be distinguished from pyogenic arthritis of the adjacent joint by the following features:

1. the point of greatest tenderness is over the bone rather than the joint
2. a good range of joint movement is retained
3. although the joint may be distended with fluid it does not contain pus (this may be confirmed by aspiration).

Acute osteomyelitis may also be confused with rheumatic fever, and, in infants, with vitamin C deficiency (scurvy) (p. 80). Whenever possible the causative organism must be identified bacteriologically. It is important that blood for culture be taken before antibiotic therapy is commenced.

Complications. The important complications are:

1. septicaemia or pyaemia
2. extension of infection to the adjacent joint with consequent pyogenic arthritis (Fig. 7.5A)
3. retardation of growth from damage to the epiphysial cartilage (Fig. 7.5B).

Acute osteomyelitis often passes into a state of chronic infection.

Treatment. Efficient treatment must be begun at the earliest possible moment.

General treatment. This is by rest in bed and systemic antibiotic therapy, started intravenously to ensure high blood levels. Initially, it is recommended that broad-spectrum antibiotics with good anti-Staphylococcus activity are used, such as a third-generation cephalosporin combined with a synthetic penicillin, but as soon as the causative organism has been identified the antibiotic to which it is most sensitive should be ordered. In cases where a multiple-resistant *Staphylococcus aureus* (MRSA) is suspected it may be appropriate to use vancomycin instead of the penicillin. Antibiotics should be continued for at least 4 weeks, even when the response has been rapid.

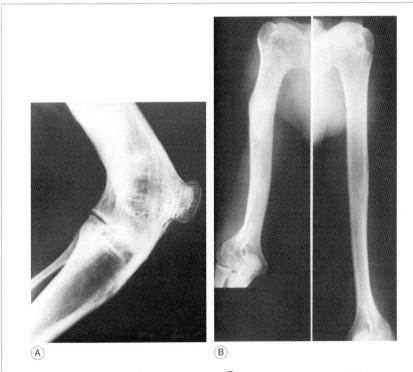

Fig. 7.5 Two complications of osteomyelitis. Ⓐ Pyogenic arthritis, which led in this case to bony ankylosis. Ⓑ Arrest of epiphysial growth, with consequent shortening. The normal humerus is shown for comparison.

Infections of bone and joints

Local treatment. The question of operation and its timing is still controversial. Operation may be unnecessary if effective antibiotic treatment can be begun within 24 hours of the onset of symptoms, and this should always be the aim. But in practice diagnosis is not always so prompt, and in that event it seems wiser to undertake early operation, in order to release pus and to relieve pain, which is often severe. This should definitely be performed if there has not been a marked improvement to the antibiotic treatment within 48 hours. Release of pus may also reduce the risk of ischaemic bone necrosis; and furthermore it allows the organism to be identified and its sensitivity to antibiotics determined. An incision at the site of maximum tenderness is made down to the bone and subperiosteal pus is evacuated. It is advisable – though not always essential – to make one or two drill holes through the cortex to improve medullary drainage. In most cases the wound may safely be sutured. Thereafter the limb is splinted until the infection is overcome.

OSTEOMYELITIS COMPLICATING OPEN FRACTURE OR SURGICAL OPERATION

When acute infection complicates open fracture or surgical operation the organisms are introduced directly through the wound. Any part of the bone may be affected, depending upon the site of injury. Suppuration and necrosis occur as in haematogenous osteomyelitis, but the pus discharges through the primary wound rather than collecting under the periosteum. The infection often becomes chronic.

Clinical features. This type of osteomyelitis may occur in children or in adults. The temperature fails to settle after the primary treatment of the wound or rises a few days later. Pain is not a prominent feature because pus is not contained under pressure. Re-examination of the wound reveals a purulent discharge.

Radiographic features. In the early stages radiographs do not help significantly. Later there may be local rarefaction, and eventually sequestrum formation may be evident.

Treatment. The main principle of treatment is to secure free drainage through the wound, which may be enlarged if necessary for the purpose. Appropriate antibacterial drugs should be ordered. Later, any bone fragment that has sequestrated should be removed.

CHRONIC OSTEOMYELITIS (Chronic pyogenic osteomyelitis)

Chronic osteomyelitis is nearly always a sequel to acute osteomyelitis. Occasionally infection is subacute or chronic from the beginning.

Cause. As with acute osteomyelitis, the *Staphylococcus* is the usual causative organism, but streptococci, pneumococci, typhoid bacilli, or other bacteria may be responsible.

Pathology. It is commonest in the long bones. It is often confined to one end of the bone, but it may affect the whole length. The bone is thickened and generally denser than normal, though often honeycombed with granulation tissue, fibrous tissue, or pus. Sequestra are commonly present within cavities in the bone. Often a sinus track leads to the skin surface: the sinus tends to heal and break down recurrently, but if a sequestrum is present it never heals permanently.

Clinical features. The main symptom is usually a purulent discharge from a sinus over the affected bone. In other cases pain is the predominant feature which brings the patient to the doctor. Discharge of pus may be continuous or intermittent. Reappearance of a sinus that has been healed for some time is heralded by local pain, pyrexia, and the formation of an abscess. This is termed a 'flare-up', or 'flare', of infection.

On examination the bone is palpably thickened, and there are nearly always a number of overlying scars or sinuses.

Imaging. *Radiographic examination*: The bone is often thickened and shows irregular and patchy sclerosis which may give a honeycombed appearance. If a sequestrum is present it is seen as a dense loose fragment, with irregular but sharply demarcated edges, lying within a cavity in the bone (Fig. 7.6). *Radioisotope scanning* may show increased uptake in the vicinity of the lesion. In diffuse disease *MRI* and *CT scanning* may be of value for localisation of abscess cavities and sequestra, thus allowing accurate planning of operative treatment.

Complications. If the bone has been much weakened by disease pathological fracture may occur. Rarely, amyloid disease may complicate long-continued chronic osteomyelitis with persistent discharge of pus. Another rare complication in cases of many years' duration is the development of squamous celled carcinoma in a sinus.

Treatment. An acute flare-up of chronic osteomyelitis often subsides with rest and antibiotics. If an abscess forms outside the bone it must be drained. If there is a persistent and profuse discharge of pus a more extensive operation is advised. The aim should be to remove fragments of infected dead bone

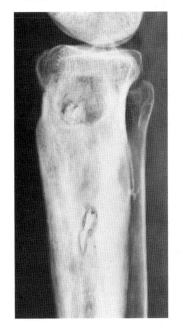

Fig. 7.6 Extensive chronic osteomyelitis of the tibia. The upper part of the shaft is thickened and shows patchy sclerosis. Two cavities are evident, each containing a sequestrum.

(sequestra) and to open up or 'saucerise' abscess cavities by chiselling away the overlying bone. Sometimes it is possible to obliterate a cavity with a flap of muscle, or to exteriorise it and line its walls directly with split-skin grafts. The principles of treatment are (1) remove dead and foreign material, (2) obliterate dead space, (3) if necessary, stabilise the skeleton, (4) obtain soft tissue cover, (5) if necessary, reconstruction of the bone defect, (6) possible appropriate antibiotic cover.

Brodie's abscess[1] (chronic bone abscess)

This is a special form of chronic osteomyelitis which arises insidiously, without a preceding acute attack. There is a localised abscess within the bone, often near the site of the metaphysis. A deep 'boring' pain is the predominant symptom.

Imaging. Radiographically, the lesion is seen as a circular or oval cavity surrounded by a zone of sclerosis (Fig. 7.7A), but the site and extent of the lesion can be shown more accurately on an MRI scan (Fig. 7.7B). The rest of the bone is normal.

Treatment is by operation. The cavity is de-roofed and the pus evacuated. Whenever possible the cavity should be filled with a muscle flap to obliterate the dead space.

TUBERCULOUS INFECTION OF BONE

Tuberculous infection of bone is uncommon except in the vertebral bodies and in association with tuberculous infection of joints. Occasionally it occurs as an isolated lesion in a long bone or in a bone of the hand or foot.

Pathology. Tubercle bacilli reach the bone either through the blood stream or by direct extension from an adjacent focus of infection in joint or soft tissue. There is a typical tuberculous inflammatory reaction. Part of the bone is destroyed and replaced by granulation tissue. A tuberculous abscess is commonly formed; it tracks beneath the soft tissues or towards the surface of the body. With treatment there is a tendency to healing, with fibrosis.

Tuberculosis of a vertebra

The infection typically affects the vertebral body. It may arise initially in the bone (Fig. 7.8A) or it may spread to the vertebra from the adjacent intervertebral disc. Tuberculous vertebral bodies collapse anteriorly but often retain their full depth behind, thereby becoming wedge-shaped (Fig. 7.8B). An abscess usually tracks downwards along the vertebral column; it may also extend backwards towards the spinal canal, where it may interfere with the function of the spinal cord.

Juxta-articular tuberculosis

The articular ends of bones are frequently eroded by tuberculosis beginning primarily in the joint. Less often there is an isolated focus of infection within the bone (Fig. 7.9). From such a lesion the infection may spread eventually to the neighbouring joint.

---

[1] Sir Benjamin Brodie (1783–1862) English surgeon at St George's Hospital London who was also President of the Royal Society. He described the clinical presentation and pathology of the lesion in 1832.

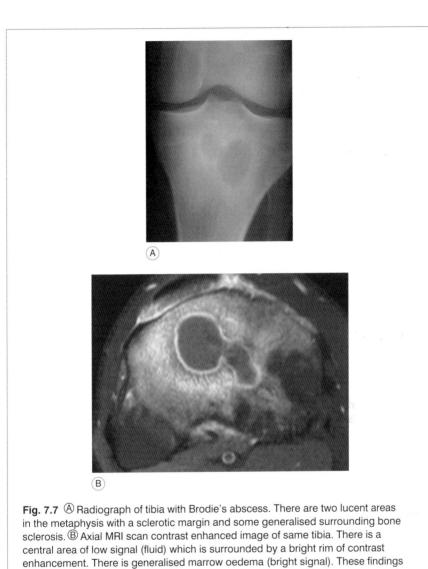

Fig. 7.7 Ⓐ Radiograph of tibia with Brodie's abscess. There are two lucent areas in the metaphysis with a sclerotic margin and some generalised surrounding bone sclerosis. Ⓑ Axial MRI scan contrast enhanced image of same tibia. There is a central area of low signal (fluid) which is surrounded by a bright rim of contrast enhancement. There is generalised marrow oedema (bright signal). These findings are diagnostic of a bone abscess.

Bony tuberculosis in the hand or foot

The metacarpals or phalanges are the bones most commonly affected (tuberculous dactylitis). Characteristically the bone is enlarged by a fusiform swelling which at first represents thickened and raised periosteum. Later, much of the original bone is destroyed, but at the same time new bone is laid down beneath the expanded periosteum, giving the affected metacarpal or phalanx a 'distended' appearance (Fig. 7.10). Similar changes may affect a bone of the foot, or occasionally a long bone.

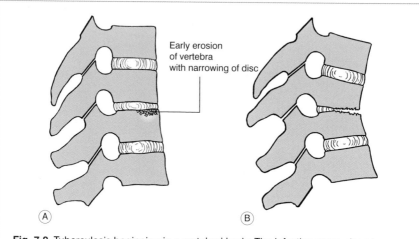

Fig. 7.8 Tuberculosis beginning in a vertebral body. The infection starts close to the anterior border and adjacent to an intervertebral disc Ⓐ. It soon involves the disc and may spread to adjoining vertebrae. The bone destruction is most marked anteriorly; so the affected vertebral bodies become wedge-shaped Ⓑ.

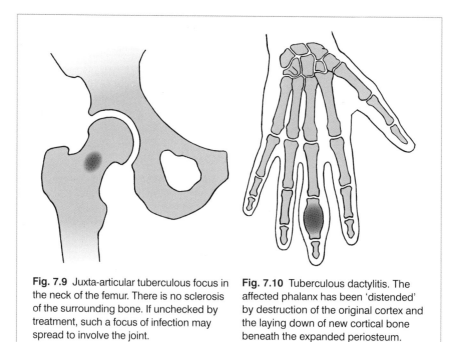

Fig. 7.9 Juxta-articular tuberculous focus in the neck of the femur. There is no sclerosis of the surrounding bone. If unchecked by treatment, such a focus of infection may spread to involve the joint.

Fig. 7.10 Tuberculous dactylitis. The affected phalanx has been 'distended' by destruction of the original cortex and the laying down of new cortical bone beneath the expanded periosteum.

Clinical features. There is usually evidence of constitutional ill health. The local symptoms and signs depend upon the site of the infection. In general, pain is the initial symptom; and at most sites it is associated with obvious swelling and often with the formation of a 'cold' abscess. When the bone lesion is associated with tuberculous joint disease the joint symptoms predominate (see sections on the individual joints).

Imaging. The typical *radiographic features* of tuberculous infection of bone are:

1. diffuse rarefaction around the site of infection
2. erosion or 'eating away' of bone, leaving a fluffy, ill-defined outline with no suggestion of a surrounding zone of sclerosis
3. in many cases a shadow in the soft tissues, denoting abscess formation.

On *radioisotope scanning* there is increased uptake of isotope in the vicinity of the lesion.

Investigations. Except in the case of quite small lesions the erythrocyte sedimentation rate is raised. The Mantoux test is positive. Aspirated pus is yellow and creamy: only occasionally can organisms be identified by direct examination, but culture may prove its tuberculous nature. Biopsy of affected bone or surrounding soft tissue will show the histological features of tuberculosis.

Diagnosis. The diagnosis can often be presumed with fair certainty from a consideration of the history, clinical features, and radiographic findings. Features that lend support are a history of contact with tuberculosis, a positive Mantoux test (particularly in children), a raised erythrocyte sedimentation rate, and evidence of a tuberculous lesion elsewhere. The diagnosis can be proved only by identifying the causative organism or by demonstration of the typical histological features in excised fragments of tissue.

Treatment. In most instances tuberculosis of bone is associated with infection of a joint, and the treatment is mainly that of the joint lesion (tuberculous arthritis, p. 98). The treatment of an isolated tuberculous focus in bone is along similar lines, main reliance being placed upon a combination of antituberculous drugs, usually rifampicin and isoniazid for a period of six months, as outlined on page 102. Local collections of pus should be removed by aspiration or, sometimes, by operative drainage followed by immediate suture of the wound. Resolution is indicated by improvement in the general health and weight, decrease of erythrocyte sedimentation rate, and improved radiographic appearance.

SYPHILITIC INFECTION OF BONE

In Western countries syphilitic infection of bone is now seen only rarely, but it is still found in some parts of the world, and it is important that the possibility of its occurrence should be borne constantly in mind. Bone changes are a late manifestation of acquired syphilis, but they may appear early in life in patients with congenital syphilis. Similar bone changes may occur in yaws, a related disease seen commonly in many tropical countries.

Syphilis of bone can take many forms, but the two commonest types are syphilitic metaphysitis of infants, and osteo-periostitis (combined osteitis and periostitis) in children or adults.

Syphilitic metaphysitis presents as severe local limb pain in young infants in the first six months of life with congenital syphilis. It can affect several epiphyses, with replacement of the adjacent metaphysis by granulation tissue. These appear as a zone of sclerosis on radiographs and the Wasserman reaction is positive, though unlike osteomyelitis there is no leucocytosis. Treatment by intensive antisyphilitic drugs is rapidly effective.

Syphilitic osteo-periostitis occurs when the diaphysis or body of a bone is infected by syphilis. There is usually a combination of osteitis and periostitis, although one or other may predominate. Osteo-periostitis often occurs with

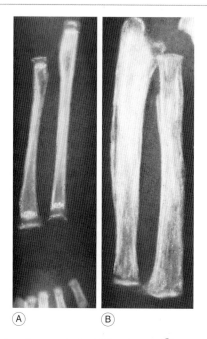

Fig. 7.11 Two examples of congenital syphilis of bone. Ⓐ Metaphysitis in an infant. Note white lines at ends of metaphyses, with adjacent zones of rarefaction. Ⓑ Osteo-periostitis in a child. New bone has been laid down in layers under the periosteum.

metaphysitis in infants (Fig. 7.11A); it may occur separately in older children with congenital syphilis (Fig. 7.11B), or in adults with acquired syphilis.

Clinical features. Deep boring pain, worse at night, and swelling are the predominant symptoms. *On examination* there is either a localised fusiform swelling over the shaft of the bone or a diffuse thickening of the whole length of the bone.

Radiographic features. Syphilitic bone disease is represented by a variety of radiographic changes ranging from severe osteoporosis to dense sclerosis and may be easily confused with a malignant bone tumour. Occasionally the predominant change is bone destruction without new bone formation.

Investigations. The Wassermann reaction is positive.

Treatment. The bone lesions usually respond well to intensive antisyphilitic measures.

PYOGENIC ARTHRITIS (Infective arthritis; septic arthritis)

In this form of arthritis a joint is infected by bacteria of one of the pyogenic groups. Typically there is acute joint infection of rapid development, but the infection may be subacute or even chronic. When pus is formed within the joint the condition is sometimes termed suppurative arthritis.

Cause. The staphylococcus, streptococcus, or pneumococcus is usually responsible – occasionally the gonococcus or other organisms.

Pathology. The organisms may reach the joint by three routes:

1. through the blood stream (haematogenous infection)
2. through a penetrating wound
3. by extension from an adjacent focus of osteomyelitis – especially when the infected metaphysis is wholly or partly within the joint cavity (as are the upper humeral metaphysis, all the metaphyses at the elbow, and the upper and lower metaphyses of the femur (Fig. 7.2, p. 87) (i.e. almost all of the physes apart from those between the knee and ankle)).

The infection causes an acute or subacute inflammatory reaction in the joint tissues. There is exudation of fluid within the joint: the fluid is turbid or frankly purulent according to the severity of the infection. The outcome varies from complete resolution, with normal function, to total destruction of the joint and fibrous or bony ankylosis (Fig. 7.12).

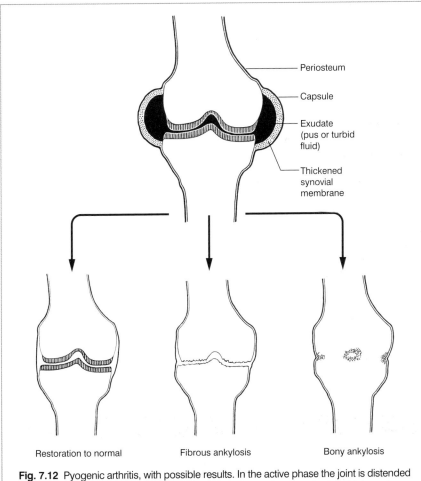

Fig. 7.12 Pyogenic arthritis, with possible results. In the active phase the joint is distended with pus or turbid fluid; the synovial membrane is inflamed and moderately thickened. The outcome varies with the intensity of the infection and the response to treatment. There may be: 1. restoration to normal; 2. fibrous ankylosis; or 3. bony ankylosis.

Clinical features. The onset is acute or subacute, with pain and swelling of the joint. There is constitutional illness, with pyrexia.

On examination the joint is swollen, partly from fluid effusion and partly from thickening of the synovial membrane. When the affected joint is super-ficial, the overlying skin is warmer than normal and it is often reddened. All movements are restricted; in severe cases they are almost totally prevented by protective muscle spasm. Attempted or forced movement increases the pain. In cases of haematogenous infection a boil or other primary focus of infection is often to be found elsewhere in the body. In other cases there may be a history of penetrating injury, or of bone infection adjacent to the joint.

Imaging. Radiographs in the early stages do not show any alteration from the normal (Fig. 7.13A), though an ultrasound scan may reveal the presence of an effu-sion in the affected joint which can then be aspirated to aid diagnosis (Fig. 7.13B). Later, if the infection persists, there may be diffuse rarefaction of bone adjacent to the joint, loss of cartilage space, and possibly destruction of bone. Radioisotope bone scanning shows increased uptake of the isotope in the region of the joint.

Investigations. There is a polymorphonuclear leucocytosis. The C-reactive protein and the erythrocyte sedimentation rate are raised. Bacteriological examination of aspirated joint fluid usually identifies the causative organism.

Diagnosis. This is from other forms of arthritis (especially tuberculous arthritis, gouty arthritis, and haemophilic arthritis), and from infections near the joint (especially acute osteomyelitis).

Prognosis. This varies widely according to the severity of the infection, the organism responsible, and the promptness with which efficient treatment is begun. Many joints can be saved intact, but many are destroyed more or less completely, with fibrous or bony ankylosis (Fig. 7.12).

Treatment. Very prompt treatment is essential if there is to be a reasonable prospect of preserving normal joint function.

Constitutional treatment. Rest in bed may sometimes be required if a major lower limb joint is affected, together with appropriate antibiotic drugs given systemically by intravenous injection until the acute symptoms subside. Whenever possible the causative organism must be identified by culture of the blood and of joint aspirate and its sensitivity to antibiotics determined, so that the most effective drug may be given. Until that information is available treat-ment should be begun with broad-spectrum antibiotics, such as a third-generation cephalosporin, that have high anti-staphylococcal activity.

Local treatment. The joint is rested, usually in a plaster splint. In the case of the hip or knee, sustained weight traction is useful in relieving spasm and pain. The fluid exudate, which is often purulent, is removed by aspiration or, if neces-sary, by incision. Aspiration is repeated daily so long as the exudate continues to form. Rest is enforced until the infection is overcome, as shown by the subsid-ence of pyrexia and retrogression of the local signs. Thereafter active movements are encouraged in order to restore the greatest possible function to the joint.

TUBERCULOUS ARTHRITIS

In Britain the incidence of tuberculous arthritis, formerly common, decreased markedly in the years following the Second World War, probably because of the general improvement in living standards and the introduction of streptomycin and other antituberculous drugs. Pasteurisation of milk and elimination of infected cattle have virtually abolished bovine infection. In some Asiatic and

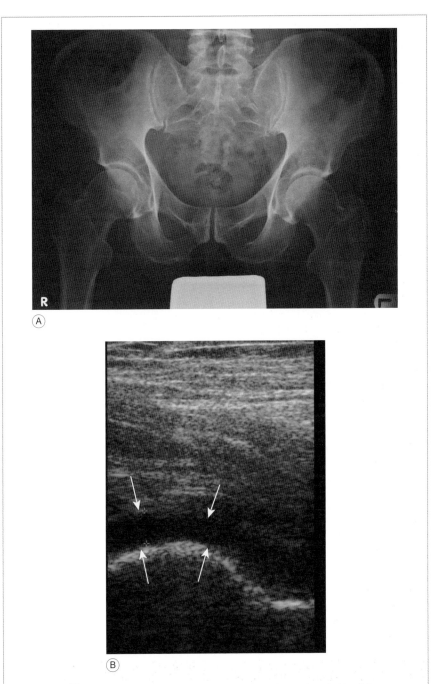

Fig. 7.13 Ⓐ Radiograph of pelvis in patient with an early septic arthritis of the right hip presenting with joint pain. There is an apparently normal radiographic appearance in both hips. Ⓑ Ultrasound scan of the same hip demonstrating a joint effusion. The fluid in the joint is seen as a dark area (between the arrowheads).The lower arrows indicate the femoral head. Ultrasound is very sensitive to the presence of joint fluid and is the investigation of first choice in joint sepsis.

African countries tuberculous infection is still common, and cases are now seen regularly among immigrants to Britain.

Whereas formerly a joint affected by tuberculosis was nearly always destroyed, with modern treatment good recovery of function may now be expected in most patients treated early.

Cause. Tuberculous arthritis is caused by infection of a joint with tubercle bacilli, human or (rarely) bovine. The infection is commonly contracted from another patient with open pulmonary tuberculosis.

Pathology. No joint is immune, but the joints most often affected are the intervertebral joints of the thoracic or lumbar spine, and next in frequency the hip and knee. The organisms reach the joint through the blood stream from a focus elsewhere. The synovial membrane is much thickened (Fig. 7.14)

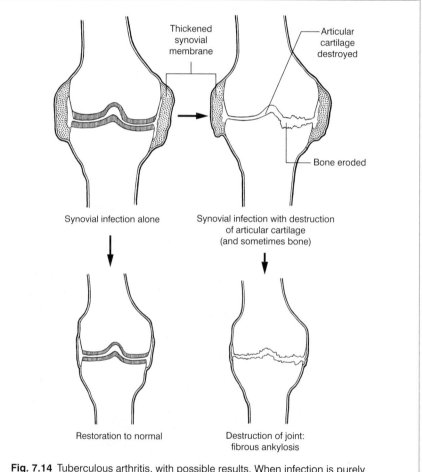

Thickened synovial membrane

Articular cartilage destroyed

Bone eroded

Synovial infection alone

Synovial infection with destruction of articular cartilage (and sometimes bone)

Restoration to normal

Destruction of joint: fibrous ankylosis

Fig. 7.14 Tuberculous arthritis, with possible results. When infection is purely synovial there is marked thickening of the synovial membrane but the articular cartilage is intact (note similarity to early rheumatoid arthritis). With efficient treatment begun at this stage restoration to normal is possible; but if neglected the disease progresses to involve the articular cartilage and bone: the joint is destroyed, and fibrous ankylosis is the natural outcome.

by the tuberculous inflammatory reaction, which is of characteristic type, with round-cell infiltration and giant-cell systems. Unless the disease is arrested the articular cartilage is soon destroyed and the underlying bone is eroded. Sometimes the infection begins in bone adjacent to a joint rather than in the joint itself; thence it extends into the joint by direct continuity. The slow formation of an abscess – a 'cold' or chronic abscess in contradistinction to the florid abscess that may accompany an acute pyogenic infection – is a common feature. The abscess often makes its way towards the skin surface and may eventually rupture, giving rise to a chronic tuberculous sinus. This may provide a route for the entry of secondary infecting organisms.

If healing occurs before the articular cartilage and bone have been damaged the function of the joint is restored virtually to normal; but if cartilage or bone has been damaged before healing is secured permanent impairment – often complete loss of function – is inevitable (Fig. 7.15).

Clinical features. Children and young adults are most commonly affected. There is often a history of contact with a patient with active pulmonary tuberculosis. In general, the predominant symptoms are pain, swelling, and impairment of function of the affected joint. There is usually some impairment of the general health. On examination the characteristic features are increased warmth of the overlying skin, swelling from synovial thickening, and painful restriction of movement in all directions. Forced movement causes sharp pain and induces protective muscle spasm. The muscles controlling the joint are usually wasted. An abscess or sinus is often apparent. A tuberculous lesion may be found elsewhere in the body.

Imaging. Radiographic features. The earliest change in tuberculous arthritis is diffuse rarefaction throughout a fairly wide area of bone adjacent to the joint. If the disease is arrested early there may be no further change; but if the

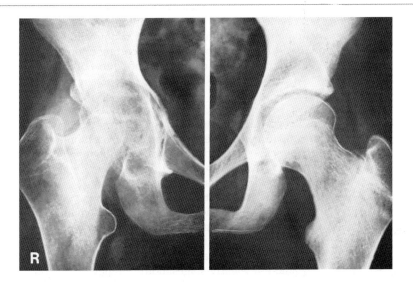

Fig. 7.15 Tuberculous arthritis of right hip. Note the rarefaction, loss of joint cartilage, and early erosion of bone surfaces. The normal side is shown for comparison.

infection progresses the cartilage space is narrowed and the underlying bone is eroded (Fig. 7.15). As the disease heals the bones harden up again – that is, the rarefaction becomes gradually less apparent until the bone density is restored to normal.

Radioisotope bone scanning shows increased uptake of the isotope in the region of the joint.

Investigations. The erythrocyte sedimentation rate is raised in the active stage. Its gradual decrease is an indication of healing. The Mantoux test is positive. Aspiration of the joint may yield a little turbid fluid, in which organisms can seldom be demonstrated, but culture may prove its tuberculous nature. Examination of pus withdrawn from an abscess often reveals tubercle bacilli. Biopsy of thickened synovial membrane shows the typical histological features of tuberculosis (caseous granulation and acid-fast bacilli).

Complications. These are:

1. sinus formation
2. secondary infection through a sinus track
3. spread of disease to another part of the body.

Other complications are peculiar to special regions – for example, compression of the spinal cord by an abscess in tuberculosis of the spinal column.

Course. This depends largely upon the conditions in which the patient lives, and upon the promptness with which treatment is begun and its efficiency. Under favourable conditions early treatment usually promotes gradual healing, with preservation of a useful or even a normal joint; but where conditions tend to be poor and the disease florid, the joint may be largely or totally destroyed.

Treatment. The principles of treatment are the same no matter which joint is affected, with antibacterial drugs as the mainstay of treatment. Variations in detail will be discussed in the sections on individual joints.

Antibacterial drugs. There is now a choice of several antituberculous drugs, including rifampicin, isoniazid, pyrazinamide, streptomycin, and ethambutol. Regimens vary: a common combination of drugs is rifampicin, isoniazid and pyrazinamide, with the addition if appropriate (depending upon the resistance of the organisms) of streptomycin or ethambutol. The course of drug treatment should continue for 6–9 months, with streptomycin or ethambutol (if used) discontinued after 2 months.

Careful watch must be kept for undesirable side effects, especially with ethambutol, which may cause optic atrophy; and with streptomycin, which may cause auditory impairment. Liver function must be monitored during treatment because rifampicin, isoniazid, and pyrazinamide may be harmful to liver cells. Streptomycin carries the additional disadvantage that it has to be administered by intramuscular injection.

Local treatment varies according to the particular joint that is affected. Tuberculosis of a large joint such as the hip or knee may demand a period of rest in bed, at any rate in the early stages; whereas a patient with disease of a smaller joint – particularly in the upper limb – may be up and about throughout the period of treatment. Immobilisation of the affected joint in a plaster or splint is usually advisable in the early stages, both to relieve pain and to provide favourable conditions for healing. Splintage should generally be continued for 2 to 4 months, depending on the severity of the disease. Meanwhile abscesses should be aspirated or drained surgically.

Subsequent management depends on progress. If cartilage and bone are pre-served intact and the local signs of inflammation subside, with improvement in the sedimentation rate, the outlook is good and activity may be progressively increased. If, however, the disease progresses to the point of eroding articu-lar cartilage and underlying bone, a further period of immobilisation may be required, and fusion of the joint – usually by operation – may become the ulti-mate objective. In selected patients it may be feasible to undertake replacement arthroplasty of larger joints following successful antibacterial treatment. This should only be considered when the disease has been quiescent clinically for at least a year with a normal erythrocyte sedimentation rate.

Infections of bone and joints

8 Bone tumours and other local conditions

Co-written by Nigel Raby

TUMOURS OF BONE

Primary bone tumours, both benign and malignant, are relatively uncommon in comparison with the malignancies arising in other tissues of the body. They are also much less common than metastatic (secondary) tumours which affect the skeleton by blood stream spread from primary carcinoma of the breast, prostate, lung or kidney.

The importance of primary bone tumours is not their frequent occurrence, but the difficulty they may present in diagnosis and treatment and the need to distinguish them from a number of tumour-like lesions that affect bone. Tumours originating in bone arise from mesenchymal tissue and if malignant are termed sarcoma. They are normally classified by the predominant cell type in the lesion, which may be bone, cartilage or fibrous tissue (Table 8.1).

Clinical features. Bone tumours may present clinically with local pain unrelated to activity, local swelling, limp, pathological fracture, or a combination of these symptoms. Many benign tumours may be asymptomatic and are detected as a chance finding on a radiograph taken for unrelated indications. To reach an accurate and rapid diagnosis may require access to a skilled multi-disciplinary team of radiologist, pathologist, and oncologist, as well as an orthopaedic surgeon. This is particularly important where a malignant tumour is suspected since this may require complex and extended management utilising adjuvant therapy as well as surgical treatment.

Imaging of bone tumours. Bone tumours are still best evaluated by plain films. MR scanning is required to identify the full extent of the tumour and its relationship to key anatomical structures. However, the differentiation of the most likely tumour type is still best undertaken by careful evaluation of the plain film findings.

In evaluating any lesion of the bone the following key observations will allow a correct diagnosis to be made in the majority of cases.

Age of the patient. Many tumours are most commonly found in specific age groups. Ewing's sarcoma and simple bone cysts occur in children and young adults. Chondrosarcoma generally affects patients over the age of 40.

Single or multiple lesions. Most true primary bone tumours are solitary lesions. The presence of multiple lesions suggests bone metastases, though less commonly these may occur in myeloma or lymphoma.

Site of tumour. The bone involved and the site of involvement; whether epiphysis, diaphysis or metaphysis is important. Certain tumours have a predilection for particular bones and some occur most typically in certain parts of the bone. Giant cell tumours are almost always found in a subarticular position, i.e. epiphyseal location.

Margin of the lesion. Slow-growing tumours have well-defined sometimes sclerotic margins and are most likely benign. Rapidly growing lesions will have ill-defined margins and appear to permeate diffusely into the surrounding

Table 8.1   Classification of primary bone tumours

Benign	Malignant
Arising from bone	
Osteoma	Osteosarcoma
Osteoid osteoma	
Osteoblastoma	
Giant-cell tumour	
Arising from cartilage	
Enchondroma	Chondrosarcoma
Osteochondroma (cartilage capped exostosis)	
Chondromyxoid fibroma	
Chondroblastoma	
Arising from fibrous tissue	
Fibrous cortical defect	Malignant fibrous
Non-ossifying fibroma	histiocytoma (MFH)
Fibrous dysplasia	
Tumours of uncertain origin	
Simple bone cyst	Ewing's sarcoma
Aneursymal bone cyst	Adamantinoma

bone. While this typically indicates a malignant process, other rapidly progressing conditions, such as acute osteomyelitis, can give a similar appearance.

Appearance of matrix. Lesions of mainly cartilage tissue will tend to show areas of calcification. A lesion arising from bone-forming cells may contain areas of ossification. If either of these findings is present then the differential diagnosis is narrowed considerably.

Periosteal reaction. If present, a periosteal reaction gives clues as to the nature of the underlying lesion. A thick well-organised periosteal reaction implies a slow-growing lesion, as for example with osteoid osteoma. A periosteal reaction consisting of layers of thin periosteum implies rapid growth and is generally indicative of a rapidly growing malignant lesion.

Breach of cortex. Destruction of the cortex indicates an aggressive invasive lesion.

Soft tissue mass. If present extension into soft tissues is also evidence of a rapidly growing aggressive lesion.

Of the above the most helpful in narrowing the differential diagnosis is the age of the patient and the site of the tumour. With these two pieces of information alone it is possible to suggest the correct diagnosis in the majority of patients.

Other investigations. Blood tests should be undertaken routinely, though these rarely provide a definitive diagnosis. A raised white cell count with an increased erythrocyte sedimentation rate and C-reactive protein suggests the possibility of a bone infection. Hypercalcaemia suggests extensive bone resorption from hyperparathyroidism, or the presence of multiple bone metastases or myeloma deposits. Multiple myeloma can be confirmed when the plasma proteins show a very high globulin level, while prostatic carcinoma spread is accompanied by a raised serum acid phosphatase.

Biopsy. In the majority of cases it is necessary to undertake a biopsy of material from the lesion for histological and bacteriological examination to reach a final definitive diagnosis. The biopsy may be an open procedure, or a closed needle or trephine technique may be used. The closed technique may be guided by CT scanning, but gives very little material for additional investigations, such as immunohistochemistry or cytogenetics. Needle biopsy should only be used where advice is available from an expert bone pathologist with the necessary technical resources for processing small tissue samples. Once diagnosed the treatment of the lesion depends on whether it is benign or malignant and will be described in more detail for the individual types of tumour.

BENIGN TUMOURS OF BONE

It would be inappropriate to give a detailed description of every type of benign tumour, but the general principles in their management will be illustrated for four of the more common types encountered in practice. These are:

1. osteoid osteoma (Fig. 8.1)
2. chondroma (Fig. 8.2)
3. osteochondroma (Fig. 8.3)
4. giant-cell tumour (Fig. 8.4).

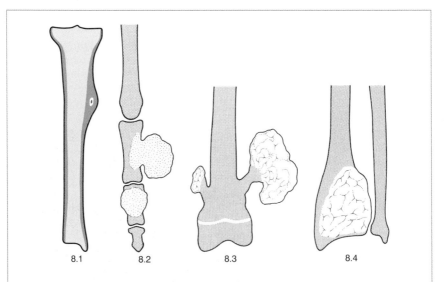

8.1   8.2   8.3   8.4

Fig. 8.1 Osteoid osteoma with central nidus surrounded by reactive sclerotic bone.

Fig. 8.2 Two types of chondroma: ecchondroma on proximal phalanx; enchondroma in middle phalanx. (See also Figs 6.4A, B)

Fig. 8.3 A small and a large osteochondroma. Originating at the growth cartilage, they have migrated away from it with growth of the bone. Each is capped by cartilage. (See also Fig. 6.3B)

Fig. 8.4 Giant-cell tumour (osteoclastoma). Note expansion of cortex and scanty fine trabeculae within the tumour. The tumour extends close up to the articular surface.

Bone tumours and other local conditions

Osteoid osteoma

This is a benign circumscribed lesion that may arise in the cortex of long bones or occasionally in the cancellous bone of the spine. It affects young patients aged 10–35 and is three-times commoner in males.

Pathology. The characteristic feature is the formation of a small nidus of osteoid tissue, usually less than 0.5 cm diameter, surrounded by a reactive zone of dense sclerotic new bone formation (Fig. 8.1).

Clinical features. They usually present with increasingly severe, but well-localised, deep aching pain and sometimes local bone tenderness. The pain is worse at night and is eased by aspirin or NSAIDs, a diagnostic feature.

Imaging. *Plain radiographs* typically show local sclerotic thickening of the shaft that may obscure the small central nidus within the area of rarefaction (Fig. 8.5). The nidus is best seen on a fine cut CT scan (Fig. 8.6) and also exhibits intense uptake on an isotope bone scan.

Treatment. In younger patients some osteomas may resolve spontaneously after several months, but most require surgical treatment. Removal of the central nidus results in resolution of the reactive bone formation and dramatic relief of symptoms. This can be achieved by open surgical excision or curettage, but increasingly less-invasive methods are being used. Where the necessary equipment is available, a CT-guided needle can be inserted into the nidus and the lesion ablated with radiofrequency coagulation.

Chondroma

This is a tumour composed of translucent hyaline cartilage, usually presenting in the 15–50 age group.

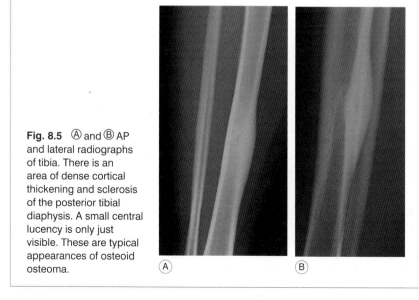

Fig. 8.5 Ⓐ and Ⓑ AP and lateral radiographs of tibia. There is an area of dense cortical thickening and sclerosis of the posterior tibial diaphysis. A small central lucency is only just visible. These are typical appearances of osteoid osteoma. Ⓐ Ⓑ

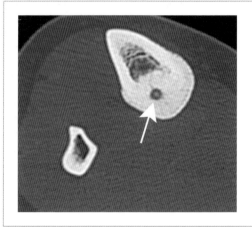

Fig. 8.6 CT scan demonstrates a central small lucency (arrow) containing a more dense central nidus within the thickened cortex. The appearance is diagnostic of an osteoid osteoma.

Pathology. There are two forms of chondroma: in the commonest type the tumour grows within a bone and expands it (enchondroma) (Fig. 8.2); in the other more rare form it grows outward from a bone (periosteal chondroma or ecchondroma). Most periosteal chondromas arise in the hands or feet, or from flat bones such as the scapula or ilium. They often reach a large size and are more prone to develop malignant change. Enchondromas are fairly common in the long bones, but over 50% occur in the small bones of the hands and feet. The affected bone is expanded by the tumour and its cortex is much thinned; so pathological fracture is common and usually the presenting feature. Many remain asymptomatic and are only discovered as chance findings on radiographs taken for other purposes.

Imaging. Central enchondromas expand the bone with thinning, but not erosion, of the cortex and exhibit a variable degree of mineralisation or speckled calcification (Fig. 8.7).

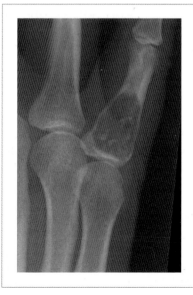

Fig. 8.7 Radiograph of metacarpophalangeal joint of the little finger with a typical enchondroma in the proximal phalanx. The lucent lesion has produced slight medullary expansion with thinning of the overlying cortex. There is some calcification within the lesion indicating a lesion of cartilage origin.

Multiple enchondromata of the major long bones occur mainly in the distinct, but rare, clinical condition known as dyschondroplasia (multiple chondromatosis or Ollier's disease) (p. 65). In this disorder, which begins in childhood, enchondromata arise in the region of the growing epiphysial cartilages (growth plates) of several bones: they interfere with normal growth at the epiphysial plate and consequently may lead to shortening or deformity (see Fig. 6.4A).

Occasionally an enchondroma undergoes malignant change, becoming a chondrosarcoma, usually in one of the major long bones rather than in the small bones of the hands or feet. Clinically this should be suspected when there is a sudden increase in size of the swelling or if the lesion becomes painful.

Treatment. A chondroma is often best left alone. If it causes a fracture or is unsightly it should be removed by curettage and the defect filled with bone graft.

Osteochondroma (osteocartilaginous exostosis)

This is the commonest benign tumour of bone, usually presenting in the 10–20 age group.

Pathology. The tumour originates in childhood from the growing epiphysial cartilage plate, but as the bone grows in length the outgrowth gets 'left behind' and tends to point away from the adjacent joint. It frequently grows outwards from the bone like a mushroom with a bony stalk in continuity with the cortex of the underlying bone (Fig. 8.3). Less commonly the lesion may be sessile with a more broad-based origin. The bony stalk has a larger cap of cartilage which continues to grow until the cessation of skeletal growth.

The ordinary osteochondroma is single; but in the condition known as diaphysial aclasis (multiple exostoses) (p. 63) the tumours affect several or many bones. The risk of malignant change to a chondrosarcoma is higher in these multiple lesions than in the solitary lesion and should be suspected if the tumour continues to enlarge or becomes painful after puberty.

Clinical features. The tumour may be noticed as a circumscribed hard swelling near a joint, but is usually painless. It may become painful due to pressure effects on adjacent nerve or vascular structures, or from the formation of an overlying pseudobursa, though increase in size and pain should always be regarded with suspicion.

Imaging. Plain radiographs show the mushroom-like stalk of the bony tumour (Fig. 8.8), but not the larger cartilaginous cap until this calcifies once skeletal maturity is reached. Patients with known lesions should be warned to seek referral for further imaging if their swelling enlarges or becomes painful.

Treatment. The tumour should be excised if it causes pain or if it enlarges after puberty and must be sent for routine histological examination to exclude any malignant change.

Giant-cell tumour (osteoclastoma)

This is an important tumour because, though generally classed as benign, it tends to recur after local removal or curettage. It occurs most commonly in young adults in the 20–40 age group. In about 10% of cases it behaves as a frankly malignant tumour, metastasising through the blood stream to the lungs.

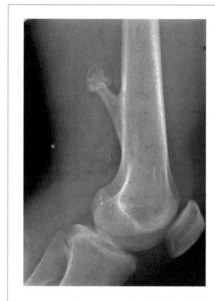

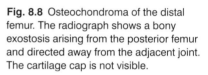

Fig. 8.8 Osteochondroma of the distal femur. The radiograph shows a bony exostosis arising from the posterior femur and directed away from the adjacent joint. The cartilage cap is not visible.

Pathology. The commonest sites are the lower end of the femur, the upper end of the tibia, the lower end of the radius, and the upper end of the humerus – that is, at those ends of the long bones at which most growth occurs. It may also occur in the spine and sacrum. Characteristically it occurs in the end of the bone, occupying the epiphysial region and often extending almost to the joint surface (Fig. 8.4). It destroys the bone substance, but new bone forms beneath the raised periosteum, so that the bone end becomes expanded and pathological fracture is common.

Histologically the tumour consists of abundant mononuclear oval or spindle-shaped stromal cells profusely interspersed with giant cells that may contain as many as fifty nuclei (Fig. 8.9), hence the name 'giant cell tumour'. The giant cells possibly represent fused conglomerations of the oval or spindle-shaped stromal cells, which may frequently show mitotic figures, though this is not necessarily indicative of malignant change.

Clinical features. The symptoms are pain at the site of the tumour and a gradually increasing local swelling. Sometimes the patient is made suddenly aware that something is wrong by the occurrence of a pathological fracture. Examination reveals a bony swelling which may be tender on firm palpation.

Imaging. *Radiographs* show lytic destruction of the bone substance, with expansion of the cortex, but no sclerotic rim or periosteal reaction (Fig. 8.10). A few bony trabeculae may remain within the tumour giving a faintly loculated appearance. The tumour tends to grow eccentrically, and often extends as far as the articular surface of the bone. Magnetic resonance imaging will help to determine the amount of soft tissue extension of the tumour (Fig. 8.11).

Treatment. This depends upon the site of the tumour. Curettage of the contents with a high-speed burr is the standard method of treatment for most giant cell tumours, though this is associated with a high rate (20–25%) of recurrence. This rate can be reduced to less than 10% by the use of adjuvant treatment

Bone tumours and other local conditions

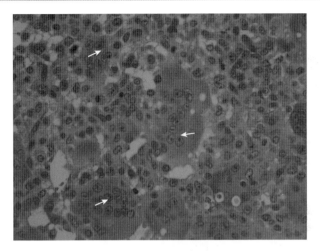

Fig. 8.9 Histology of giant cell tumour showing large osteoclastic multinucleate giant cells (arrows) with interspersed mononuclear tumour cells. The nuclei of the two cell types are very similar. (Haematoxylin and eosin ×400.)

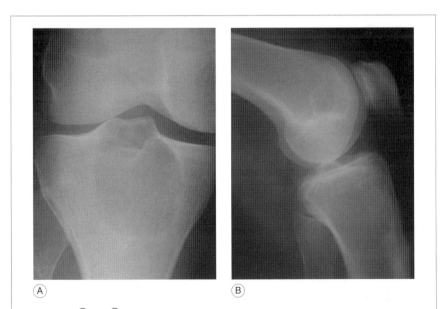

Ⓐ Ⓑ

Fig. 8.10 Ⓐ and Ⓑ Radiographs of giant cell tumour in the proximal tibia. There is a lucent lesion in the metaphysis, with extension into the epiphyseal region extending to the articular surface of the knee. In a patient with fused epiphyses the most likely diagnosis is a giant cell tumour.

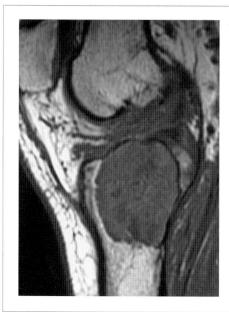

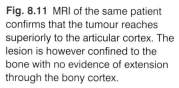

Fig. 8.11 MRI of the same patient confirms that the tumour reaches superiorly to the articular cortex. The lesion is however confined to the bone with no evidence of extension through the bony cortex.

applied to the lining of the cavity after curettage. Methods used include the chemical phenol, freezing with liquid nitrogen, or the insertion of poly-methylmethacrylate bone cement. In addition to its exothermic reaction on any residual cells, the cement has the added advantage of providing support to the subchondral bone and cartilage of the articular surface of the joint. In some bones, or after multiple recurrences, it may be possible to excise the tumour and replace it with allograft bone or a metal prosthesis, without undue functional compromise. Sites where this is possible include the distal radius, distal femur, and proximal tibia.

Radiotherapy is sometimes used and is capable of bringing about per-manent cure, but there is a risk that it may itself induce malignant change, perhaps many years later. It should therefore be confined to tumours at sites that are inaccessible to operation, particularly in the spinal column and sacrum.

Chondromyxoid fibroma and chondroblastoma

Both of these benign bone tumours are extremely rare and readers should consult larger textbooks for details of their clinical presentation, imaging and treatment.

MALIGNANT TUMOURS OF BONE

In this brief review only the five commonest primary malignant tumours of bone will be described together with the secondary or metastatic tumours.

1. osteosarcoma (osteogenic sarcoma) (Fig. 8.12)
2. chondrosarcoma of bone
3. malignant fibrous histiocytoma of bone
4. Ewing's tumour (Fig. 8.13)
5. myeloma (plasmacytoma) (Fig. 8.14)
6. secondary (metastatic) tumours (Fig. 8.15).

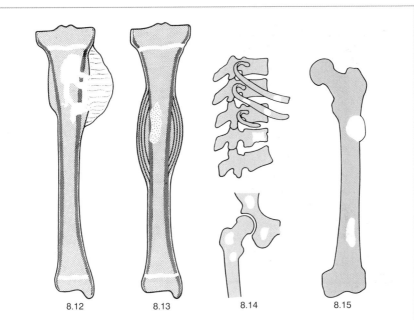

Fig. 8.12 Osteosarcoma. It arises in the metaphysis. Note the destruction of bone, the raising of the periosteum with new bone formed beneath it, and disruption of the cortex by the tumour. The appearance is variable, and the formation of neoplastic bone by the tumour may be profuse or scanty.

Fig. 8.13 Ewing's tumour. It arises in the diaphysis. Note the central area of destruction and concentric layers of subperiosteal new bone giving an 'onion-peel' appearance.

Fig. 8.14 Multiple myeloma. Small 'punched-out' osteolytic tumours are scattered throughout the skeleton, especially in bone containing abundant red marrow.

Fig. 8.15 Metastatic tumours in bone, as found in disseminated carcinoma. Note the circumscribed destruction of bone without any periosteal reaction. Metastatic tumours in bone are very much more common than primary malignant bone tumours.

Osteosarcoma (osteogenic sarcoma)

This is predominantly a tumour of childhood or adolescence, occurring most commonly in the 10–25 age group. When it occurs in later life it is often a complication of Paget's disease (osteitis deformans) (p. 66).

Pathology. An osteosarcoma arises from primitive bone-forming cells. The commonest sites are the lower end of the femur, the upper end of the tibia, and the upper end of the humerus – that is, in those areas in which, prior to epiphysial fusion, most active growth is occurring. The tumour begins in the metaphysis – that is, the part of the shaft that is adjacent to the epiphysial plate. It destroys the bone structure and eventually bursts into the surrounding soft tissues, though it seldom crosses the epiphysial cartilage into the epiphysis itself (Fig. 8.12). The histological appearance varies widely, because any type of connective tissue may be represented. Thus the tumour may be composed largely of fibrous tissue, of cartilage or of myxomatous tissue; but characteristically there will always be found, in some parts of the tumour, areas of neoplastic new bone or osteoid tissue that indicate the

Bone tumours and other local conditions

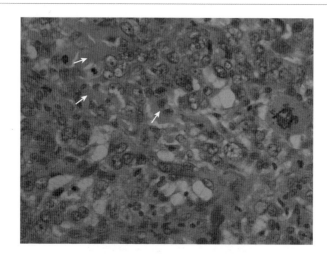

Fig. 8.16 Histological appearance of a typical osteosarcoma with areas of immature bone osteoid formation (arrows) and numerous atypical malignant stromal cells showing nuclear pleomorphism and mitotic activity. (Haematoxylin and eosin ×400.)

true nature of the lesion, and in some cases newly formed bone is abundant (Fig. 8.16). The tumour metastasises early by the blood stream, especially to the lungs and sometimes to other bones.

Clinical features. The usual presentation is local bone pain associated with a gradually increasing swelling. Examination reveals a diffuse firm thickening near the end of a bone, close to the joint. The overlying skin is warmer than normal because of the vascularity of the tumour; and the part may be so distended by tumour that the skin appears stretched and shiny.

Imaging. *Plain radiographs* show irregular medullary and cortical destruction of the metaphysis. Later the cortex appears to have been 'burst open' at one or more places by the soft tissue extension (Fig. 8.17), but there are always vestiges of the original cortex. *MR scanning* allows accurate delineation of the tumour size and the extent of invasion of the soft tissues (Fig. 8.18). There is usually evidence of new bone formation under the corners of the aggressive periosteal reaction (Codman's triangle) (Fig. 8.17B). Occasionally well-marked radiating spicules of new bone are seen within the tumour ('sun-ray' appearance) (Fig. 8.17A). In a parosteal osteosarcoma, a variant that may occur in older patients with a better prognosis, there may be profuse formation of new bone on the surface of the cortex.

Radioisotope (technetium) scanning will show increased uptake at the site of the tumour and can provide additional information on the intramedullary spread by any 'skip' lesions, though these are normally detected by MRI scanning.

A chest radiograph may show pulmonary metastases (Fig. 8.19), but *CT scanning* of the lung fields (Fig. 8.20) is now mandatory for pre-treatment staging as it can detect small pulmonary metastases before they are apparent in plain radiographs.

Diagnosis. In atypical cases an osteosarcoma may be confused with subacute osteomyelitis, or with other bone tumours such as chondrosarcoma, malignant fibrous histiocytoma, giant-cell tumour, Ewing's tumour, or even

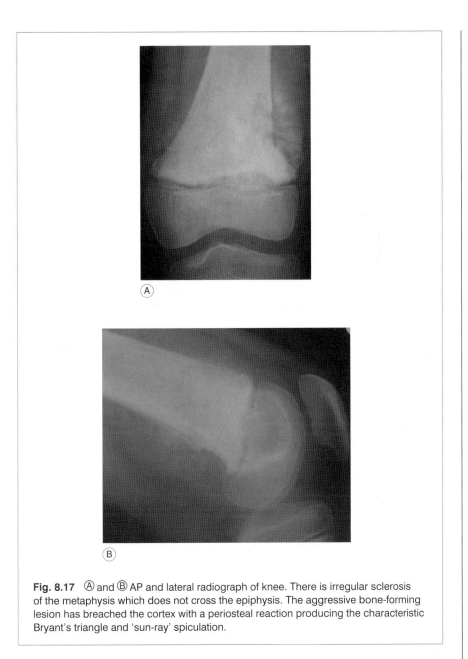

Fig. 8.17 Ⓐ and Ⓑ AP and lateral radiograph of knee. There is irregular sclerosis of the metaphysis which does not cross the epiphysis. The aggressive bone-forming lesion has breached the cortex with a periosteal reaction producing the characteristic Bryant's triangle and 'sun-ray' spiculation.

metastatic tumour. A representative piece of the tumour should always be removed by closed needle or open biopsy and sent for histological examination.

Prognosis. Prior to the introduction of effective chemotherapy, when surgical excision or amputation was the only treatment, the mortality was in the region of 80%. Recent advances in adjuvant treatment added to surgical ablation have changed the prognosis markedly for the better, with increased survival time and often lasting cure.

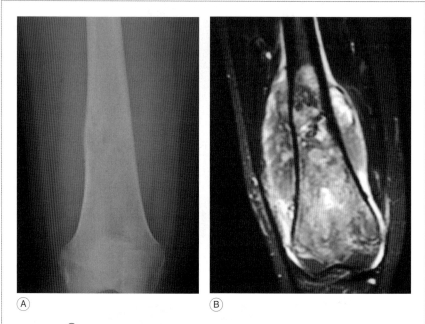

(A) (B)

Fig. 8.18 Ⓐ Radiograph of osteosarcoma of the femur. There is an area of ill-defined lucency in the mid shaft associated with some periosteal reaction. Ⓑ MR of same patient. The area of marrow abnormality is seen to be extending far into the distal femur with a large soft tissue mass surrounding the femur not evident on the plain film.

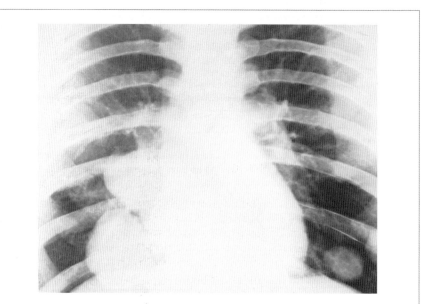

Fig. 8.19 Pulmonary metastases in a case of osteosarcoma of the tibia. Such metastases are the usual cause of death.

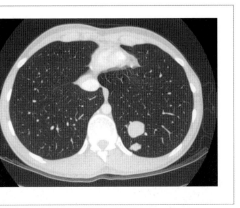

Fig. 8.20 CT of chest showing two intrapulmonary metastases posteriorly in the left lung.

Treatment. The introduction of new powerful cytotoxic drugs for adjuvant chemotherapy has revolutionised the treatment of these tumours, because of their ability to prevent or delay the appearance of pulmonary micrometastases. The drugs currently used include high-dose methotrexate, doxorubicin, cisplatin, and ifosfamide in combinations which are the subject of multi-centre controlled trials. They all have major side effects and should only be used at treatment centres skilled in their use. Chemotherapy is usually commenced before surgical treatment, and is continued intermittently for 6 months to a year after ablation of the tumour. Commencing chemotherapy before operative treatment allows the pathologist to assess the response of the tumour to the drugs by histological examination of the resected specimen. The ability of chemotherapy to control local recurrence and distant metastatic spread has permitted the increasing use of 'limb salvage surgery' as an alternative to amputation. In selected cases, based on accurate surgical staging from biopsy and modern imaging techniques, it is possible to undertake radical resection and replacement with a metallic prosthesis or a massive bone graft. Recent reports have shown over 70% disease-free survival after 5 years by this approach in patients with osteosarcoma, with no increase in local recurrence rates when compared with amputation.

Chondrosarcoma of bone

A chondrosarcoma is a malignant tumour derived from cartilage cells, and it tends to maintain its cartilaginous character throughout its evolution.

Pathology. It may develop in the interior of the bone (central chondrosarcoma) or upon its surface (peripheral chondrosarcoma). A *central chondrosarcoma* occurs most commonly in the femur, the tibia, or the humerus. It may arise *de novo*, without there having been a pre-existing lesion (Figs 8.21 and 8.22), or it may arise from malignant transformation of a previously existing enchondroma (especially in the condition known as dyschondroplasia, Ollier's disease or multiple chondromatosis (p. 65).

A *peripheral chondrosarcoma*, on the other hand, tends usually to affect a flat bone such as the innominate bone (Figs 8.23 and 8.24), the sacrum, or the

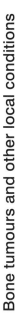

Bone tumours and other local conditions

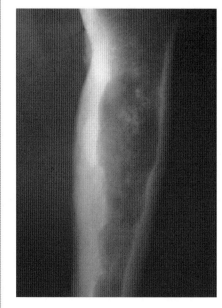

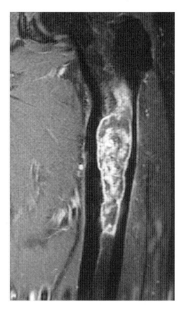

Fig. 8.21 Radiograph of proximal femur with a central chondrosarcoma. The lytic lesion has produced endosteal scalloping, indicating an aggressive lesion, and shows calcification indicating a chondroid matrix.

Fig. 8.22 MR of same patient. Demonstrates the extent of the femoral lesion which is similar to that seen on the plain film and is still confined to bone.

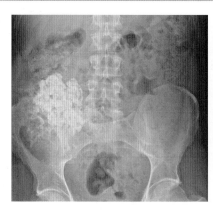

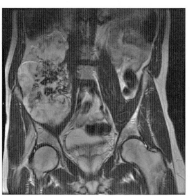

Fig. 8.23 Plain radiograph of the pelvis showing a large lobulated calcified mass arising from the right iliac wing, which proved to be a low-grade peripheral. chondrosarcoma.

Fig. 8.24 MR of same patient as in Fig. 8.23 shows a much larger mass than is apparent on the plain film . This consists of non-calcified cartilage and suggests that the chondrosarcoma has developed in a cartilage-capped exostosis arising from the pelvis.

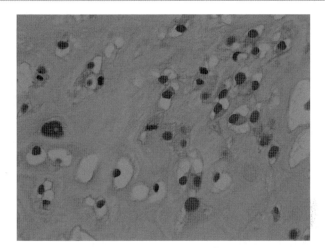

Fig. 8.25 Histological appearance of chondrosarcoma with an extensive chondroid matrix, containing scattered atypical chondrocytes with nuclear pleomorphism and some spindle cell morphology. (Haematoxylin and eosin ×400.)

scapula, and it generally arises from malignant transformation of a previously existing osteochondroma (especially in the condition of diaphysial aclasis or multiple exostoses (p. 63)).

Histologically, a chondrosarcoma may be highly cellular (Fig. 8.25). The cartilage cell nuclei tend to be swollen, and double nuclei may be seen. These features, suggestive of malignancy, may be found in only a few microscopic fields, the remainder of the tissue appearing relatively benign.

Clinical features. The patient is usually in the 30–60 age group, who complains of pain and local swelling, often in an area where there was known to be a previous lesion, such as multiple exostoses or Ollier's disease. The tumour grows slowly and may attain a large size.

Imaging. *Radiographically*, a central chondrosarcoma is seen to grow at the expense of the cortical bone with endosteal scalloping and may result in pathological fracture (Fig. 8.21). In contrast a peripheral chondrosarcoma shows as a large mass growing outwards from the surface of the bone (Fig. 8.23). Both types characteristically show blotchy areas of calcification within the tumour mass. *Magnetic resonance scanning* is essential to define the soft tissue extension of the tumour (Figs 8.22 and 8.24).

Prognosis. A chondrosarcoma grows slowly and does not metastasise early; so the prognosis, depending on the grade of the tumour, is somewhat more favourable than it is for osteosarcoma. Because of the variable grades and slow growth of chondrosarcoma the overall survival rate may be over 75%, though in high-grade lesions this may fall to 20%.

Treatment. Since adjuvant chemotherapy is not effective against chondrosarcoma, surgery must remain the treatment of choice. Wide surgical margins must be achieved to permit complete resection, though in some low-grade lesions or borderline malignancy it may be possible to undertake local excision or even curettage. In very large high-grade tumours or following local recurrence, amputation may still be required.

Malignant fibrous histiocytoma of bone

This rare highly malignant tumour includes many of the lesions once classified as fibrosarcoma, because their histology shows a predominance of fibroblast-type cells mixed with primitive histiocytes. It affects adults in the 20–60 age group, mainly occurring in the diaphysis of long bones, presenting with pain, swelling and sometimes pathological fracture.

Imaging with radiographs and MR shows permeative bone destruction from a large soft tissue mass with no sclerosis or periosteal reaction.

Treatment is similar to osteosarcoma, requiring radical surgery and adjuvant chemotherapy.

Ewing's[1] tumour (endothelial sarcoma of bone)

Ewing's tumour (endothelial sarcoma of bone) is an uncommon but highly malignant sarcoma that arises in bone marrow.

Pathology. The tumour is commonest in the shaft of the femur, tibia, or humerus. Unlike osteosarcoma, it arises in the diaphysis rather than the meta-physis of a bone. It probably develops from endothelial elements within the bone marrow, though the precise cell of origin is not known. The tumour tissue is soft and vascular. As it expands it gradually destroys the bone substance. There is a striking reaction beneath the periosteum, where abundant new bone is formed in successive layers (Fig. 8.13). Histologically the tumour consists of sheets of uniform small round cells (Fig. 8.26). The tumour metastasises early through the blood stream, especially to the lungs, and sometimes to other bones.

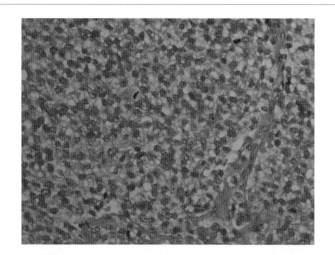

Fig. 8.26 Histological appearance of Ewing's sarcoma with sheets of cells, containing round or oval nuclei, but with very little intercellular stroma. (Haematoxylin and eosin ×400.)

[1]James Ewing (1866–1943) American pathologist who was founder and Director of Memorial Sloan-Kettering Cancer Center in New York and described the tumour in 1920.

Clinical features. Children and adolescents in the 5–20 age group are the usual victims. Typically, there is local pain with rapidly increasing firm swelling over one of the long bones, usually near the middle of the shaft (in contrast to osteosarcoma which arises at the metaphysis). Local symptoms may be accompanied by fever, weight loss and general malaise. On examination the swelling is diffuse or fusiform, and of firm consistency. The overlying skin becomes stretched and warmer than normal due to the large size and vascularity of the tumour mass.

Imaging. *Plain radiographs* show destruction of bone substance with concentric layers of subperiosteal new bone ('onion-peel' appearance) (Fig. 8.27). *MR scanning* will reveal the extent of the large soft tissue mass of the tumour (Fig. 8.28). An isotope bone scan is also required in staging to detect any multifocal lesions. A radiograph or CT scan of the chest may show pulmonary metastases.

Diagnosis. In atypical cases there may be confusion with subacute osteomyelitis, because of the systemic disturbance and raised ESR. In particular, it may be confused histologically with a metastasis from a suprarenal neuroblastoma. A percutaneous needle biopsy should be undertaken when the tumour is suspected.

Prognosis. Until recent years Ewing's tumour was uniformly fatal – usually from pulmonary metastases, with fewer than 15% of patients surviving beyond 5 years. The advent of adjuvant chemotherapy and improved radiotherapy has changed this gloomy outlook, and now 5-year survival rates can be expected in 50–60% of cases.

Treatment. Chemotherapy differs from that used for osteosarcoma and a number of different drug combinations have been used and continue to

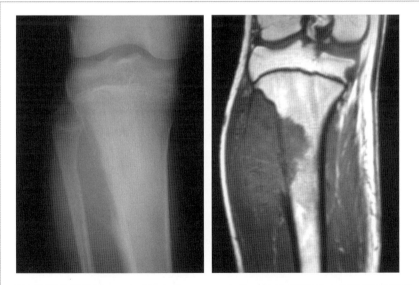

Fig. 8.27 (left) Radiograph of Ewing's sarcoma in the proximal tibia in a child. The lateral cortex is destroyed and there is periosteal elevation at the lower margin of the lesion.

Fig. 8.28 (right) MR of the same patient as in Fig. 8.27. This shows there is extensive involvement of the tibial shaft, the cortex is breached and there is a large associated soft tissue mass.

evolve. A combination of vincristine, cyclophosphamide, dactinomycin, and doxorubicin is commonly recommended and is commenced as adjuvant therapy prior to any operative treatment. The tumour itself may be treated by radical operative excision with prosthetic replacement, or by amputation. Radiotherapy may be used as an alternative to operation, since the tumour is radiosensitive. Surgical excision with a special prosthesis adjustable for progressive limb growth is preferred for lower limb lesions, particularly in young children where leg length discrepancy and joint contractures may follow radiotherapy. Radiotherapy is usually reserved for upper limb tumours and for tumours at inaccessible sites such as the pelvis or spine.

Myeloma (myelomatosis; plasmacytoma)

This is a tumour of bone marrow, occurring in older adults aged 50–70, often presenting as a single lesion but later spreading to involve the bone marrow at other sites. It is usually ultimately fatal, though modern treatment regimens may produce very long-term remission for up to 10 years.

Pathology. It arises from the plasma cells of the bone marrow and is disseminated to many parts of the skeleton through the blood stream, so that by the time the patient seeks advice the tumour foci are usually multiple, affecting chiefly the bones that contain abundant red marrow. Less commonly the tumour may present as a solitary bone plasmacytoma (Fig. 8.29) with spread to other skeletal sites only after months or years. The lesions are mostly small and circumscribed (Figs 8.14 and 8.30) but occasionally large: the bone is simply replaced by tumour tissue and there is no reaction in the surrounding bone. Pathological fracture is common, especially in the spine (Fig. 8.30). Histologically the tumour consists of

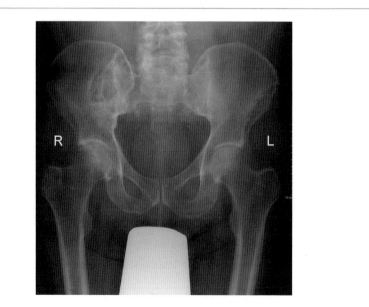

Fig. 8.29 Radiograph of pelvis. There is a large lytic lesion of the right iliac wing. The imaging findings are non-specific, but biopsy indicated this to be a solitary plasmacytoma.

Bone tumours and other local conditions

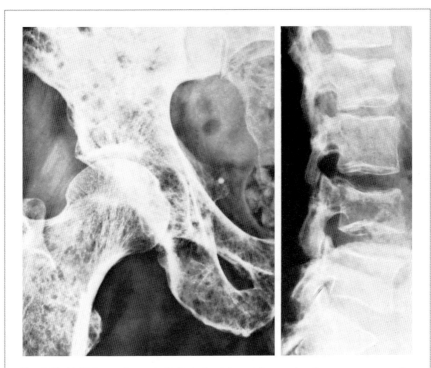

Fig. 8.30 Multiple myeloma. *Left*: Part of pelvis and femur, showing numerous small tumour foci. *Right*: Spine, showing diffuse rarefaction, with partial collapse of the bodies of the second and fourth lumbar vertebrae.

a mass of small round cells of plasma-cell type: the cells may be somewhat larger than normal plasma cells, and less uniform (Fig. 8.31).

Clinical features. In most cases the tumour affects adults past middle age. There is general ill health, with local pain at one or more of the tumour sites, or sometimes a pathological fracture. On examination the patient is pale from the associated anaemia due to suppression of red marrow function. There is often local tenderness over the affected bones, but there may be no obvious swelling or deformity unless pathological fracture has occurred. The patient is prone to develop infections due to the suppression of normal antibody production.

Imaging. *Radiographs* show multiple punched out lytic lesions, especially in bones containing red marrow, such as ribs, vertebral bodies, pelvic bones, skull, and proximal ends of femur and humerus (Fig. 8.30). Sometimes there is diffuse rarefaction of bone (Table 6.2, p. 77).

MRI scanning is potentially useful for imaging multiple skeletal lesions, particularly in suspected spinal involvement because of the superior soft tissue resolution it provides.

Investigations. There is microcytic anaemia. The erythrocyte sedimentation rate is increased. Bence Jones protein is present in the urine in more than half the cases. Serum globulin is increased, often so much that the albumin–globulin ratio (normally 2:1) is reversed. Marrow biopsy usually shows a profusion of plasma

Bone tumours and other local conditions

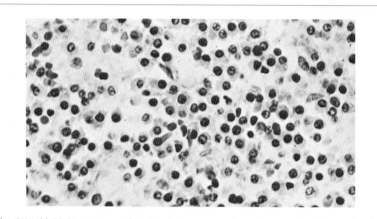

Fig. 8.31 Multiple myeloma. Sheets of cells resembling plasma cells. (Haematoxylin and eosin ×400.)

cells which can be characterised by immunohistochemistry and cytogenetics to give more help in planning treatment and predicting prognosis.

Diagnosis. Iliac or sternal marrow biopsy will often confirm the diagnosis when the clinical and radiographic features are equivocal.

Prognosis. The tumour is usually fatal, though its progress can often be checked for several years by the improving treatment regimens.

Treatment. The tumour foci respond to radiotherapy for a while, and pain is well relieved. The mainstay of chemotherapy in the past has been melphalan, an alkylating agent, which was sometimes used in conjunction with prednisolone. Newer drug combinations are showing improved results using thalidomide, or one of its analogues, with dexamethasone and a proteasome inhibitor, bortezomib. In a favourable case remission for up to 4 years may be gained. The possible place of bone marrow stem cell transplantation is also under trial. When hypercalcaemia is a problem treatment with bisphosphonates to inhibit excessive bone resorption may be required.

Secondary (metastatic) tumours in bone

Secondary malignant tumours in bone are much more common than primary tumours; but whereas most primary malignant bone tumours occur in children or young adults, secondary tumours generally occur in later life.

Pathology. The tumours that metastasise most readily to bone are carcinomas of the lung, breast, prostate, thyroid, and kidney (hypernephroma). Metastases occur most commonly in the parts of the skeleton that contain vascular marrow, especially the vertebral bodies, ribs, pelvis, and upper ends of the femur and humerus. The bone structure is simply destroyed and replaced by tumour tissue (Fig. 8.15). Pathological fracture is therefore very liable to occur.

Clinical features. Pain is the usual main symptom, but sometimes the disability is insignificant until a pathological fracture occurs. The spine is frequently involved, often with progressive neurological symptoms as well as local pain, from pressure on nerve roots or the spinal cord. In advanced widespread metastatic disease the patient may develop symptoms of hypercalcaemia, with nausea, vomiting, dehydration, and even coma. The primary tumour can usually be demonstrated.

Analysis of the different types of clinical presentation has shown that 50% of patients present initially with bone pain, 25% with pathological fracture, 15% with paraplegia or paraparesis, and 10% with local swelling.

Imaging. In *plain radiographs* the bone appears to have been eaten away so that there is a clear circumscribed area of lysis, without any reaction in the surrounding bone (Fig. 8.32). Exceptionally, new bone is laid down within the metastasis, causing marked sclerosis – the exact opposite to the usual osteolytic lesion. This type is almost confined to secondary deposits from prostatic carcinoma. In cases of diffuse infiltration there may be widespread osteoporosis (Table 6.2, p. 77). A radiograph or CT scan of the chest should always be obtained because of the possibility that metastases may be present in the lungs.

Technetium isotope scanning is the best technique for detecting occult metastatic deposits in the skeleton, as areas of increased uptake (Fig. 2.14B). These may be apparent long before the lesions are visible in plain radiographs, making it a very sensitive screening method. *Magnetic resonance imaging* is an even more sensitive method of screening, particularly for the detection of spinal metastases.

Investigations. In prostatic metastases the content of acid phosphatase in the plasma is usually increased above the normal range. The increase is specifically in the tartrate labile or 'prostatic' phosphatase. Hypercalcaemia may sometimes occur when there is excessive bone resorption from widespread bone metastases.

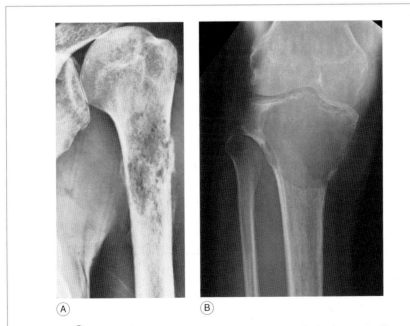

Fig. 8.32 Ⓐ Typical appearance of a metastatic carcinoma in the humerus. The primary tumour was in the lung. With increasing destruction of bone, pathological fracture is likely to occur. Ⓑ AP radiograph of tibia showing a solitary renal metastasis. There is a lytic expansile lesion in the proximal tibia with breach of the medial cortex indicating an aggressive lesion and the patient has a known renal carcinoma.

Bone tumours and other local conditions

Treatment. Radiotherapy is a valuable palliative treatment, particularly in more localised disease. Chemotherapy is sometimes appropriate (see p. 117). Radio-active iodine is valuable for metastases from carcinoma of the thyroid. Hormone analogue therapy may be appropriate for metastases from the breast or prostate, and in selected cases adrenalectomy and hypophysectomy have proved worthwhile in slowing the progress of the disease when other measures have failed. In the presence of life-threatening hypercalcaemia, treatment by bisphosphonates is valuable in that it inhibits further bone resorption and may also relieve bone pain. Local splintage may be required, but metallic internal fixation, or even custom prosthetic replacement of bone, is used increasingly for the treatment of impending or pathological fracture of the long bones as a means of maintaining independent function. Strong analgesics and sedatives may be required and a multi-disciplinary team is essential for the overall management of severe intractable pain.

Bone changes in leukaemia and lymphoma

This is a convenient place to note that changes may occur in the skeleton in leukaemia and in Hodgkin's disease or related lymphomas. In *leukaemia* the changes are due to infiltration of bone by proliferating white cells, and they are seen most commonly in subacute lymphatic leukaemia in children. Characteristically there are zones of rarefaction with delicate subperiosteal new bone formation in the metaphysial regions of the femur or humerus, or in the spine or pelvis. Leukaemia is also an occasional cause of diffuse widespread rarefaction of the skeleton (Table 6.2, p. 77).

In *Hodgkin's disease* or the related *lymphomas* there may be osteolytic lesions in the proximal limb bones or in the spine or pelvis, denoting destruction and replacement by tumour tissue.

TUMOUR-LIKE LESIONS OF BONE

SIMPLE BONE CYST (Solitary bone cyst; unicameral bone cyst)

Simple bone cysts occur mostly in the long bones of children or adolescents, commonly affecting the metaphysis of the proximal humerus or femur. They also occur occasionally in the small bones of the adult carpus, especially in the scaphoid or lunate bone.

Pathology. The cyst begins as a spherical lesion, but as it enlarges it tends to become oblong with its long diameter in the axis of the bone. In the long bones it tends to lie centrally in the shaft rather than to grow eccentrically, and the remaining cortex may appear expanded equally in all directions. The cyst contains clear fluid. It weakens the bone and often leads to pathological fracture. It is often stated that after a fracture through the wall of a cyst spontaneous filling in of the cyst may occur, but in fact this is by no means always the case.

Histologically, a bone cyst has only a very thin connective-tissue lining. Its wall contains abundant osteoclasts, a fact that has led to confusion with giant-cell tumour.

Clinical features. Solitary bone cysts seldom cause symptoms unless a pathological fracture occurs and are usually a chance radiological finding.

Imaging. Plain radiographs show a circumscribed area of lucency with only a thin surrounding zone of sclerosis (Fig. 8.33A). The cyst may appear faintly

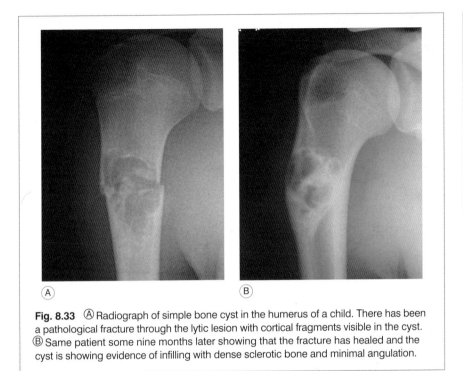

Fig. 8.33 Ⓐ Radiograph of simple bone cyst in the humerus of a child. There has been a pathological fracture through the lytic lesion with cortical fragments visible in the cyst. Ⓑ Same patient some nine months later showing that the fracture has healed and the cyst is showing evidence of infilling with dense sclerotic bone and minimal angulation.

loculated and the overlying cortex may be thinned, or if fractured, a cortical fragment may drop into the cyst ('fallen fragment').

Diagnosis. A cyst must be differentiated from other osteolytic lesions. It may be confused with a bone abscess, with a lipoid or eosinophilic granulomatous deposit, with localised fibrous dysplasia, or occasionally with a tumour. It should be remembered also that cyst formation in bones may be a feature of hyperparathyroidism, which must therefore be considered in differential diagnosis. A solitary bone cyst is distinct from an aneurysmal bone cyst (see below).

Treatment. Small uncomplicated cysts do not require treatment, since they tend to heal after skeletal maturity (Fig. 8.33B), but they should be kept under periodic observation. A large cyst may be curetted and packed with bone chips, but percutaneous aspiration and injection of corticosteroid solution or autogenous bone marrow into the cyst have now replaced operative treatment as the principal method of management. If fracture occurs each case must be treated on its merits: most heal with conservative treatment, but if internal fixation is required it should be combined with bone grafting.

ANEURYSMAL BONE CYST

Aneurysmal bone cysts also occur in children or young adults, usually before epiphyseal closure, but they are distinct from the simple bone cysts described above. Their origin is unknown: the term 'aneurysmal' signifies no more than a seeming 'blown-out' distension of one surface of the bone. There is no relationship to arterial aneurysm. The cyst may bulge into the soft tissues, contained only by periosteum and a thin shell of newly formed cortex. The lining consists of connective tissue with numerous vascular spaces and some giant cells; the cyst contains fluid blood.

Imaging. Plain radiographs show the cyst to be situated eccentrically in the bone; it presents a characteristic 'blown-out' appearance, as already mentioned (Fig. 8.34). These features distinguish it from the ordinary simple bone cyst, which is placed more centrally in the shaft and expands the bone uniformly without periosteal reaction. CT or MRI scanning may provide additional information on the extent of cortical destruction and may also demonstrate the multiple fluid levels that are typical of aneurysmal bone cysts.

Treatment. At most accessible sites the cyst should be curetted out and filled with bone chips. However, if the bone that is affected can be removed without consequent disability – for instance the fibula or a rib – the relevant part of the bone may be excised together with the cyst.

LOCALISED FIBROUS DYSPLASIA OF BONE
(Monostotic fibrous dysplasia)

In this condition a solitary area of bone is partly replaced by fibrous tissue, in which scanty bone trabeculae may persist. The cause is unknown, as also is its relationship to polyostotic fibrous dysplasia (p. 68). It is not related to the fibroblastic changes seen in association with the 'brown cysts' of hyperparathyroidism (p. 73).

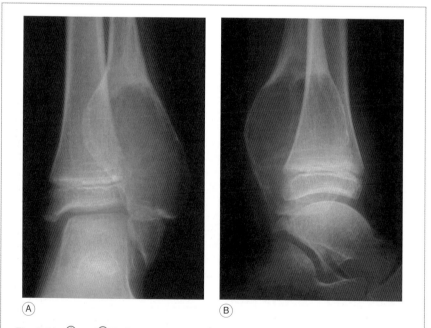

(A) (B)

Fig. 8.34 Ⓐ and Ⓑ Radiographs of aneurysmal bone cyst in the ankle of a child. There is an abnormal 'blown-out' appearance of the distal fibula in the metaphysis, but the epipyhseal plate is not crossed. These features make aneurysmal bone cyst the most likely diagnosis.

Pathology. One of the limb bones is usually the site affected, commonly the central fibrous lesion expands the medullary cavity at the expense of the bone, which is weakened and may fracture.

Clinical features. The lesion occurs in children and young adults who may present with local pain in the affected bone, though in many there are no symptoms and diagnosis may be on the basis of a coincidental X-ray finding.

Imaging. Plain radiographs show a zone of lucency within the bone, often with a homogeneous 'ground-glass' appearance and a thick sclerotic rim (Fig. 8.35). In larger lesions softening of the bone and repeated microfractures may result in progressive deformity, such as the 'shepherd's crook' of the proximal femur.

Treatment. This depends on the bone affected and the extent of the lesion. Simple curettage and autogenous bone grafting is ineffective, but for larger lesions cortical bone grafts with internal fixation may sometimes be required to control deformity.

METAPHYSIAL FIBROUS DEFECT (Fibrous cortical defect, non-ossifying fibroma)

This is a benign fibrous tissue defect in the metaphysial region of the cortex of a long bone, found accidentally from time to time in a child or young adult undergoing radiological examination for injury or for some other unconnected reason. The lesion is symptomless.

Imaging. Radiographs show a characteristic, well-defined notching of the cortex of the affected long bone (Fig. 8.36). Typically it has a scalloped, sclerotic border.

Treatment. Other than observation for a period, treatment is not required, but if the diagnosis is in doubt the lesion should be excised.

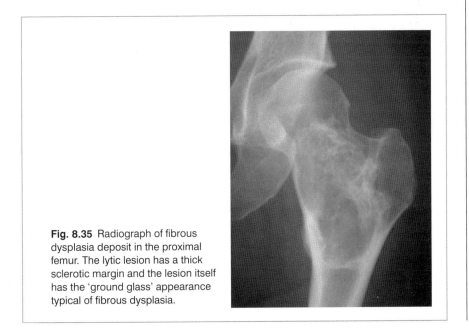

Fig. 8.35 Radiograph of fibrous dysplasia deposit in the proximal femur. The lytic lesion has a thick sclerotic margin and the lesion itself has the 'ground glass' appearance typical of fibrous dysplasia.

Bone tumours and other local conditions

Bone tumours and other local conditions

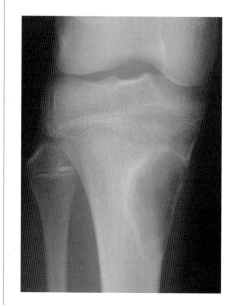

Fig. 8.36 Radiograph of tibia of an adolescent with an asymptomatic fibrous cortical defect. There is a lytic lesion with a sclerotic rim which is eccentrically placed in the metaphysis. The cortex is intact and there is no expansion of the bone.

OTHER LOCAL AFFECTIONS OF BONE

There is a miscellaneous group of solitary lesions of bone that do not fall into the category of infection or tumour. The most important members of the group are osteochondritis juvenilis and localised fibrous dysplasia of bone.

OSTEOCHONDRITIS JUVENILIS (Osteochondrosis)

The term osteochondritis juvenilis, or simply osteochondritis, is used to describe certain obscure affections of developing bony nuclei in children and adolescents. The term has also been used, wrongly, for some other affections of epiphyses or apophyses that are more likely traumatic in origin. Typically, a bony centre affected by osteochondritis becomes temporarily softened, and while in the softened state it is liable to deformation by pressure. The disease runs a course of variable length (often about 3 years), but eventually spontaneous rehardening occurs. The precise cause of the disease is unknown, but it is widely believed that temporary interruption of the blood supply to the affected epiphysis is the predominant factor. It should be noted that osteochondritis juvenilis is entirely distinct from osteochondritis dissecans (p. 153).

Sites. Osteochondritis juvenilis is recognised at the following sites (Table 8.2), though the pathology may not be identical at each site:

1. the upper epiphysis of the femur (Perthes' or Legg–Perthes' disease, p. 366)
2. Kienböck's disease of the lunate bone (p. 310) presents similar features and may be included in this group despite the fact that it occurs in fully developed adult bone
3. the nucleus of the navicular bone (Köhler's disease, p. 445)

4. the disorder of the head of the second or third metatarsal known as Freiberg's disease (p. 462) may possibly fall into the category of osteochondritis juvenilis, but there is a tendency now to ascribe it instead to osteochondritis dissecans.

A similar radiographic change in the central epiphysis of a vertebral body (Calvé's disease, p. 235) is now generally ascribed to eosinophilic granuloma rather than to osteochondritis. And the affection of the 'ring' epiphyses of the vertebral bodies in the thoracic region of the spine known as Scheuermann's disease or adolescent kyphosis (p. 232), again formerly thought to be an example of osteochondritis, is also now believed to be of different pathology. In brief, only the sites shown in Table 8.2 are now regarded as those where true osteochondritis commonly occurs.

Radiological appearances that bear some resemblance to the changes of osteochondritis are also seen in cases of pain at the apophysis of the tibial tubercle (Osgood–Schlatter's disease, p. 415) and at the apophysis of the calcaneus (Sever's disease, p. 448). These conditions were formerly thought to be examples of osteochondritis, but it is now recognised that they are traumatic in origin. There is simply a chronic strain of the apophysis from the pull of the tendon that is inserted into it. This type of lesion is now usually termed *apophysitis*.

Pathology. In a typical example of osteochondritis the histological and radiological evidence suggests that the affected bony centre undergoes partial necrosis, possibly from interference with its blood supply. The necrotic bone is invaded by granulation tissue, broken up, and eventually removed by osteoclasts. During

Table 8.2 Common sites of osteochondritis or related changes.

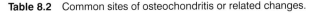

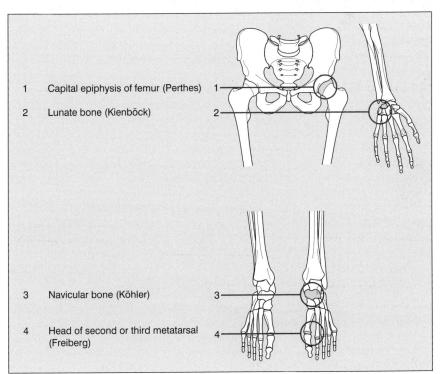

1	Capital epiphysis of femur (Perthes)	1
2	Lunate bone (Kienböck)	2
3	Navicular bone (Köhler)	3
4	Head of second or third metatarsal (Freiberg)	4

Bone tumours and other local conditions

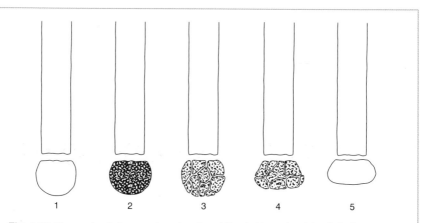

Fig. 8.37 The cycle of changes in osteochondritis. 1. Normal epiphysis before onset. 2. The bony nucleus undergoes necrosis, loses its normal texture, and becomes granular. 3. The bony nucleus becomes fragmented during the process of removal of dead bone. 4. If subjected to pressure the softened epiphysis becomes flattened. 5. Re-ossification with restoration of normal bone texture, but deformity may persist. The cycle occupies 2–3 years.

this stage of fragmentation the centre is liable to deformation if subjected to pressure (Fig. 8.37). The dead tissue is gradually replaced by new living bone trabeculae and eventually the bone texture is restored to normal; but if deformation has been allowed to take place there is permanent alteration of shape.

Clinical features. The age at which the condition arises varies according to the particular bone affected. In general, it occurs during the stage of active development of the bony nucleus. The main symptom is local pain. If the affected epiphysis forms part of a joint, the function of the joint is disturbed and joint movement aggravates the pain. The general health is not impaired.

Imaging. *Radiographic examination*. The cycle of changes can be followed in serial radiographs taken at intervals of a few months. First there is a slight and often patchy increase in density of the bony nucleus. Next the patchy appearance passes to one of fragmentation, representing irregular absorption of dead bone by osteoclasts and the commencing deposition of new bone. At this stage some flattening of the nucleus may be apparent by comparison with the normal side. Later there is a gradual return to normal bone texture, but any flattening that has occurred will remain. *Radioisotope bone scanning* may show absence of uptake of the isotope ('cold scan') during the stage at which the epiphysis is avascular.

Prognosis. Osteochondritis in itself is harmless to the general health, but if it leads to distortion of a joint surface it predisposes to osteoarthritis which, in the case of a large joint such as the hip, may cause serious disability in later years.

Treatment. The treatment depends largely upon the site of the affection. When the bony nucleus is relatively unimportant (as for instance that of the navicular bone) treatment may be unnecessary, or it may be sufficient to protect the part in a plaster for six or eight weeks while the pain is severe. But in the case of osteochondritis involving a major joint such as the hip every effort must be made to prevent distortion of the softened epiphysis.

Further details of these disorders will be found in the chapters dealing with individual regions.

9 | Arthritis and other joint disorders

ARTHRITIS

The term arthritis is used here to include both inflammatory and degenerative lesions of a joint.[1] It implies a diffuse lesion affecting the joint as a whole. It does not include localised mechanical disorders such as loose body formation or tears of the menisci of the knee, which are better designated as internal derangements. Nor should it embrace acute injuries of joints.

Clinically, arthritis is generally characterised by pain and restriction of movement at a joint, arising spontaneously; in superficial joints these features are usually accompanied by obvious swelling or thickening. If a joint is not swollen and if it moves freely and painlessly through its normal range it is very unlikely that it is affected by arthritis.

Types of arthritis

For convenience the infective types of arthritis, specifically pyogenic and tuberculous arthritis, have been dealt with in Chapter 7 together with the bone infections caused by the same organisms. Although other types of arthritis, particularly rheumatoid arthritis, have a major inflammatory component they have not been shown to be associated with a specific infective organism or virus. They are therefore considered here together with degenerative osteoarthritis and the less common types of arthritis associated with metabolic disturbances such as gout.

The incidence of different types varies greatly from country to country and from continent to continent, racial influences often being important. Thus osteoarthritis is very common in the white races, but is relatively uncommon among Africans and Asians.

The types of non-infective arthritis that are common, taken worldwide, are:

1. rheumatoid arthritis and juvenile chronic arthritis
2. osteoarthritis
3. gouty arthritis
4. haemophilic arthritis
5. neuropathic arthritis (Charcot's osteoarthropathy)
6. the arthritis of rheumatic fever
7. ankylosing spondylitis.

[1]The term arthrosis is sometimes used to denote a degenerative lesion of a joint, arthritis being used only for inflammatory lesions. But the use of the word 'arthrosis' to denote degeneration is without valid etymological grounds, and can be justified only on the basis of common usage.

RHEUMATOID ARTHRITIS (Rheumatoid polyarthritis)

Rheumatoid arthritis is a chronic inflammation of joints, often associated with mild constitutional symptoms. It nearly always affects several joints at the same time (polyarthritis). Joint changes of a similar nature also occur in a number of other conditions such as juvenile chronic arthritis (Still's disease), Reiter's syndrome, psoriasis, lupus erythematosus, and other connective tissue or collagen diseases.

Cause. The cause is unknown. At present only two possibilities attract serious consideration:

1. that the disease is due to auto-immunity
2. that it is caused by infection.

The hypothesis of auto-immunity, possibly to type II collagen, is based mainly on the observation that the serum of many patients with rheumatoid arthritis contains an antibody known as rheumatoid factor, which reacts with the body protein gamma globulin. When the antibody is present the disease is termed 'sero-positive', as contrasted with sero-negative arthritis when the antibody is absent. The source of the antigen, and many other details of the mechanism by which rheumatoid factor is formed, are unknown.

The hypothesis of infection is likewise without sure foundation. Infection – possibly by a virus or by organisms of the mycoplasma or diphtheroid group – may result in liberation of antigenic type II collagen from the patient's own articular cartilage.

Pathology. The synovial membrane is thickened by chronic inflammatory changes: characteristically it is infiltrated with macrophage-like cells and T-cell lymphocytes (Fig. 9.1). Later the articular cartilage is gradually softened and eroded, and the subchondral bone may also be eroded, characteristically at the joint margins – probably from the action of lytic enzymes and inflammatory mediators produced in the thickened synovial membrane. The eroded surfaces become covered by a soft membrane of inflammatory tissue known as 'pannus'.

The pathological changes are not confined to joints. The synovial lining of tendon sheaths may be similarly inflamed and thickened, both in the hands and in the feet. The contained tendons may become softened and may rupture, aggravating any existing deformity. Inflammatory nodules may form in the soft tissues.

After months or years of activity the disease process tends to become less active, usually leaving a number of joints that are permanently damaged, with consequent deformity, instability, or ankylosis.

Clinical features. The patient is usually a young or middle-aged adult, and is more likely to be a woman than a man. Any joint may be affected, but the incidence is higher in the more peripheral joints such as the hand joints, wrists, feet, knees, and elbows than in the lumbar or thoracic spine, shoulders, or hips. The onset is gradual, with increasing pain and swelling of a joint. Soon a number of other joints are similarly affected. Pain and stiffness are often worst when activity is resumed after resting. Often there is constitutional disturbance, with tiredness and anaemia, and occasionally fever.

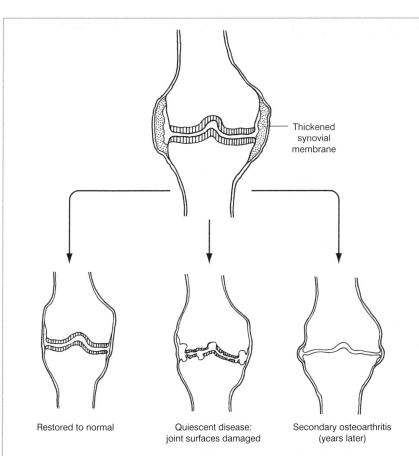

Fig. 9.1 Rheumatoid arthritis, with possible results. In the active phase there is marked thickening of the synovial membrane. Later, the articular cartilage is often eroded and in severe cases there may be some destruction of bone. The possible results are: 1. restoration to normal (only after mild disease of short duration); 2. continuing mildly active disease with permanently damaged joint surfaces and restricted movement; and 3. secondary osteoarthritis from wear-and-tear degeneration of the damaged joint surfaces.

On examination the affected joints are swollen from synovial thickening. The overlying skin is warmer than normal. The range of joint movements is restricted, and movement causes pain, especially at the extremes. These clinical features are often more severe in sero-positive disease than when rheumatoid factor is absent from the serum.

It is important always to study the condition of the cervical spine, which is commonly affected. Despite relatively minor symptoms, destruction of ligaments and bone may sometimes lead to subluxation of an intervertebral joint of such degree that the spinal cord is endangered, and it is important always to be wary of this possibility.

Extra-articular features may include enlargement of lymph nodes, muscle wasting, subcutaneous rheumatoid nodules, and anaemia.

Imaging. Radiographic features: At first there is no alteration from the normal. Later, there is diffuse rarefaction in the area of the joint. Eventually destruction of joint cartilage may lead to narrowing of the cartilage space and, in severe cases, to localised erosion of the bone ends (Fig. 9.2) especially in periarticular sites. Radioisotope bone scanning shows increased uptake of the isotope in the region of affected joints.

Investigations. Both the erythrocyte sedimentation rate and C-reactive proteins are raised during the active phase. The rheumatoid factor is present in the serum of 80% of patients with rheumatoid arthritis and is detected by the latex fixation or Rose-Waaler sheep cell agglutination tests.

Diagnosis. For a diagnosis of rheumatoid arthritis four of the following seven criteria must be present.

1. Morning stiffness in and around joints lasting more than 1 hour
2. Arthritis of three or more joints simultaneously
3. Arthritis in at least one area in a wrist, metacarpal or proximal interphalangeal joint
4. Symmetrical arthritis
5. Rheumatoid nodules
6. Positive rheumatoid factor
7. Radiological changes typical of RA on hand and wrist X-rays.

The clue to the diagnosis is the simultaneous involvement of several joints, with raised sedimentation rate. The presence of rheumatoid factor in the blood is highly suggestive, though the tests are not specific for rheumatoid arthritis; and rheumatoid factor may be absent in about 20% of patients even in well-established rheumatoid arthritis.

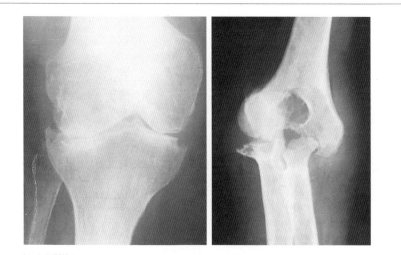

Fig. 9.2 Joint damage in rheumatoid arthritis. *Left*. Long-established rheumatoid arthritis of the knee. Note the rarefaction and loss of cartilage space. *Right*. Destruction of the elbow joint in a case of severe rheumatoid arthritis of long duration.

A search should always be made for evidence of one of the distinct clinical entities that may be associated with joint changes of a rheumatoid type. The most important of such conditions are:

1. psoriasis
2. Reiter's syndrome (urethritis, arthritis, conjunctivitis, and hyperkeratotic eruptions on the skin)
3. lupus erythematosus (scaly erythema of face or other parts)
4. scleroderma.

These conditions are all sero-negative, and they may be associated with ankylosing spondylitis.

Course. There is a tendency for rheumatoid arthritis to become quiescent after remaining active for months or years. In most cases there is permanent impairment of joint function. In certain joints – especially in the knees – degenerative changes are often superimposed upon the previous rheumatoid condition, and lead to increasingly severe disability even though the original rheumatoid affection is no longer active.

Treatment. The treatment of rheumatoid arthritis is still evolving, but no specific cure has been found. Innumerable drugs have been tried, but it is by no means certain that any of them has an influence on the duration of the disease or on its eventual outcome in a particular case. Undoubtedly some drugs can mitigate the symptoms, particularly the group of non-steroidal anti-inflammatory drugs (NSAIDs) which also have an analgesic effect in addition to their action in reducing synovial inflammatory changes.

Methods of treatment may be classified into the following categories:

1. rest and constitutional treatment
2. drugs, which include mainly the various non-steroidal anti-inflammatory agents; the 'second-line' drugs such as gold salts, sulfasalazine, and penicillamine; and (rarely) the 'third-line' corticosteroids
3. intra-articular injections of hydrocortisone
4. physiotherapy
5. occupational therapy
6. operation.

Rest and constitutional treatment. Rest is thought to be beneficial, especially in the early stages of the disease and during an exacerbation. At many centres patients are admitted to hospital at the outset for a period of rest, and sometimes this temporary removal from the home environment, with skilled nursing, regular food, and proper sleep, has a remarkably good effect on the general health, which is often impaired in these cases. Rest for individual joints is also helpful during the initial active stage of inflammation, provided it is not enforced for too long. Convenient light splints for this purpose may be made from expanded polystyrene, or plaster of Paris may be used. Splintage is seldom required for more than a few weeks and should be followed by graduated exercises under the supervision of a physiotherapist.

Drugs. Drugs used in rheumatoid arthritis fall mainly into the categories of the NSAIDs, and the potent anti-inflammatory agents grouped under the heading of corticosteroids. A logical plan is to use aspirin since it has both analgesic and mild anti-inflammatory properties, but to be effective it may have to be given in fairly large doses. Alternative first-line drugs should probably be chosen from the group of NSAIDs, which includes indometacin, ibuprofen, naproxen, phenoprofen and piroxicam. Due regard must be paid to the risk of side effects: gastric pain is a common complaint with most of these drugs, and more serious complications, such as gastric bleeding, are seen occasionally.

A different class of anti-rheumatic agents, to be regarded as second-line drugs, includes the potentially toxic group of compounds containing gold salts, usually given by intra-muscular injection. These must be used with care, but they are thought to be sometimes beneficial and therefore justified in severely afflicted patients who have failed to respond to the first-line drugs. Sulfasalazine, a derivative of sulphapyridine, is now also used increasingly as a second-line drug. Its mode of action is uncertain, but it has the advantage over gold salts of oral administration and fewer side effects. Another drug in this second-line category is penicillamine, the effect of which is comparable to that of gold. This also is potentially toxic for the kidneys and must be used with caution. Also included in this category are certain immuno-suppressive agents, such as azathioprine and methotrexate.

Newer developments in drug therapy have centred on biological molecules manufactured by genetic engineering that can block or reduce the production of destructive cytokines and enzymes from the cells of the rheumatoid synovium. The first of these, anti-tumour necrosis factor (TNF) has given very encouraging results in modifying the disease, but no long-term results are yet available.

The place of corticosteroids in rheumatoid arthritis is still controversial. There is wide agreement that because of their serious side effects they should be avoided altogether in the great majority of patients. There may be a small proportion of severely afflicted patients in whom the advantages outweigh the hazards.

Intra-articular injections. Injections of corticosteroids (usually hydrocortisone) into an affected joint can produce worth-while relief, but the disadvantages have precluded their widespread use. The main disadvantages are:

1. risk of infection, especially with repeated injections
2. risk of accelerating a degenerative reaction, the mechanism of which is not yet clear
3. the short duration of the relief obtained
4. repeated injections at several sites may become so irksome to the patient as to be unacceptable.

In general, it is wise to avoid repeated injections.

Physiotherapy. Physiotherapy is widely used and generally beneficial, even though some of the benefit may result from suggestion or 'placebo effect' rather than from a direct effect on the disease process. Heat in the form of infra-red radiation or short-wave diathermy is commonly used, but probably the most useful contribution of physiotherapy is active exercises including hydrotherapy, designed both to keep joints as mobile as possible and to maintain useful function in the muscles that control them.

Occupational therapy. Occupational therapy is useful mainly in helping seriously disabled patients to find ways in which they can more easily carry out the various activities of everyday life – bathing, toilet, cooking, feeding, boarding public transport, and many others. Many useful aids for the disabled are available, and those that are appropriate should be brought to the patient's notice.

Operation. Operation has an important place in treatment, but each operation must be considered as a component in the overall plan of management and not as a substitute for other measures. Operation may be applicable to the early stages of the disease, or it may be used in the later stages to salvage a joint that has been permanently damaged and remains a source of persistent pain.

In the early stages the operation most commonly used is synovectomy – excision of thickened and inflamed synovial membrane from joint or tendon sheath. As well as relieving pain, this may possibly slow down the inflammatory process and so help to preserve articular cartilage in an affected joint. It is undertaken mainly in the knee and wrist, and in the small joints and tendon sheaths of the hand.

Operation may also be required in the hand for repair or replacement of ruptured tendons, or for correction of finger deformities. In the painful elbow there is often a place for excision of the diseased radial head, and at the wrist excision of the lower end of the ulna may bring worthwhile relief in selected cases.

Operations used in the later stages of joint disease are arthroplasty and arthrodesis. Arthroplasty is applicable particularly to the hip and knee, and sometimes to the shoulder or elbow, and to the joints of the fingers and toes. Arthrodesis is usually the operation of choice for the joints of the spine, the wrist and the ankle.

Further details are given in the sections on individual joints.

JUVENILE CHRONIC ARTHRITIS (Juvenile rheumatoid arthritis; Still's disease)

Juvenile chronic arthritis is uncommon. In the past the general term 'Still's disease' was often used broadly to cover all its manifestations, but almost certainly the disease is not a single entity. Rather it comprises a number of conditions that are more or less distinct, though features common to all are pain, swelling and stiffness of joints. Recognised types include:

1. sero-positive polyarthritis (adult type occurring in children)
2. classical Still's disease
   (a) with systemic manifestations
   (b) with polyarthritis, and
   (c) with pauciarticular arthritis (i.e. minimal joint involvement)
3. sero-negative polyarthritis with sacro-iliitis
4. arthritis associated with psoriasis, ulcerative colitis or Crohn's disease.

These subgroups vary in age of onset, sex incidence, course, complications, and prognosis.

Sero-positive juvenile rheumatoid arthritis is similar in all respects to the same disease in adults. It tends to begin rather late in childhood and affects girls more often than boys.

Classical Still's disease begins in early childhood. In the systemic type there is swinging pyrexia with enlargement of lymph glands and of the spleen, with joint involvement simultaneously or later. The eventual outlook is favourable, as it is with the sero-negative polyarticular and pauciarticular variants – though the pauciarticular disease is complicated rather frequently by iridocyclitis necessitating local or systemic steroid therapy.

The sero-negative disease with sacro-iliitis is commoner in boys than in girls and tends not to begin until late in childhood: it may lead on to ankylosing spondylitis in early adult life. Most such patients show a positive test for HLA-B27 antigen and there is often clinical overlap between these patients and relatives with ankylosing spondylitis, Reiter's disease, ulcerative colitis, or Crohn's disease. It is thus probable that there is a hereditary factor in the causation.

Treatment. This is similar to that for rheumatoid arthritis in adults, with reliance on aspirin in the first instance and resort later if necessary to non-steroidal anti-inflammatory agents and possibly – in florid sero-positive disease – to gold therapy or penicillamine. Corticosteroid therapy should usually be avoided except for patients with iritis or iridocyclitis. General management includes adequate rest, temporary splinting of inflamed joints, graduated exercises with the physiotherapist, and occasionally operation – for instance, correction of fixed deformity or arthroplasty of the hip.

OSTEOARTHRITIS (Degenerative arthritis; arthrosis; osteoarthrosis; hypertrophic arthritis; post-traumatic arthritis)

Osteoarthritis is a degenerative wear-and-tear process occurring in joints. The joints may have been impaired by congenital defect, vascular insufficiency, or previous disease or injury. It is by far the commonest variety of arthritis.

Cause. It is caused by wear-and-tear that exceeds the capacity of the articular cartilage to renew and repair itself. If a joint were never put under stress it would never become osteoarthritic. Hence the relatively lightly stressed joints of the upper limb are, in general, less prone to osteoarthritis than the heavily stressed joints of the lower limb. Nearly always, however, there is a predisposing cause that accelerates the wear-and-tear process and there is now evidence that this may have a genetic basis. Almost any abnormality of a joint may be responsible, indirectly, for the development of osteoarthritis – often many years later. The main predisposing factors are:

1. congenital failures of normal development, such as hip dysplasia
2. irregularity of joint surfaces from previous fracture
3. internal derangements, such as a loose body or a torn meniscus
4. previous disease, leaving a damaged articular cartilage (for example, rheumatoid arthritis or haemophilia)
5. mal-alignment of a joint from any cause (for example, bow leg)
6. obesity.

Age alone is not a cause of osteoarthritis, though it may be associated with an impaired capacity for tissue repair after injury, and this may be an indirect causative factor.

Pathology. Any joint may be affected, the lower limb joints more often than the upper. The articular cartilage is slowly worn away until eventually the underlying bone is exposed (Fig. 9.3). This subchondral bone becomes hard and glossy ('eburnation'), though it may also show the presence of degenerative cysts. Meanwhile the bone at the margins of the joint hypertrophies to form a rim of projecting spurs known as osteophytes. There is no primary change in the capsule or synovial membrane, but the recurrent strains to which an osteoarthritic joint is subject often lead to slight thickening and fibrosis.

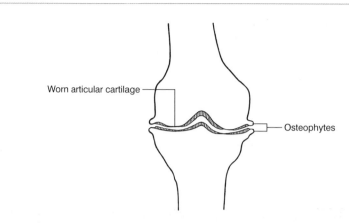

Fig. 9.3 Osteoarthritis. The main changes are in the articular cartilage and underlying bone. The cartilage is gradually worn away, disappearing first at the points of greatest pressure. The subchondral bone becomes sclerotic, and at the joint margins it hypertrophies to form osteophytes.

Clinical features. Most patients with osteoarthritis are past middle age. When it occurs in younger patients there is usually a clear predisposing cause such as previous injury or disease of the joint. The onset is very gradual, with pain that increases almost imperceptibly over months and years. Movements slowly become more and more restricted. In some joints (notably the hip) deformity is a common feature in the later stages. This means that the joint cannot be placed in the neutral (anatomical) position.

On examination slight thickening is often found on palpation; it is mainly a bony thickening caused by the marginal osteophytes. There is no increased warmth. Movements are impaired slightly or markedly according to the degree of arthritis; in the larger joints movement is accompanied by palpable or audible crepitation of a rather coarse type. Fixed deformity (that is, inability of the joint to assume the neutral anatomical position) is often found in the hip, and sometimes at the knee and in other joints.

Radiographic features. The characteristic features of osteoarthritis are:

1. diminution of cartilage space
2. subchondral sclerosis
3. subchondral cysts
4. spurring or 'lipping' of the joint margins from the formation of osteophytes (Figs 9.3 and 9.4).

Diagnosis. This is usually made clear by the history, clinical findings, and radiographic features. Osteoarthritis is not easily confused with inflammatory forms of arthritis, because there is no synovial thickening, no increased local warmth, and no muscle spasm; radiographs show sclerosis rather than rarefaction, and the erythrocyte sedimentation rate is not increased.

Course. Osteoarthritis usually increases slowly year by year. In many cases the disability never reaches the stage at which treatment is required. In others increasing pain, stiffness, or deformity drives the patient to demand measures for its relief.

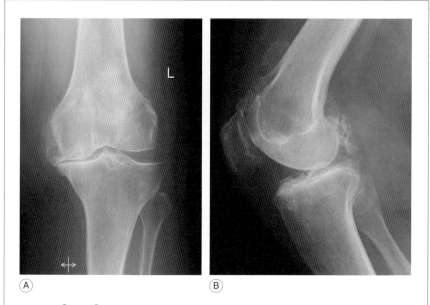

Fig. 9.4 Ⓐ and Ⓑ Radiographs of knee showing advanced osteoarthritis. There is marked joint space narrowing on the medial side and in the patello-femoral joint. Sclerosis of the sub-chondral bone and osteophyte formation at the joint margins are all typical features of osteoarthritis.

Treatment. The management of osteoarthritis exemplifies well the three categories of treatment that should be considered in every orthopaedic problem – namely:

1. no treatment, but advice and reassurance only
2. conservative treatment
3. operative treatment.

In many cases treatment is not required. The patient may have sought advice only because of anxiety lest some grave disease be present. Reassurance, with advice to restrict excessive stresses on the affected joint with weight reduction where appropriate, is all that is required.

When more active treatment is called for, conservative measures should usually be tried first. The methods available include physiotherapy (often by local heat and muscle-strengthening exercises), analgesic drugs, supportive bandages or orthoses to normalise stresses, and, in selected cases, local (intra-articular) injections of hydrocortisone or hyaluronate. However, repeated steroid injections are of questionable benefit in osteoarthritis and may accelerate joint degeneration. In addition, the stress that is put upon the affected joint should be reduced – for instance, in the case of the joints of the lower limb, by restricting the amount of walking or by the use of a stick (cane) or crutch.

When severe disability, particularly rest or night pain and limitation of function, is unrelieved by conservative treatment, operation may be justified. Among the operations available are osteotomy to realign a joint; arthroplasty (the construction of a new joint) (p. 40); and arthrodesis (elimination of the joint by fusion) (p. 39). Osteotomy is useful mainly at the knee to correct varus or valgus deformity, and is occasionally used at the hip, but will only provide pain relief for a period of a few years. Arthroplasty has become the operation of choice in the majority of patients particularly when osteoarthritis affects the hip and knee, where it can provide good painless function in 95% of patients after 10–15 years. For a few joints, particularly in the hands and feet, arthrodesis may still be the operation of choice. Further details of treatment will be given in the sections on individual joints.

GOUTY ARTHRITIS (Podagra; urate crystal synovitis)

Gout is the clinical manifestation of a disturbed purine metabolism. It is characterised by deposition of uric acid salts – especially sodium biurate – in connective tissues such as cartilage (of joints, or of the ear), the walls of bursae, and ligaments.

Cause. The precise cause of the disturbance of metabolism is unknown. There is an inherited predisposition to the disease. In susceptible persons an attack may be induced by excessive consumption of purine-rich foods such as liver, kidneys, sweetbreads, shellfish, beer, or heavy wines. An attack may also be precipitated by recent injury or operation.

Pathology. The primary fault is an impaired excretion of uric acid by the kidneys. In consequence the level of urate in the plasma is increased, sometimes to 0.5 mmol/litre or more (normal = 0.1–0.4 mmol/litre (2.0–7.0 mg/100 ml)). In the blood the uric acid is in solution in a loose combination with proteins; it comes readily out of solution as a sodium salt (sodium biurate) to be deposited in the form of crystals in certain connective tissues, especially those that have been injured or those that have a sluggish blood supply, such as the articular cartilage of the joints of the foot. The deposited crystals set up an inflammatory reaction. In acute gout the deposit is microscopic in amount and is soon reabsorbed, with restoration of the tissue to normal. In chronic gout, however, widespread deposits of sodium biurate in joint cartilages, ligaments and the articular ends of bones lead to considerable disorganisation of affected joints. Gouty deposits, known as tophi, are also common at other sites, notably in the olecranon bursa and in the cartilage of the ear, where they may form prominent rounded nodules.

Clinical features. The patient is nearly always over 40, and is more likely to be a man than a woman, in the ratio of 10:1. The chief clinical manifestations are arthritis and bursitis.

Arthritis. Gout affects principally the peripheral joints such as the joints of the toes, tarsus, and ankle, and the small joints of the hands. It occurs in recurrent attacks. The first attack is usually in the great toe; later attacks may affect other joints. In an acute attack the onset is sudden – often during the night. The affected joint is swollen, red, and glossy. Pain is very severe. Movements are greatly restricted because of the pain. The attack subsides after a few days and the joint is normal between attacks.

In chronic gout several joints may be affected together. They are thickened and nodular, and painful on movement.

Bursitis. The bursa most commonly affected by gout is the olecranon bursa. It becomes distended with fluid, and there may be palpable deposits of uric acid salts.

Other manifestations. Deposits of uric acid salts (tophi) are common in the ear cartilages, where they form palpable nodules. Similar tophi may also occur at other sites.

Radiographic features. In acute attacks of articular gout the joints do not show any radiographic change. In chronic gout the deposits of uric acid salts in the bone ends show as clear-cut erosions adjacent to the articular surfaces, for the deposits are transradiant (Fig. 9.5).

Investigations. There is sometimes a mild leucocytosis and the erythrocyte sedimentation rate may be increased. The plasma uric acid content is raised. Aspiration of swollen joints may yield a small quantity of turbid fluid, but never organisms. Polarised light microscopy of synovial fluid usually reveals needle-shaped crystals showing negative birefringence.

Diagnosis. Acute gout has to be distinguished from other forms of arthritis of acute onset, especially from acute pyogenic arthritis, acute 'pseudogout' (see below), haemophilic arthritis, and rheumatic fever. Features suggestive of gout are: a history of previous attacks, with symptom-free intervals; a raised plasma urate content; the presence of tophi in the ears or elsewhere; detection of crystals in synovial fluid; and a favourable response to treatment.

Chronic gout involving several joints may simulate rheumatoid arthritis.

Course. Gout usually occurs in recurrent acute attacks. Early attacks subside in a few days, leaving the joint clinically normal. In chronic gout the affected joints are gradually disorganised, and permanent disability is inevitable.

Treatment. For acute attacks reliance is usually placed upon a non-steroidal anti-inflammatory drug such as indometacin or naproxen. Colchicine is also effective. The affected joint should be rested until the attack has subsided.

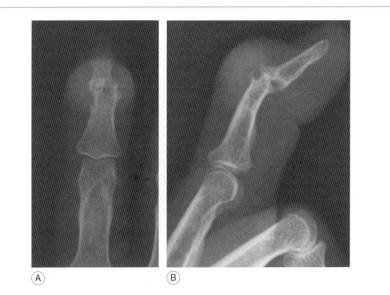

(A)   (B)

Fig. 9.5 Ⓐ and Ⓑ Radiograph of finger showing gouty arthritis in the distal interphalangeal joint. There is marked soft tissue swelling from the deposit of urate crystals and well-defined 'punched out' juxta-articular erosions.

A large effusion in a major joint such as the knee should be aspirated and replaced by an instillation of hydrocortisone.

For patients with frequent attacks or with chronic gout, especially if the plasma urate level is persistently raised, long-term drug therapy to reduce the plasma urate level may be required. The two types of drug available are represented by:

1. probenecid, which paralyses renal tubular reabsorption of urates and thus increases their excretion in the urine
2. allopurinol, which reduces the formation of uric acid by inhibiting the enzyme xanthine oxidase.

Provided its long-term use is not associated with toxic reactions, allopurinol is probably to be preferred because it does not increase the load of urate in the urine, with its hazard of stone formation.

PYROPHOSPHATE ARTHROPATHY (Pseudogout)

With the general acceptance of the idea that joint manifestations in gout are caused by the presence of urate crystals, it has more recently come to be appreciated that similar manifestations may be induced by the crystals of other salts. In most such cases the crystals are composed of calcium pyrophosphate showing positive birefringence, and characteristically calcification of articular cartilage or of menisci is demonstrable radiologically (Fig. 9.6). Arthritis of this type has been termed 'pseudogout'. It usually presents as a chronic arthritis with characteristic calcification of cartilage, but it may occur in an acute form mimicking a joint infection, from the shedding of crystals into the synovial fluid. The diagnosis can be confirmed by the finding of pyrophosphate crystals in the aspirated joint fluid. Treatment of an acute attack should be by rest, aspiration of joint fluid with intra-articular steroid injection, and a non-steroidal anti-inflammatory agent.

HAEMOPHILIC ARTHRITIS

Joint manifestations are common in haemophilia, but examples are seen only infrequently because haemophilia is itself an uncommon disease.

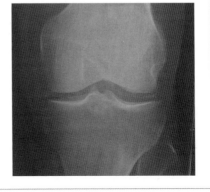

Fig 9.6 AP radiograph of knee with pseudogout or pyrophosphate arthropathy. There is a characteristic line of calcification within the joint space due to crystal deposition within the menisci and deeper layers of the articular cartilage.

Pathology. The term 'haemophilia' is used loosely to embrace a group of different defects in the process of coagulation of the blood. Classical haemophilia, the commonest of the group, occurs in males but is transmitted by females. There is an inherited deficiency of a specific clotting factor known as antihaemophilic factor (Factor VIII). In consequence the clotting time of the blood is prolonged and there is a tendency to undue bleeding, external or internal, when even quite small vessels are cut or torn. Joint manifestations are caused by haemorrhage into a joint, occurring after a minor strain or even without any known injury. The joints most commonly affected are those most vulnerable to strain – especially the knee, elbow, and ankle. The joint cavity is distended with blood (haemarthrosis), which is later slowly reabsorbed if the joint is rested. Recurrent haemarthroses lead eventually to degenerative changes in the articular cartilage and to fibrosis of the synovial membrane.

Clinical features. The patient, often a young boy, may be a known sufferer from haemophilia or can recall previous episodes of bleeding. He suddenly finds that a joint has become painful and swollen. On examination the findings vary according to the phase and duration of the arthritis. In the absence of specific treatment the joint remains swollen for several weeks after the acute onset – partly from effused blood and partly from the synovial thickening that results from interstitial extravasation. The overlying skin is abnormally warm. Joint movements are restricted and very painful.

In the quiescent phase between attacks of haemarthrosis there is moderate thickening of the joint from synovial fibrosis, movements are slightly impaired, and often there is some degree of fixed deformity – for instance, inability to straighten the knee fully.

Diagnosis. Because of the synovial thickening, increased warmth of the skin, and restriction of joint movements, haemophilic arthritis is easily mistaken for acute or chronic infective arthritis. The history of previous episodes of bleeding, the sudden onset, and the recurrent nature of the attacks are important diagnostic features: the prolonged clotting time of the blood is confirmatory evidence.

Imaging. In the later stages of the disease, particularly in those patients who have multiple bleeds from poor control of their clotting factor, the joints may show extensive surface erosions, juxta-articular bone cysts, with bone destruction and deformities (Fig. 9.7).

Treatment. When the necessary facilities are available, the correct treatment for a recent acute incident is to promote coagulability of the blood by the administration of antihaemophilic factor in the form of Factor VIII concentrate or of cryoprecipitate, and then to treat the joint as for ordinary traumatic haemarthrosis by aspiration and temporary support in a plaster splint. Early treatment on these lines should reduce the incidence of irreversible fibrosis of the synovial membrane, hitherto a cause of serious permanent disability.

Failing adequate supplies of antihaemophilic factor, resort must be had to prolonged splintage.

In the chronic degenerative phase that follows repeated haemarthroses it is often necessary to give permanent support to the joint by means of a moulded plastic splint or other appliance. Operation must be avoided whenever possible, though it may if necessary be undertaken safely, provided that adequate cover by antihaemophilic factor can be provided.

The future outlook for haemophilic patients is much improved by the new-found ability to manufacture Factor VIII in commercial quantities by genetic

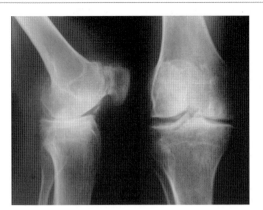

Fig. 9.7 AP and lateral radiograph of knee in chronic haemophiliac arthropathy. There are marked joint abnormalities in all three joint compartments with oversized epiphyses, build-up of osteophytes and reactive sclerosis.

engineering technology. If such a product can be developed to the point of being effective when taken by mouth the advantage will clearly be even greater.

NEUROPATHIC ARTHRITIS (Charcot's osteoarthropathy)

In neuropathic arthritis a joint is disorganised by repeated minor injuries because it is insensitive to pain.

Cause. The underlying cause is a neurological disorder interfering with deep pain sensibility, although in a third of patients no demonstrable neurological deficit is present. In patients with involvement of joints of the lower limb the commonest cause in the past was tabes dorsalis, a manifestation of syphilis; but tabes is now uncommon, and there has been a corresponding decline in the incidence of neuropathic arthritis in the lower limb. Other causes are diabetic neuropathy, cauda equina lesion, and in some countries leprosy. In those with upper limb involvement the usual cause, apart from leprosy, is syringomyelia.

Pathology. Any of the large joints may be affected, including the joints of the spine. The knee, ankle, and subtalar joint are most commonly affected in the lower limb, and the elbow in the upper limb. In a normal joint harmful strains are prevented by a protective reflex whereby muscle contraction is evoked by incipient pain. When joint sensibility is destroyed the protective function of pain is lost. Strains are unrecognised and, cumulatively, they lead to severe degeneration of the joint. The changes may be regarded as a much exaggerated form of osteoarthritis. The articular cartilage and subchondral bone are worn away, but at the same time there is sometimes massive hypertrophy of bone at the joint margins. The ligaments become lax and the joint is unstable. Indeed it is often subluxated or even dislocated.

Clinical and radiographic features. The patient is usually in adult life. The main symptoms are swelling and instability of the affected joint. Since the joint is insensitive pain is slight or, sometimes, absent. On examination the joint is thickened,

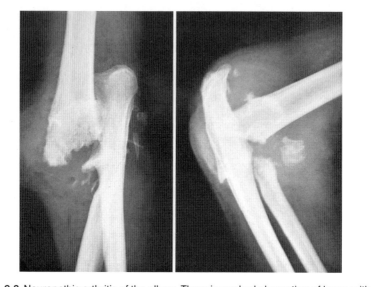

Fig. 9.8 Neuropathic arthritis of the elbow. There is marked absorption of bone, with pathological dislocation. The underlying cause was syringomyelia.

mostly from irregular hypertrophy of the bone ends. The range of movement is moderately restricted, and there is marked lateral laxity leading to instability. In extreme cases the joint may be dislocated. Further examination will reveal evidence of the underlying neurological disorder. Radiographs show severe disorganisation of the joint (Fig. 9.8). The changes are basically those of osteoarthritis, but enormously exaggerated. There is a loss of cartilage space and some absorption of the bone ends, often with considerable hypertrophy of bone at the joint margins.

Treatment. In most instances the best treatment is simply to provide support for the joint by a suitable appliance. Sometimes operation may be undertaken to fuse the joint, but fusion may be difficult to achieve. The primary neurological disorder will usually demand appropriate treatment.

ARTHRITIS OF RHEUMATIC FEVER

In adolescent children and young adults arthritic manifestations are a prominent feature of rheumatic fever. This has now become an uncommon disease in Western countries; so joint manifestations from this cause are hardly ever seen except in under-developed parts of the world.

Cause. Rheumatic fever is ascribed to a sensitivity reaction associated with infection by a haemolytic streptococcus. There may be an inherited predisposition to the disease.

Pathology. Any joint may be affected. The synovial membrane is acutely inflamed, but there is no suppuration. Clear fluid is effused into the joint.

Clinical features. The patient is usually a child over 10, or a young adult. There is constitutional illness, with malaise and pyrexia. A joint becomes painful and swollen, and soon afterwards other joints are likewise affected. On examination an affected joint is swollen, partly from contained fluid and partly from synovial thickening. The overlying skin is warmer than normal. Movements are markedly restricted, and painful if forced. Other features of rheumatic fever, such as carditis and chorea, should be looked for. Radiographs of affected joints do not show any alteration from the normal.

Investigations. There is a mild leucocytosis. The erythrocyte sedimentation rate is increased.

Diagnosis. Arthritis of rheumatic fever has to be distinguished from other forms of arthritis – especially from acute pyogenic arthritis, rheumatoid arthritis, gout, and haemophilic arthritis – and from acute osteomyelitis. Features suggestive of rheumatic fever are: onset in adolescence; affection of several joints together or in succession; severe pain with signs of acute inflammation, but without suppuration; a mild rather than a marked leucocytosis; a concomitant cardiac lesion; and a rapid favourable response to salicylates.

Treatment. For joint involvement alone salicylates are adequate, but prednisolone or a related steroid may be required if the heart is affected. A therapeutic course of penicillin should also be given to eliminate streptococci, and thereafter twice-daily oral penicillin should be continued well into adult life to reduce the risk of recurrent attacks.

ANKYLOSING SPONDYLITIS (Spondylitis ankylopoietica; Marie–Strümpell arthritis)

As the name implies, ankylosing spondylitis is primarily a disease of the spine, though in a few cases the arthritic changes involve also the proximal joints of the limbs, especially the hips. Briefly, it is a chronic inflammatory affection of the joints and ligaments of the spine, beginning in the sacro-iliac joints. It progresses slowly, the changes gradually creeping up the spinal column from below. The natural outcome is bony ankylosis of the affected joints (Fig. 9.9) but the disease may be arrested at any stage short of this.

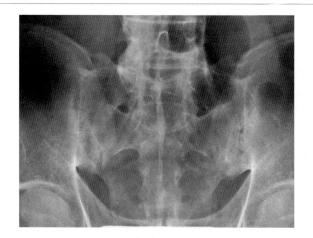

Fig. 9.9 AP radiograph of sacroiliac joints in advanced ankylosing spondylitis showing typical complete fusion of the joints.

Typically, ankylosing spondylitis affects men in early adult life, with a strong hereditary link to the HLA-B27 gene. After remaining active for several years it tends eventually to become quiescent, always leaving some degree of permanent stiffness of the spine. A fuller description is given in Chapter 13 (p. 229).

DISLOCATION AND SUBLUXATION OF JOINTS

The cause of dislocation or subluxation of a joint may be congenital, spontaneous, traumatic, or recurrent. By definition, a joint is subluxated when its surfaces are partly displaced but retain some contact one with the other (Fig. 9.10B). A joint is dislocated or luxated when its articular surfaces are wholly displaced one from the other, so that all apposition between them is lost (Fig. 9.10C).

CONGENITAL DISLOCATION OR SUBLUXATION

The most important representative of this group is congenital (developmental) dislocation of the hip (p. 343). Congenital club foot (talipes equino-varus) (p. 434) may be regarded as congenital subluxation of the talo-navicular joint. Congenital displacement of other joints is rare: an example that is seen occasionally is congenital dislocation of the head of the radius.

TRAUMATIC DISLOCATION OR SUBLUXATION

Injury is by far the commonest cause of dislocations. Traumatic dislocations are described in textbooks of fractures and joint injuries, and they will not be considered further here.

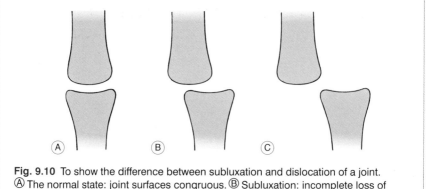

Fig. 9.10 To show the difference between subluxation and dislocation of a joint. Ⓐ The normal state: joint surfaces congruous. Ⓑ Subluxation: incomplete loss of contact between the joint surfaces. Ⓒ Dislocation: total loss of contact between the joint surfaces.

SPONTANEOUS (PATHOLOGICAL) DISLOCATION OR SUBLUXATION

Displacement may occur spontaneously at any joint in consequence of a structural defect or of destructive disease. It is encountered frequently in the spine, where the stability of the intervertebral joints may be impaired by structural defects, by previous injury, or by destructive arthritis (pyogenic, rheumatoid, or tuberculous). In the foot, it is common for a phalanx to become dislocated dorsally at the metatarso-phalangeal joint in cases of severe clawing of the toes; and in the hands interphalangeal subluxation may occur in rheumatoid arthritis. Another example is the dislocation of the hip that sometimes complicates severe tuberculous arthritis or pyogenic arthritis. Spontaneous subluxation or dislocation is also a common feature of neuropathic arthritis (p. 147).

RECURRENT DISLOCATION OR SUBLUXATION

Certain joints are liable to repeated dislocation or subluxation. Usually, but not always, there has been an initial violent dislocation which causes permanent damage to the ligaments or articular surfaces. The joints most often affected are the shoulder (p. 263), the patello-femoral joint (p. 409), and the ankle (p. 433).

INTERNAL DERANGEMENTS OF JOINTS

The term internal derangement implies a localised mechanical fault which interferes with the smooth action of a joint. An internal derangement is distinct from arthritis, which is nearly always a diffuse lesion involving the joint as a whole (see p. 133).

Internal derangements will be considered in three groups:

1. interposition of soft tissue
2. loose body formation
3. osteochondritis dissecans.

INTERPOSITION OF SOFT TISSUE IN JOINTS

The smooth action of a joint may be obstructed by a displaced mass of soft tissue within it. The soft tissue most often responsible is an intra-articular fibrocartilage, especially a meniscus in the knee (p. 399). As a rule a fibrocartilage can be displaced only when it is torn. Other soft tissues that are occasionally interposed are synovial fringes and ligamentous tags.

Clinical features. Disorders of this type are common only in the knee. The characteristic features are recurrent sudden 'locking' or giving way of the joint, with later an effusion of clear fluid within it.

LOOSE BODIES IN JOINTS

Intra-articular loose bodies may be derived from bone, cartilage, or synovial membrane. They may be entirely free within the joint or they may retain a pedicle of soft tissue.

Causes. The commonest causes of loose bodies are:

1. osteochondritis dissecans (1 to 3 loose bodies)
2. osteoarthritis (1 to 10 loose bodies)
3. chip fracture of the articular end of a bone (1 to 3 loose bodies)
4. synovial chondromatosis (50 to 500 loose bodies).

Pathology. *Osteochondritis dissecans* (see below). The loose body is derived from a part of the articular surface that undergoes necrosis and separates.

Osteoarthritis. The bodies may be derived from marginal osteophytes, in which case they often retain firm soft-tissue attachments and may cause little trouble. Free bodies may be derived from shed flakes of articular cartilage: nourished by synovial fluid, these gradually enlarge.

Fracture of articular margin (osteochondral fracture). Fractures only occasionally cause intra-articular loose bodies. A well-recognised example is a fracture-separation of the medial epicondyle of the humerus, which may be sucked into the elbow joint while still retaining its muscle attachments.

Synovial chondromatosis (osteochondromatosis). This is a rare but well-recognised disease of synovial membrane. A large number of villous folds become pedunculated and their bulbous extremities undergo metaplasia to cartilage. Eventually they separate from their pedicles to become free mobile bodies, and many of them become calcified. The disease may affect any joint – or even the synovial lining of a bursa.

Clinical features. Loose bodies do not necessarily cause symptoms unless they become caught between the joint surfaces. In that event the characteristic feature is sudden painful but usually momentary locking of the joint, succeeded after some hours by an effusion of clear fluid within it.

Imaging. A radiograph of the affected joint will reveal the presence of multiple loose bodies, characteristically surrounding the margins of the articular surfaces (Fig. 9.11).

Treatment. When a loose body causes trouble it should be removed. In synovial chondromatosis this may be combined with subtotal synovectomy.

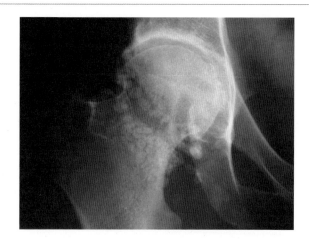

Fig. 9.11 AP radiograph of hip in synovial chondromatosis. There are multiple small calcified bodies within the distribution of the joint capsule.

OSTEOCHONDRITIS DISSECANS

Osteochondritis dissecans is a localised disorder of convex joint surfaces in which a segment of subchondral bone becomes avascular and, with the articular cartilage that covers it, may slowly separate from the surrounding bone to form a loose body.

Common sites. The only joints commonly affected are the knee and the elbow. In the knee the site of the lesion is nearly always the medial femoral condyle, and in the elbow, the capitulum of the humerus. Rarely the hip joint (femoral head) and the ankle joint (talus) are affected. The disorder of a metatarsal head known as Freiberg's disease (p. 462) is thought by some to be an example of osteochondritis dissecans and by others to represent osteochondritis juvenilis. It shows some features common to both conditions.

Cause. The precise cause is unknown. Impairment of blood supply to the affected segment of bone and cartilage – possibly by thrombosis of an end artery – has been postulated. The significance of injury is uncertain. There is probably an inborn susceptibility to the disease, for it may occur in several joints of the same patient, or in several members of a family.

Pathology. A segment of the articular surface of a bone becomes avascular (Fig. 9.12A), and a line of demarcation slowly forms between the avascular segment and the surrounding normal bone (Fig. 9.12B). The affected segment varies in size: in the knee it often measures about one to three centimetres in diameter and half a centimetre in depth. It is always on the convex joint surface. If the segment is small it is sometimes re-attached spontaneously, especially in adolescents; but in most cases it finally separates to form a loose body in the joint, still covered by its articular cartilage (Fig. 9.12C). The resulting cavity in the articular surface of the bone fills with fibrous tissue, but there is inevitably some irregularity of the joint surface which predisposes to the later development of osteoarthritis.

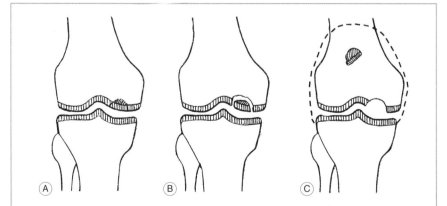

Fig. 9.12 Evolution of osteochondritis dissecans. Ⓐ Segment of articular surface of medial femoral condyle deprived of blood supply. Ⓑ A line of demarcation has formed and the avascular fragment is separating from the surrounding healthy bone. Ⓒ Fragment loose in joint. A cavity remains in the articular surface.

Clinical features. The patient is an adolescent or a young adult. The early symptoms and signs are those of a mild mechanical irritation of the joint – namely a tendency to aching after use, with recurrent effusion of clear fluid. After separation of a fragment from the articular surface the clinical features are those of an intra-articular loose body: recurrent sudden locking of the joint accompanied by sharp pain and followed by effusion.

Radiographs show a clearly defined shallow excavation in the articular surface of the bone, with a discrete bone fragment lying either within the cavity or elsewhere in the joint. However, the osteochondral fragment may only appear on X-ray as a small thin flake of bone. Earlier changes can be seen more clearly on MRI scans and allow the clinician to monitor the progress of any healing or separation of the fragment.

Treatment. Until a loose body has separated or appears 'ripe' for separation, treatment should be expectant. In the case of a small lesion in early adolescence rest in plaster for two months may allow spontaneous re-attachment of the fragment. When a fragment has separated it should usually be removed, though in the case of a large fragment it may be practicable to fix it back in position with a pin. Further details will be found in the appropriate sections on the knee (p. 405), the elbow (p. 286), and the foot (p. 445).

10 Soft tissue tumours and other diseases

Co-written by Nigel Raby

SWELLINGS AND TUMOURS OF SOFT TISSUE

Soft tissue swellings are a common presentation to primary care physicians and a cause of great anxiety to patients when they discover a lump in their limb or trunk which they interpret as a cancer. In fact malignant tumours are very rare and benign tumours are much more common in a ratio of more than 100:1. These tumours frequently cause problems in diagnosis and treatment because of the difficulty in differentiating them from other, much commoner, causes of lumps and swellings in the limbs. These include cysts and ganglia around joints, normal muscle variants, muscle rupture, haematoma, vascular aneurysm, and myositis ossificans.

Normal muscle variants

These can present as a clinically palpable mass. They have presumably been present for years but for some reason the patient has only just noticed the swelling. One of the commonest sites is at the ankle where an accessory soleus muscle may mimic a soft tissue mass. Knowledge of the normal anatomy will assist in making the diagnosis along with the observation that the area of interest has identical signal to adjacent muscle on all MR sequences. The palmar aspect of the wrist is another area where anomalous developments in the flexor tendons may sometimes result in compression of the ulnar or median nerves in their fibro-osseous tunnels.

Muscle tears

Symptomatic muscle tears are not usually a problem since there is typically a history of trauma and painful onset of swelling. Clinically there is therefore no suggestion that this is a soft tissue mass. However some patients, particularly in an older age group, present with a painless swelling with no clear history of any single incident to account for it. Characteristically this is seen in the anterior thigh. The reason is spontaneous rupture of rectus femoris muscle. The proximal muscle can contract unopposed with a resulting soft tissue mass palpable in the thigh. In cases of clinical doubt an MRI scan will confirm that the swelling is muscle and demonstrate the defect at the site of rupture (see Fig. 18.29, p. 414).

Haematoma

An acute tissue haematoma, whether from injury or post-surgery, should not pose a problem for clinical diagnosis. Difficulty can occur when a large deep haematoma does not resolve and enters a chronic phase that may mimic the swelling from a recurrent lesion. The MRI scan should aid diagnosis showing a peripheral dark rim from the presence of iron-containing haemoglobin breakdown products (Fig. 10.1).

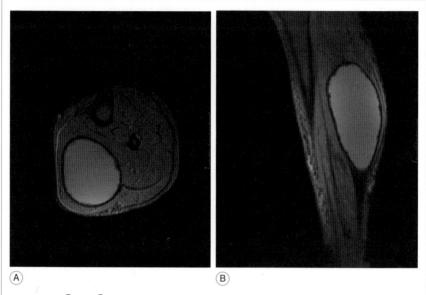

Fig. 10.1 Ⓐ and Ⓑ T2 weighted axial and sagittal MR scans of a chronic haematoma in the calf. There is a well-circumscribed mass which is of high signal in the posterior compartment. The rim is very low (dark) signal indicating haemosiderin deposition seen with breakdown of blood.

Aneurysm

Occasionally an aneurysm originating from a deep vessel may mimic a soft tissue tumour, but careful clinical examination will normally identify arterial pulsation. Imaging with MR and digital arteriography can confirm the nature of the lesion and the vessel of origin.

Synovial cysts and ganglia

Ganglia are of unknown origin situated typically around joints and contain mucoid tissue. Trauma and synovial herniation are suggested as causative factors. They do not usually have a demonstrable connection with the underlying joint. They are seen most commonly around the wrist and ankle, but also occur near the knee arising from the proximal tibio fibular joint (Fig. 10.2).

Synovial cysts are a synovial lined outpouching which connects with the underlying joint space.

These therefore occur around joints most commonly and are typically seen especially in the knee. Popliteal (Baker's) cysts (Fig. 18.32A, p. 418) and cysts associated with meniscal tears can present as palpable soft tissue masses. Ultrasound is the easiest method of confirming that these are cystic and not solid lesions.

Myositis ossificans (heterotopic ossification)

This is an uncommon but troublesome lesion because of its apparent malignant behaviour. It presents as a painful and tender lump in a limb muscle, with or without a history of recent trauma to the site. Imaging is crucial to obtain the correct diagnosis and MRI and ultrasound are the most useful in the

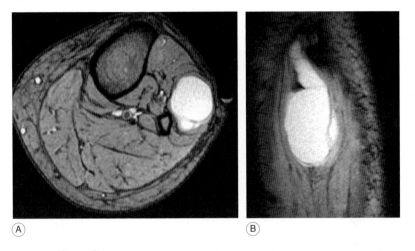

(A)   (B)

Fig. 10.2 Ⓐ and Ⓑ T2 weighted axial and sagittal MR scans showing a large ganglion arising from the proximal tibio-fibular joint. The high signal of the well-circumscribed mass in the anterior compartment suggests a fluid content. The sagittal image demonstrates the long thin proximal extension from the joint.

very early stages as they can detect the presence of calcification in the lesion which is the key to diagnosis (Fig. 10.3A). Later imaging with CT scanning will reveal a diagnostic rim of ossification at the periphery of the well-circumscribed lesion. Plain radiographs after several weeks will show some calcification in the muscle which should indicate the correct diagnosis (Fig. 10.3B). However, in some patients where the early changes are not recognised these appearances may be misinterpreted and may lead to a presumed diagnosis of soft tissue osteosarcoma. This assumption may be reinforced if a biopsy is performed, as this will show a very active lesion containing immature mesenchymal cells with atypical nuclei and osteoid formation. No active treatment is required, other than careful observation, as the lesion will resolve in 2–3 months.

TUMOURS OF SOFT TISSUE

The soft-tissue tumours that are met with in orthopaedic practice arise from the connective tissues or blood vessels of the limbs or trunk. They may be benign or malignant. They usually present clinically as painless soft-tissue lumps, and cause symptoms only when quite large.

BENIGN TUMOURS OF SOFT TISSUE

Benign peripheral nerve sheath tumours

Tumours arising from nerves are of two types: schwannomas and neurofibromas.

Schwannoma

These are just a little less common than neurofibromas. They are slow growing and painless with no neurological symptoms. They are typically less than

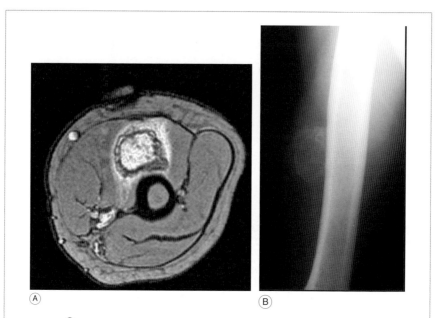

Fig. 10.3 Ⓐ T2 weighted axial MR scan of the arm with myositis ossificans in the biceps muscle. Inside the mass of high signal there is a ring of low signal representing calcification. MR or ultrasound will detect calcification long before it is visible on plain films. Ⓑ Radiograph of humerus in the same patient as Fig. 10.3A. This was obtained several weeks after the MR scan and the calcification within the muscle is now evident and a diagnosis of myositis ossificans is most likely.

5 cm in size. The tumour usually lies eccentric to the nerve which is displaced. Surgical excision can thus be undertaken with sparing of the nerve.

Neurofibroma
These are a little commoner and present as a soft, circumscribed, rounded, and slightly tender swelling in the skin or deeper tissues. They are more often associated with neurological symptoms. Pathologically they are not separate from the nerve which can be seen entering and leaving the tumour. Thus resection of the tumour requires sacrifice of the involved nerve.

Histologically the tumour is composed of cellular fibrous tissue arranged in whorls. The tumour may be solitary; but in the condition known as multiple neurofibromatosis (von Recklinghausen's disease) (p. 70) numerous tumours are associated with pigmented areas in the skin. A neurofibroma growing within the spinal canal is an important cause of compression of the spinal cord or cauda equina.

Imaging with MR scanning can identify the nature of the lesion and sometimes its neural origin (Fig. 10.4).

Lipoma
A lipoma is a common tumour that may arise in almost any part of the body. It usually occurs in the subcutaneous tissues, but may also develop more deeply as an intramuscular lesion. It forms a soft, often large, lobulated mass enclosed within a thin capsule. It consists of fat, usually with little connective tissue

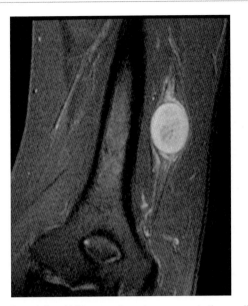

Fig. 10.4 Coronal T2 weighted MR scan of a schwannoma in the medial aspect of the arm, just proximal to the elbow. The high signal in the round lesion suggests nerve tissue and this extends as a 'tail' at the superior and inferior ends making it likely that this is most likely a nerve sheath tumour.

stroma. When the lesion is deep to fascia and of a large size it may be difficult to differentiate on clinical grounds from malignant liposarcoma. Imaging by MRI may be diagnostic of lipoma if it shows a homogeneous white lesion on the T1 weighted image with the same density as the subcutaneous and intramedullary fat (Fig. 10.5). However where there is less than 75% of fat in the lesion, or if the septation is nodular rather than linear, there is a possibility of malignancy and a biopsy is required prior to surgical excision.

Treatment, if required, is by local excision and the specimen when removed must always be sent for histological examination.

Haemangioma

Haemangioma is a benign tumour of blood vessels, usually present at birth. A **capillary haemangioma** forms a dark red, irregular, slightly raised blotch on the skin ('port wine stain'). It is usually congenital. A **cavernous haemangioma** is composed of widely dilated vascular channels with intervening connective tissue. It forms a localised or diffuse tumour within the skin, subcutaneous tissue, or muscle. A characteristic feature of diagnostic importance is that the tumour is compressible and may vary in size from day to day. It may cause symptoms from its cosmetic appearance, or from the complication of thrombosis, which may be associated with local pain and swelling. When a cavernous haemangioma occurs in a massive form in a limb it may lead to marked increase in growth of the limb as a whole (elephantiasis).

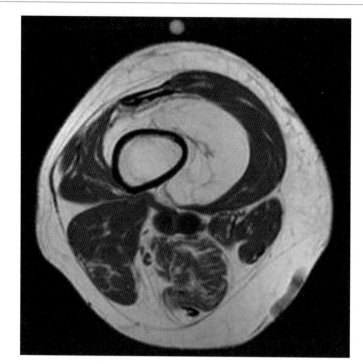

Fig. 10.5 Axial T1 weighted scan of thigh showing a large mass deep to the quadriceps muscles wrapped around the femur. This high signal, which is the same as subcutaneous and marrow fat, confirms that this is a lipoma.

Imaging by MR scanning shows characteristic clusters of abnormal dilated blood vessels giving a variegated serpiginous appearance.

Treatment. Superficial capillary haemangiomata fall within the province of the plastic surgeon or dermatologist. Some are amenable to laser ablation therapy. A localised deep cavernous haemangioma is usually amenable to excision. Extensive diffuse tumours cannot be eradicated, but improvement may follow transcutaneous arterial embolisation. In the worst cases amputation may be required.

Musculo-aponeurotic fibromatosis (desmoid tumour)

This rare tumour occurs mostly in young adults as a slowly growing hard swelling in the musculo-aponeurotic tissues, particularly in the trunk and shoulder regions. When it involves the abdominal wall or arises intra-abdominally it is known as an abdominal desmoid tumour. It is important because of its histological resemblance to malignant sarcoma and the characteristic infiltrative growth locally. Imaging by MRI scans will show a variable degree of heterogeneity (Fig. 10.6), which is not diagnostic, but will show the extent of the lesion and any involvement of neuro-vascular structures. Biopsy and histological examination will differentiate it from sarcoma and fortunately it has a more benign course and never metastasises. However, there is a high 30–40% risk of local recurrence, even after radical wide-margin excision, suggesting that it may arise from multicentric foci in the same limb.

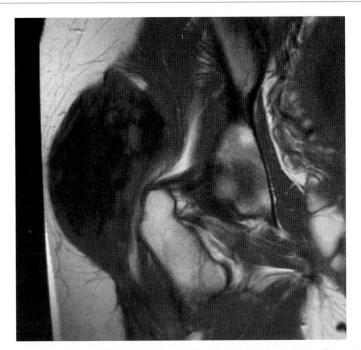

Fig. 10.6 Coronal T1 weighted scan of right hip affected by fibromatosis. There is an ill-defined mass of mostly low (dark) signal overlying the greater trochanter and infiltrating the gluteal muscle. The low signal indicates either calcification, or as in this case dense fibrous tissue. This suggests fibromatosis, but a biopsy is still required for definitive diagnosis.

MALIGNANT TUMOURS OF SOFT TISSUE

Malignant tumours of soft tissue (soft-tissue sarcomas) are uncommon, comprising 1% of adult malignant neoplasms. Of mesenchymal origin, they arise from connective tissues such as fascia, aponeurosis, tendon sheath, intermuscular septa, voluntary muscle, and synovial membrane. Such a tumour presents difficulties both in diagnosis and in treatment. It may be hard to distinguish from its benign counterpart, presenting as a progressively enlarging but usually painless swelling. It is of firm consistency and may appear to be well localised, though this is usually a false impression. It may spread widely within the soft tissues and the surrounding pseudocapsule forms no barrier. Metastasis occurs through the blood stream, mainly to the lungs.

Investigation of these tumours is aided by magnetic resonance imaging (MRI). MRI scans provide good definition of the anatomical extent of the tumour and of its relationship to the neurovascular structures (Fig. 10.7), thereby allowing correct planning of surgical treatment. However the scans cannot reliably differentiate between benign and malignant lesions, which must ultimately depend on expert histological examination from a representative biopsy.

Biopsy must be planned in such a way as to minimise the spillage of malignant cells. It may be by needle aspiration or localised incision, but never by local excision of the tumour (excision biopsy).

Soft tissue tumours and other diseases

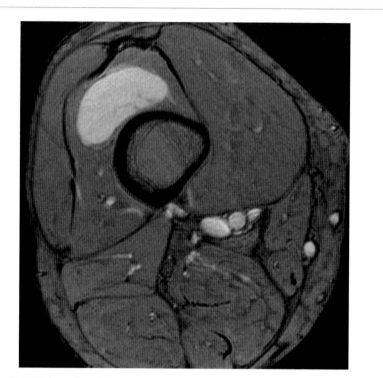

Fig. 10.7 High-grade soft tissue sarcoma of the thigh seen in an axial T2 weighted scan. The mass of high signal lies within the vastus intermedius, but has no features which allow a specific diagnosis to be made and a biopsy is required.

The results of the surgical treatment of most types of soft-tissue sarcoma have been improved by adjuvant therapy with radiation or potent chemotherapeutic agents used in combination as for bone sarcomas. Radiotherapy may be used after operative excision, to reduce the risk of local recurrence, but does not remove the need for adequate surgical treatment, which demands excision with wide margins of healthy tissue rather than simple local excision or enucleation.

Malignant fibrous histiocytoma

This tumour is composed predominantly of histiocytic-type cells, but may also include spindle cells resembling fibroblasts. It was formerly included under the diagnosis of fibrosarcoma. It is now regarded as the commonest malignant soft-tissue tumour in older adults. It has a poor prognosis, with local recurrence or metastasis to the lungs in more than half the patients.

Liposarcoma

This is the second commonest of the soft-tissue sarcomas, usually occurring in the deep tissues. It grows as a lobulated mass, usually in the buttock or thigh, and may often attain an enormous size (Fig. 10.8). It has a wide range of behaviour, depending upon its histological appearance and the amount of myxomatous

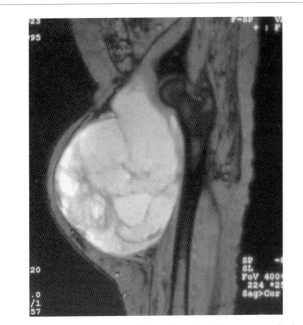

Fig. 10.8 Magnetic resonance image of large low-grade liposarcoma in the buttock, showing typical lobulated appearance of the soft tissue mass.

content. Tumours showing predominantly pleomorphic and round cells have a poor prognosis, but the presence of myxoid tissue improves the outlook.

Imaging with MRI scans is not diagnostic. These lesions do not contain macroscopic fat despite their name. MR scanning is generally non-specific and there is no fat signal from most of these lesions. Treatment is by radical excision or amputation, with the possible addition of adjuvant radiotherapy or chemotherapy in selected cases. Recurrence or metastasis is generally slow.

Synovial sarcoma (malignant synovioma)

This highly malignant but rare tumour was once thought to arise from the synovial lining of joints or tendon sheaths because of its proximity to these structures. Pathologically it forms a solid, whitish, fleshy mass with a slow but insidious invasion of the soft tissues. It is most common in young and middle-aged adults. It has a poor prognosis, with early pulmonary metastases or spread to local lymph nodes. Histologically the tumour is composed of masses of fusiform cells, but the picture is characterised by the formation of spaces or clefts lined by cuboidal cells which suggest the formation of a synovial cavity – hence the name given to this tumour. Treatment is by wide excision if this is practicable, with pre-operative and post-operative radiotherapy. When the tumour involves a joint amputation offers the best hope of survival.

Rhabdomyosarcoma

This rare variety of soft-tissue sarcoma which arises from skeletal muscle occurs mainly in children or young adults. It affects particularly the trunk or lower limbs. It forms a rapidly growing mass. Histologically it is characterised by cells showing longitudinal and cross striations typical of primitive myoblasts. It metastasises early, mainly to the lungs.

MANAGEMENT OF SOFT TISSUE SWELLINGS

While the above descriptions and classification of lesions is helpful, in clinical practice it is likely that after taking a history and examining the patient a definitive diagnosis is not possible.

It is often stated that small superficial lesions are likely to be benign and that larger >5 cm lesions, especially if deeply placed, are likely to be malignant. While this is statistically correct there are far too many lesions that break this rule of thumb to make it a sensible basis for clinical management.

It is now mandatory to proceed to some sort of imaging to confirm the suspected diagnosis. Ultrasound scanning is the quickest and easiest way of determining the nature of the majority of soft tissue swellings. Cystic lesions, haematomas, muscle tears and some lipomas can be identified this way. For the rest an MRI scan will be needed. When a definite diagnosis cannot be made then a biopsy is required.

The practice of removing lesions without going through these steps leads unfortunately to the rare but disastrous occasions when a lesion is excised and this turns out on histology to be a malignant sarcoma. The patient's best chance of a surgical cure is then seriously compromised.

OTHER SOFT TISSUE DISEASES

Soft tissues constitute a much larger part of the locomotor system than the bony skeleton, but the disorders that affect them receive much less attention from orthopaedic surgeons. In the past they were regarded as the province of the rheumatologist or sports medicine specialist and attracted little surgical interest. This is now changing with the introduction of more sophisticated investigations, particularly laboratory tests utilising molecular biology techniques and improved imaging with ultrasound and MRI. Today's surgeons require a greater understanding of the diseases that affect muscles, tendons, ligaments, and connective tissue to enable them to work as part of the multi-disciplinary team needed for their management.

INFLAMMATORY LESIONS OF SOFT TISSUE

Bursitis

Inflammation may occur in a normally situated bursa or in an adventitious bursa. It may arise from mechanical irritation or from bacterial infection.

Irritative bursitis

This is caused by excessive pressure or friction, occasionally by a gouty deposit. There is a mild inflammatory reaction in the wall of the bursa, and there is usually an effusion of clear fluid within the sac. Examples are the common 'bunion' that forms over a prominent metatarsal head in hallux valgus, prepatellar bursitis or 'housemaid's knee', olecranon bursitis (sometimes caused by gout), and subacromial bursitis.

Treatment. In many cases the inflammation subsides with rest if continued pressure or friction is prevented. If the sac is distended the fluid may be aspirated, and the instillation of hydrocortisone through the aspiration needle may help to prevent recurrence. In resistant cases cure can be effected only by operative excision of the bursa.

Infective bursitis

There may be acute inflammation from infection by an organism of the pyogenic group, or chronic inflammation as in tuberculous bursitis. Examples of acute pyogenic bursitis are infected bunion, infected prepatellar bursitis, and infected olecranon bursitis. A bursa that is sometimes affected by tuberculosis is the trochanteric bursa.

Treatment. Treatment of acute suppurative bursitis is by surgical drainage and antibacterial drugs. In chronic bursitis excision of the bursa is required.

Tenosynovitis

The term tenosynovitis implies inflammation of the thin synovial lining of a tendon sheath as distinct from its outer fibrous sheath. Like bursitis, tenosynovitis may be caused by mechanical irritation or by bacterial infection.

Irritative (frictional) tenosynovitis and peritendinitis

This is caused by excessive friction from over-use. The synovial sheath is mildly inflamed and there is an exudate of watery fluid within it, visible on ultrasound scanning (Fig. 10.9). A similar traumatic inflammation may affect the flimsy paratenon surrounding those tendons that are devoid of synovial sheaths. This is termed paratendinitis and is a common problem around the wrist and hand. The controversial condition known as repetitive stress syndrome comes into this category (p. 327).

Infective tenosynovitis

Bacterial infection of a tendon sheath may be acute or chronic. Acute infective (suppurative) tenosynovitis is caused by an organism of the pyogenic group. There is an acute inflammatory reaction in the wall of the sheath, with a purulent exudate from it. It is an uncommon condition, but it is well recognised in the flexor tendon sheaths in the hand (p. 316).

In chronic bacterial tenosynovitis, also an uncommon lesion in Western countries, the infection is often tuberculous. The synovial wall is much thickened and there is a fibrinous exudate. The flexor sheaths of the forearm and hand are the usual sites (compound palmar ganglion, p. 317).

Tenovaginitis

In tenovaginitis there is a mild chronic inflammation or thickening of the fibrous wall of a tendon sheath as distinct from the synovial lining. The cause is unknown: it is not due to bacterial infection. The only common sites are the mouths of the

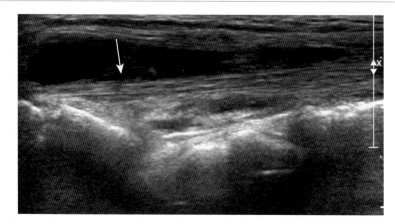

Fig. 10.9 Sagittal ultrasound scan showing tenosynovitis of the wrist. The arrow indicates a flexor tendon and the dark area above this represents excessive fluid within the tendon sheath.

fibrous flexor sheaths in the fingers or thumb ('trigger' finger, p. 329), and the sheaths of the extensor pollicis brevis and abductor pollicis longus tendons at the radial side of the wrist (de Quervain's syndrome, p. 328).

POLYMYALGIA RHEUMATICA

This connective tissue disorder has been recognised with increased frequency in older patients presenting with pain and stiffness in the muscles of the neck and shoulder girdle, or sometimes the low back and buttock regions. Because of these features it may be confused with degenerative disc disease, though characteristically the associated symptoms of malaise, low-grade fever, night sweats, and loss of weight should lead to the diagnosis. It tends to be commoner in women than in men, usually affecting patients over the age of 60 years, and in about one-third of cases it is associated with the condition of giant-cell arteritis. This is a more serious disease as it may lead to sudden blindness because of involvement of the cranial arteries.

The clinical features are ill-defined muscle pain around the shoulders or low back, with associated stiffness, and the characteristic features of systemic disturbance. When giant-cell arteritis is also present there may be marked tenderness over the temporal arteries. There may be marked elevation of the erythrocyte sedimentation rate, but the rheumatoid factor is negative. When associated giant-cell arteritis is suspected on clinical grounds, urgent administration of prednisolone in high doses is advisable pending confirmation of the diagnosis by biopsy, in order to reduce the risk of blindness. Both conditions show a good response to steroid therapy, usually in a dose of 15 mg of prednisolone daily. Once the clinical features have subsided this may be reduced to a maintenance dose of 5 mg daily.

FIBROMYALGIA (FIBROSITIS)

Fibromyalgia, formerly termed fibrositis, is a clinical rather than a pathological entity. Some deny its existence. Certainly its nature is obscure. Nevertheless the term is a useful label for a common clinical condition that at present lacks a complete explanation. The main features are pain in certain muscles, with tenderness when they are gripped or squeezed. Small firm nodules may be felt. Joint movements are full and there are no other objective signs. The condition is commonest in the muscles of the upper back, especially in the trapezius area, and affects women more frequently than men. There may be associated tiredness, sleep disturbance, and depression. Treatment, if required, is by non-steroidal anti-inflammatory medication and active exercises.

11 Neurological disorders

CEREBRAL PALSY (Spastic paralysis: spastic paresis; Little's disease)

The term cerebral palsy embraces a number of clinical disorders, mostly arising in childhood, the feature common to all of which is that the primary lesion is in the brain. The incidence of these disorders is such that cerebral palsy constitutes a major social and educational problem.

Cause. There is no single cause. Any event that results in damage to the brain may be responsible. Thus the causes may be classified into three groups: pre-natal, natal, and post-natal. Pre-natal causes include congenital defective development of the nervous system, and erythroblastosis leading to icterus gravis in the child, with consequent damage to the basal nuclei (kernicterus). Natal causes include damage to the brain and intracranial bleeds from birth injury, and anoxaemia with consequent cerebral anoxia. Prematurity is believed to be an important factor. Post-natal causes include infections such as pertussis, encephalitis, and meningitis, head injuries, and, in later life, cerebrovascular accidents (stroke). In children it is not always easy to ascribe the fault in a given case, but probably the commonest causes are damage to the brain during difficult labour and cerebral anoxia during birth.

Types. A number of clinical types may be recognised, of which the most important are:

1. spastic paresis
2. athetosis.

Mixed types also occur.

SPASTIC PARESIS

Pathology. Part of the motor cortex of the brain is replaced by areas of gliosis. There is degeneration of the pyramidal tracts.

Clinical features. Usually within the first year it is noticed that the child has difficulty in controlling the movements of the affected limbs, and there is delay in sitting up, standing and walking. Commonly the upper and lower limbs of one side are affected (hemiplegia). Less often there is involvement of a single limb (monoplegia), of both lower limbs (paraplegia), or of all four limbs (tetraplegia[1]). The trunk and face muscles may also be affected. On examination the features that are found constantly are weakness, spasticity, and imperfect

---

[1] Also termed (though less correctly because Latin is mixed with Greek) diplegia or quadriplegia.

voluntary control of movement. Usually there is also deformity, and in some cases there may be mental deficiency, impaired vision, or deafness. These various features are best considered separately.

Weakness. There is no true paralysis, but there may be fairly marked weakness of muscles. The weakness seldom affects all the muscles of a limb equally; often there is marked muscle imbalance which may lead to deformity.

Spasticity. The muscles are 'stiff': they resist passive movement of the joints, but when steady pressure is applied for some time they slowly relax, allowing the joint to be moved. When the pressure is released the spasm immediately returns. The tendon reflexes are exaggerated and muscle clonus may be elicited.

Lack of voluntary control. This is a striking feature, especially in severe cases. When the patient attempts to move a single group of muscles, other groups contract at the same time.

Deformity. When spasm and muscle imbalance are pronounced they lead eventually to the development of fixed deformity. The stronger muscles hold the limb constantly in an unnatural position, and secondary adaptive changes take place in the muscles and periarticular tissues. The commonest deformities in the upper limb are flexion contracture of the elbow, pronation deformity of the forearm, flexion of the wrist, and adduction of the thumb. In the lower limb the common deformities are adduction of the hip, flexion of the knee, and equinus of the ankle.

Mental deficiency. Impairment of mental capacity is sometimes present, but usually intelligence is normal. Lack of control of the facial and speech muscles may suggest mental impairment when in fact none exists. It is important that the medical advisers be not misled in this respect. Defective vision and deafness may also retard the child's progress.

The severity of the disability varies widely from case to case. In the mildest examples the child is able to lead a normal active life with very little handicap, whereas in the worst cases the patient is almost helpless.

Prognosis. Since an essential part of the brain is destroyed and cannot be replaced, complete cure is impossible. All that can be hoped for is improvement. To achieve even this requires endless patience on the part of the patient and the attendants. Yet perseverance is nearly always well rewarded, and there are few cases in which worth-while improvement cannot be gained. Thus a patient formerly dependent upon others in many daily activities may often gain independence, and many who were previously unable to work become capable of earning their own living.

Treatment. Up to the age of about 5 years treatment may be carried out at non-residential centres, but after the age of 5 a child who is considerably disabled should be admitted to a special residential school where adequate facilities and trained staff are available.

The methods of treatment available are muscle training, corrective splinting, speech therapy, and operations on tendons, bones, or nerves.

Muscle training. This is an important part of the management of all except the mildest cases, and it is best carried out by a physiotherapist with experience of this very demanding work. The principles of muscle training are to teach the child to relax spastic muscles, to develop the use of individual muscle groups, and to improve coordination. Repetitive rhythmic movements are valuable. Stage by stage the child is instructed in dressing, toilet, feeding, walking.

Corrective splinting. Splints or plasters are especially useful in overcoming the deformities induced by spastic muscles. Deformity is first corrected by gradual stretching of the contracted muscles, if necessary under anaesthesia. The limb is held by plaster in the over-corrected position for 6–8 weeks. Thereafter removable braces or splints (orthoses) may be used indefinitely to prevent recurrence of the deformity.

Speech therapy. Many spastic children have a speech defect which, with constant grimacing and salivation, may lead one to suppose that there is mental deficiency when in fact this is not so. In these cases the speech therapist is sometimes able to achieve a marked improvement.

Operative treatment. Operations for spastic paralysis should be approached with caution: striking benefit may be achieved in appropriate cases, but injudicious operation in unsuitable cases has often led to disappointing results. Operation may be upon tendon, joint, or nerve.

Tendon division or elongation. Division or lengthening of the tendon of a spastic muscle reduces its mechanical advantage and improves muscle balance. Examples are lengthening of the calcaneal tendon in a case of spastic equinus deformity, and tenotomy of the adductors of the hip for adduction deformity.

Tendon transfer. At certain sites transfer of the insertion of a muscle that is aggravating deformity may so modify the muscle's action that it acts beneficially instead of as a deforming force. An example is the transfer of the insertion of the hamstring tendons from the tibia to the back of the femoral condyles in a case of flexion deformity of the knee: this eliminates the undesirable action of the spastic hamstrings in flexing the knee, while enhancing their desirable action as hip extensors.

Arthrodesis. When skeletal growth is complete it is sometimes of benefit to fuse a joint in a position of function, to eliminate persistent deformity from the pull of spastic muscles. Thus a wrist that lies constantly flexed may be fused in a neutral or slightly extended position, with consequent improvement in function.

Osteotomies. Division of the bone to correct angular and rotational deformities may be of value especially in the lower limb.

Neurectomy. The principle is to divide part or the whole of a nerve that supplies an overacting spastic muscle. An example is division of the anterior branch of the obturator nerve to overcome spastic adduction at the hip.

ATHETOSIS

Pathology. The main damage is in the basal nuclei.

Clinical features. The principal feature is the occurrence of generalised overlaid involuntary movements which have no pattern and which interfere with the performance of normal movements. Any part or the whole of the muscular system may be affected.

In mild cases the child is able to lead a fairly normal life, but in the worst examples the patient may be unable to sit up, walk, feed himself, or express himself in words, even though the mental state may be good.

Treatment. The first essential in treatment is to teach the child general relaxation. Once this has been achieved, purposeful voluntary movements can be taught. Splints and appliances may be required, but in pure athetosis there is no place for operations on the limbs. In some cases of severe athetosis improvement has been reported after surgical ablation of the globus pallidus.

SPINA BIFIDA

The term spina bifida implies a failure of the enfolding of the nerve elements within the spinal canal during early development of the embryo. The defect varies in degree and in its site (Fig. 11.1). In the mildest cases there is no more than a failure of fusion of one or more of the vertebral arches posteriorly, in the lumbo-sacral region. This is often of no clinical significance. Less often, the posterior bony deficiency is marked on the surface by an abnormality of the overlying skin, in the form of a dimple, a tuft of hair, a lipomatous mass, or a dermal sinus. In these cases there may be an underlying abnormality involving nerves of the cauda equina. These relatively minor varieties of spina bifida, in which the defect is not obvious at the skin surface, are termed spina bifida occulta. This contrasts with spina bifida aperta, in which there is a major defect of enfolding of the nerve elements, involving not only the bony vertebral arches but also the overlying soft tissues and skin, and often the meningeal membranes enclosing the spinal canal, so that the neutral tube itself is exposed and open. This major variant of spina bifida may occur anywhere in the spine but is commonest in the thoraco-lumbar region, and it is attended by grave impairment of nerve function.

SPINA BIFIDA OCCULTA (Occult spinal dysraphism)

As noted above, the bony defect is simply a failure of fusion of the vertebral arches posteriorly (Fig. 11.1A). When there is neurological involvement the overlying skin nearly always shows an abnormality, as already described.

Impairment of nerve function may be caused in some such cases by tethering of the dura, and through this the spinal cord, to the skin surface by a fibrous membrane. Traction on the cord becomes gradually worse as the spinal column elongates disproportionately to the spinal cord: this can cause slow progression of the neurological deficit. A rather similar effect is caused by tethering of the distal end of the spinal cord by the filum terminale. Rarely, too, a bifid cord is transfixed by a delicate bar of bone crossing the spinal canal in the antero-posterior plane (diastematomyelia) with consequent tethering and progressive neurological impairment. In yet other cases the neurological fault may be a consequence of myelodysplasia, a congenital defect of development of nerve tissue.

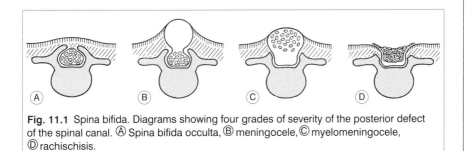

Fig. 11.1 Spina bifida. Diagrams showing four grades of severity of the posterior defect of the spinal canal. Ⓐ Spina bifida occulta, Ⓑ meningocele, Ⓒ myelomeningocele, Ⓓ rachischisis.

In cases of occult spinal dysraphism there is no close correlation between the severity of the bony defect and the degree of neurological impairment. Often there is no neurological involvement; but on the other hand it may be severe. Clinically, the common manifestation of nerve involvement is muscle imbalance in the lower limbs, often with selective muscle wasting and deformity of the foot which often takes the form either of equino-varus or of cavus.

Investigation and treatment. The patient may be brought for advice because of an abnormality of the skin over the lumbo-sacral region, because of abnormality of the feet or perhaps just a limp, or because of urinary incontinence. A plain radiograph will show the extent of the bony deficiency.

If evidence of neurological impairment is lacking, treatment is not required. If neurological impairment or incontinence is present – and especially if there has been progressive deterioration – further investigations, including MR scanning and radiculography, are required. These may point to the presence of one of the structural lesions mentioned above, and in such a case neurosurgical intervention may be required: its object is to prevent further deterioration rather than to promote complete recovery.

SPINA BIFIDA APERTA (Overt spinal dysraphism; variations include rachischisis, myelomeningocele and meningocele)

The neurological deficit that complicates the more severe forms of spina bifida leads to varying degrees of motor, sensory, and visceral paralysis, and the consequent orthopaedic disability in the lower limbs may be complex. The number of children demanding orthopaedic care for such disabilities has increased in recent years because a far higher proportion of children born with myelomeningocele survived when the associated hydrocephalus was controlled by a ventriculo-cardiac or ventriculo-peritoneal shunt. Nevertheless the incidence is likely to fall dramatically since the advent of antenatal screening for alpha-fetoprotein, high-resolution ultrasound, and amniocentesis, with the option of termination of pregnancy in positive cases. It is also to be hoped that the incidence of spina bifida will be substantially reduced by the administration of folic acid to women before or at the commencement of pregnancy.

The cause is unknown: genetic factors may play a part but environmental factors are also probably involved. In particular, the influence of certain drugs – notably anti-epileptic drugs such as sodium valproate – has been recognised. Folic acid in a dosage of 5 mg daily taken before the commencement of pregnancy, or very early in pregnancy, offers some protection against the disorder.

Pathology. The basic structural defect – failure of total closure of the embryonal neural tube or of mesodermal tissue to invest it – varies in degree. In the most serious defect, rachischisis, the neural tube is open and exposed on the surface (Fig. 11.1D). Cerebrospinal fluid leaks from the exposed upper end of the central spinal canal. In myelomeningocele the neural tube is closed by a membrane but the skin covering is deficient. The spinal cord and the nerve roots are displaced posteriorly into the sac and are outside the line of the vertebral canal (Fig. 11.1C). In meningocele the bulging sac consists of meninges and fluid only, the nerve elements being normally situated (Fig. 11.1B). The skin may or may not be intact.

The distinction between closed lesions, with intact skin, and open lesions in which skin is deficient and nerve tissue is exposed on the surface of the body, is fundamental because open lesions may demand operation within a few hours of birth to close the defect, if indeed active intervention is deemed advisable.

The neurological lesion. Neurological deficit may be primary or secondary. Primary paralysis is present at birth and implies failure of development of part of the spinal cord (myelodysplasia). This varies widely in degree. In a fairly common example there may be normal innervation down to the level of the fourth lumbar segment and failure of development below that level. But the lesion may be either less extensive or more extensive than this.

Secondary paralysis develops after birth, either from drying or infection of exposed nerve tissue when closure of an open lesion has been delayed; from stretching of tethered nerve fibres as growth occurs; or from compression of nerve tissue within the abnormal spinal canal.

Clinical assessment. It is difficult in small infants to assess accurately the extent of motor and of sensory paralysis, and particularly to determine the state of bladder function. Nevertheless the important objective at the outset is to determine the level at which normal function of the spinal cord ceases. This is done by observing what movements the child makes, and correlating these with the root level. Sensibility can be determined by stimulating the skin lightly with a pin moved upwards from the limbs to the trunk until the child is awakened.

Motor paralysis. Motor paralysis affects mainly the lower limbs and to some extent the trunk. The extent of limb paralysis corresponds to the degree of dysplasia or of secondary damage in the spinal cord. It varies from the very mild, in which there may be no more than minor weakness of a single muscle group, to the very severe, in which there is total paralysis of the limbs. In the instance quoted above of normal cord function down to the fourth lumbar segment with loss of function below that, motor power is present only in the flexors and adductors of the hips, the quadriceps and the tibialis anterior: the remaining muscles are paralysed. This is a fairly common distribution but only one of an almost infinite variety. This uneven paralysis, with consequent muscle imbalance, leads commonly to secondary contractures with fixed deformity of hips, knees, or feet. It may also lead to dislocation of the hip, a common sequel to gluteal and abductor paralysis in the presence of strong flexors and adductors.

Sensory paralysis. Motor paralysis is nearly always accompanied by sensory paralysis of approximately the same distribution. This makes treatment more difficult because the use of corrective splints is hampered by the risk of pressure sores on the insensitive skin.

Visceral paralysis. Incontinence of bladder and bowel is present in a high proportion of patients.

Hydrocephalus. Associated hydrocephalus, usually due to the Arnold–Chiari malformation of the hind-brain, is common and was formerly largely responsible for the poor rate of survival among children with severe spina bifida.

Treatment. Every child with major neurological or visceral dysfunction from spina bifida should be admitted immediately to a special centre where a team of experienced specialists – including paediatrician, paediatric surgeon, neurosurgeon, and orthopaedic surgeon – may cooperate in deciding upon a programme that is best suited to the child. The team must first decide whether or not any surgical treatment, including closure of an open defect, is to be advised. This selective approach arose from review of large series where closure was universal: in the worst cases, with gross neurological deficit or

Neurological disorders

hydrocephalus, the results were disastrous. In these it is probably better to adopt an expectant attitude, accepting the situation and relying simply on careful nursing and feeding. It has to be taken as inevitable that many of these badly affected infants will fail to survive.

The problems that are to be tackled when more active treatment is undertaken are often very complex. No firm rules can be laid down because there is so much variation between individual cases. It is sufficient here to indicate the main principles of orthopaedic treatment. These are:

1. to correct deformity
2. to maintain correction
3. to promote the best possible function in the affected.

In general, orthopaedic treatment should be deferred until the age of 1 to 3 years, to ensure that the child is thriving well and that the problems of hydrocephalus and renal function are satisfactorily controlled. This may have required a ventriculo-cardiac or ventriculo-peritoneal shunt to drain the excess cerebrospinal fluid, and urinary diversion to an artificial bladder for reasons of hygiene.

Correction of deformity. Deformity, whether of the hip, knee, or foot, should be corrected in the simplest way possible with the object of providing a limb that is straight, mobile, and with a plantigrade foot – that is, a limb that is best suited for weight bearing. This may be achieved by a combination of splintage and surgical treatment, depending on the level of paralysis and the joints affected. Splints and plasters are useful for controlling flail joints and for maintaining correction after operative procedures, but they must be fitted and used with care because of the risk of pressure sores involving the insensitive skin. When fixed deformity is present as a result of unbalanced or spastic muscle action operation is needed to divide or elongate tight structures – tendon, muscle, ligament, or joint capsule – in order to achieve a neutral anatomical position. Paralytic dislocation of the hip is common and may necessitate posterior transfer of the iliopsoas muscle to the greater trochanter (to act as a hip abductor), sometimes combined with femoral or pelvic osteotomy, to maintain stability. In the more severe lesions, where wheelchair locomotion is inevitable, it may be better to leave the dislocation unreduced while preserving mobile hips. Spinal deformity, often a combination of kyphosis and scoliosis, may require surgical correction and fusion, but the complications of pseudarthrosis and pressure sores are common.

Development of limb function. Even when lower limb paralysis is severe it is often possible to get the child walking with crutches once deformities have been overcome. In many cases external bracing in the form of limb calipers or swivel walkers is also required, and prolonged training by a skilled physiotherapist is essential if maximal function is to be achieved.

POLIOMYELITIS (Anterior poliomyelitis; infantile paralysis)

Poliomyelitis is a virus infection of nerve cells in the anterior grey matter of the spinal cord, leading in many cases to temporary or permanent paralysis of the muscles that they activate. In many countries the incidence of the disease increased so much in the years succeeding the Second World War that its management – or rather the management of the paralytic disabilities that it produces – became one of the foremost problems of orthopaedic surgery.

However, in the 1950s the incidence decreased very markedly in Western countries, in consequence of nationwide programmes of prophylactic vaccination; so much so that the disease has now been virtually eliminated. Nevertheless it is still encountered in certain countries of Asia and Africa.

Cause. It is caused by infection with a virus, of which at least three types have been identified.

Pathology. After gaining access to the body through the nasopharynx or the gastro-intestinal tract, the virus finds its way to anterior horn cells of the spinal cord (Fig. 11.2) and sometimes to nerve cells in the brain stem. According to the virulence of the infection the cells may escape serious harm, or they may be damaged or killed. If cells are damaged there is paralysis of the corresponding muscles but recovery is possible; if the cells are killed paralysis is permanent. The extent and distribution of the lesions vary widely from case to case.

Clinical features. Although it is still commonest in children, poliomyelitis often attacks young adults. For descriptive purposes the disease is conveniently divided into five stages.

Stage of incubation. This is the interval between infection and onset of symptoms. It is thought to be about 2 weeks. There are no symptoms.

Stage of onset. This lasts about 2 days. The symptoms are like those of influenza: headache, pains in the back and limbs, and general malaise. Examination may show mild pyrexia, often with neck rigidity if flexion is attempted, and tenderness of muscles. Lumbar puncture may show an increase of round cells in the cerebrospinal fluid. In many cases the disease does not progress beyond this stage, the patient making a rapid and complete recovery.

Stage of greatest paralysis. This stage, when it occurs, lasts about 2 months. Paralysis develops rapidly and is usually at its greatest within a few hours, thereafter remaining unchanged throughout this stage. The extent and distribution of the paralysis vary enormously. There may be no paralysis at all, or it may be total. In this stage muscle pain continues, and unparalysed muscles are often painful if stretched. If the respiratory muscles are paralysed preservation of life will be dependent upon the use of a ventilator.

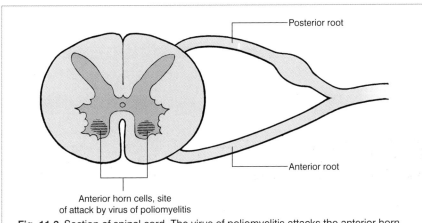

Posterior root

Anterior root

Anterior horn cells, site
of attack by virus of poliomyelitis

Fig. 11.2 Section of spinal cord. The virus of poliomyelitis attacks the anterior horn cells. If the cells are killed there is permanent paralysis of the corresponding muscle fibres. If the cells are damaged but not killed the paralysis is recoverable.

Stage of recovery. When any recovery of power occurs it may continue for about 2 years.[1] The degree of recovery varies within the widest limits. There may be complete recovery or there may be none.

Stage of residual paralysis. Paralysis or weakness persisting after two years is permanent. Its degree and extent vary from insignificant local weakness to almost total paralysis of the trunk and all four limbs. Weakness or paralysis is accompanied by obvious wasting of the affected muscles. This in turn is associated with defective growth of the bones and consequent shortening if the disease occurs in childhood.

Prognosis. In round figures, it may be stated that half of all patients clinically infected with poliomyelitis have no paralysis at any time. Of those with paralysis, 10% die (usually from respiratory paralysis); 30% recover fully; 30% have moderate permanent paralysis; and 30% have severe permanent paralysis.

Prophylaxis. In Britain prophylactic vaccination is by an attenuated living virus, taken by mouth.

Treatment. No specific treatment is available. In few diseases is the doctor so powerless to influence recovery: the patient either will or will not recover his muscle power, depending upon the severity of the neurological damage; and there is very little that the doctor can do about it. The main duties of the orthopaedic team are to prevent deformity, to assist returning muscle power by graduated exercises, and to reduce residual disability in the final stage by the provision of appropriate appliances or by operations on joints or muscles. The treatment appropriate to each stage of the disease is best considered separately.

Stage of onset. The patient should rest in bed and may be given sedatives as required.

Stage of greatest paralysis. In this stage artificial respiration by a ventilator may be necessary to preserve life if the respiratory muscles are paralysed. Paralysed limbs may have to be supported by splints in a neutral position to prevent the development of contractures with consequent deformity. Fixed equinus deformity of the ankle and foot is particularly liable to develop in cases of paralysis of the anterior leg muscles unless the foot is maintained at a right angle to the leg. Joints should be put through a full range of movement daily, so far as pain allows. Muscle pain may be eased by warmth, as from hot packs. Whether or not the patient must remain in bed in this stage will depend upon the degree and distribution of the paralysis.

Stage of recovery. The patient should be under the close supervision of a skilled physiotherapist. Any muscle that is seen to be regaining power must be exercised, gently and patiently at first, but later very strenuously, to encourage the greatest possible redevelopment. It should be remembered that power may improve partly as a result of recovery of the damaged nerve cells, but partly also from hypertrophy of muscle fibres that have escaped paralysis. When possible, walking should be resumed at this stage, if necessary with the aid of appliances, crutches, or sticks.

Stage of residual paralysis. The disability in this stage can often be reduced either by the provision of suitable external appliances (orthoses), or by operation.

Appliances (orthoses). The purpose of external appliances or orthoses is to support joints that are no longer adequately controlled by muscles. They are

---

[1] It will be observed that the figure 2 appears in the stated duration of each of the first four stages – 2 weeks, 2 days, 2 months, 2 years. These are only very approximate figures, but they are easily memorised.

required more often for the lower limbs and spine than for the upper limbs. The following are commonly prescribed:

1. spinal brace, to support a weakened spine
2. abdominal support, to check abdominal protrusion when the abdominal muscles are weak
3. knee caliper (Fig. 11.3), to hold the knee extended in cases of severe quadriceps paralysis
4. below-knee brace to stabilise a flail ankle or foot (Fig. 11.4)
5. ankle foot orthosis (Fig. 11.5), to hold the foot up when the dorsiflexor muscles are paralysed.

Operative treatment. Two main groups of operations are available:

1. arthrodesis of joints
2. muscle or tendon transfers.

Arthrodesis is a valuable method of stabilising joints that have lost their controlling muscles. It is particularly applicable to the shoulder, elbow, wrist, spine, ankle, and foot.

In *muscle* or *tendon transfer* operations the object is to use a healthy muscle to replace the function of one that is paralysed. The method finds its chief application in the upper limb. Examples are the transfer of part of the pectoralis major muscle to replace the function of paralysed elbow flexors, transfer of wrist flexors to serve as extensors of the fingers, and transfer of a flexor digitorum superficialis tendon to replace a paralysed opponens muscle.

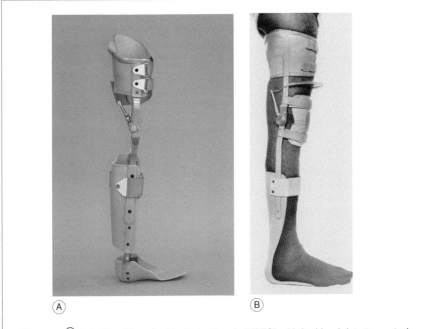

(A) (B)

Fig. 11.3 Ⓐ Articulated knee ankle foot orthosis (KAFO) with locking joints to control an unstable knee and ankle joint. Ⓑ Patient wearing knee ankle foot orthosis.

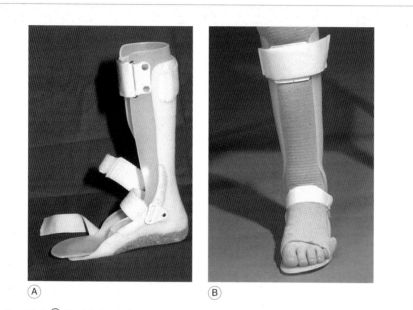

Fig. 11.4 Ⓐ Moulded polythene ankle foot orthosis (AFO) to control ankle instability. Ⓑ Patient wearing ankle foot orthosis.

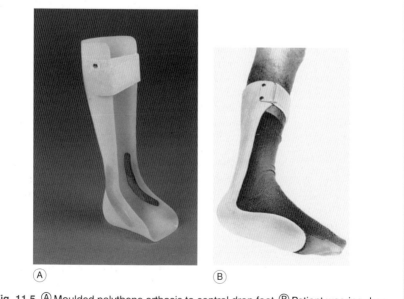

Fig. 11.5 Ⓐ Moulded polythene orthosis to control drop foot. Ⓑ Patient wearing drop foot splint which is worn inside a shoe.

PERIPHERAL NERVE LESIONS

Disorders of the peripheral nerves come largely within the sphere of the neurologist, but the orthopaedic surgeon is concerned with lesions that have a mechanical basis and with those that lend themselves to reconstructive surgery.

Pathology. Nerves may be damaged by laceration, contusion, traction, compression, friction, burns, or ischaemia. According to its severity, a nerve lesion may be classified as neurapraxia, axonotmesis, or neurotmesis. In neurapraxia the damage is slight and it causes only a transient physiological block. Recovery occurs spontaneously within days or weeks. In axonotmesis the internal architecture of the nerve is preserved, but the axons are so badly damaged that peripheral degeneration occurs. Recovery can occur spontaneously, but it depends upon regeneration of the axons and may take many months (1 mm/day is the usual speed of regeneration). In neurotmesis the structure of the nerve is destroyed by actual division or by severe scarring. Recovery is possible only after excision of the damaged section and end-to-end suture of the stumps, or after nerve grafting.

Clinical features. The effects of complete loss of conductivity of a nerve are motor, sensory, and autonomic. They are localised to the distribution of the nerve affected. Motor changes: The muscles are paralysed and wasted. Changes occur in the electrical reactions, but they take between two and three weeks to develop. These changes were described on page 27. Sensory changes: There is loss of cutaneous, deep, and postural sensibility. Autonomic changes: These include loss of sweating, loss of pilomotor response to cold ('goose-skin'), and temporary vasodilation with increased warmth, which, however, is followed later by vasoconstriction and coldness.

Complications. Injury to a peripheral nerve trunk is occasionally followed by severe burning pain in the distribution of the nerve. This is termed causalgia. It is a complication of incomplete rather than of complete lesions, and with few exceptions it is confined in the upper limb to the brachial plexus or the median nerve, and in the lower limb to the sciatic nerve or the tibial nerve. Relentless pain makes this a very disabling complication, the only effective treatment of which is by sympathetic denervation of the limb.

Treatment. *Open injuries*. If a nerve is believed to have been divided – for example, by a penetrating injury – the wound should be explored and the nerve identified. If the nerve is severed the ends should be examined carefully to determine the extent to which they have been damaged by laceration or bruising. Only in the case of a clean-cut division with minimal damage to the severed ends should primary suture be carried out. If these criteria are not satisfied it is better simply to tack the ends together with one or two sutures and to delay definitive repair – preferably with a magnification technique – until 2 or 3 weeks after the injury. At that time the extent of the scarring, and consequently the length of nerve to be resected, can be determined accurately, and thickening of the nerve sheath makes suture technically easier.

Closed injuries. In closed injuries complicated by nerve paralysis it is usually assumed that the nerve is in continuity, and expectant treatment is adopted at first. If signs of recovery are not observed within the expected time (calculated from the site of injury and length to be regenerated) exploration is advised. Evidence of muscle re-innervation may be derived from electromyography at an earlier stage than from clinical examination. Such exploration should seldom be delayed for more than 3 or 4 months, because long delay prejudices successful repair if the nerve has been divided.

Neurological disorders

When a nerve lesion has been caused by stretching, compression, or ischaemia the essential principle of treatment is to ensure that the harmful conditions are relieved, if necessary by operation to free the nerve or to remove a compressing agent.

Nerve grafting. When the gap to be bridged between healthy neurones proximally and distally is large, nerve grafting is preferable to attempted direct suture under tension. A thick nerve may be bridged by multiple grafts from a thinner nerve – for example the sural nerve. By microsurgical techniques it is also now possible to transfer a nerve complete with its blood supply, to bridge a major defect. Freeze-thawed muscle grafts have been used experimentally as an alternative to nerve grafts. They may provide a chemotactic stimulus for nerve regeneration as well as providing a microskeleton to guide axonal fibres across the gap, which should not exceed 3 cm.

BRACHIAL PLEXUS INJURIES

Injuries of the brachial plexus are a major cause of partial or complete loss of function of the upper limb. Most of such injuries are caused by forcible distraction of the upper extremity away from the neck by violent depression of the shoulder. The main injury is sustained by the upper roots of the plexus, which may be stretched, torn, or even avulsed from the spinal cord. There is consequent paralysis of the muscles supplied through the upper roots – chiefly the abductor and lateral rotator muscles of the shoulder and the flexors of the elbow (Erb type of paralysis). A less common type of brachial plexus injury is caused by forcible elevation of the arm and shoulder. This tends to drag on the lower roots of the plexus, with consequent motor and sensory paralysis mainly in the forearm and hand (Klumpke type of paralysis). In the most severe injuries the whole plexus is torn or avulsed and there is total paralysis of the upper limb.

Brachial plexus lesions in infants

In infants, brachial plexus injuries are usually caused during delivery (obstetrical palsy), and the risk is greatest in difficult breech deliveries. The upper arm type (Erb's palsy) is the more common. Soon after birth it is noticed that the child does not move the arm as he normally should. Unopposed action of the unparalysed muscles tends to bring the arm into a position of adduction and medial rotation, and secondary contracture of the soft tissues may lead to fixed deformity in that position.

Prognosis depends upon the severity of the stretching injury. If this was mild full recovery may occur, though it may take many months; but in a severe case there may be permanent loss of power and sensibility. The prognosis is less favourable in the rare lower arm type of lesion (Klumpke type) than in the commoner upper arm type.

Treatment. In a mild case the mother should be taught to move the limb frequently through the full range, to prevent fixed contracture. In a severe case seen early it may be possible, if the requisite expertise is available, to restore continuity of the damaged nerves by early operation. In late cases with permanent paralysis and deformity there is a place for late reconstructive operations such as corrective (rotation) osteotomy of the humerus, arthrodesis of the shoulder or tendon transfer operations.

Brachial plexus lesions in adults

In adults brachial plexus injuries are usually caused by forcible depression of the shoulder. By far the commonest cause is a motorcycling accident.

It is important to distinguish between preganglionic lesions, in which the nerve roots are avulsed from the spinal cord, and postganglionic lesions, in which the nerves are torn more distally. Preganglionic lesions are irrecoverable, whereas there is potential for some recovery in postganglionic lesions. Clinical and electrical tests may indicate the approximate site of the lesion, but special investigations are needed for more accurate assessment. Initially, spinal root imaging by radiculography may show dural pouches at the sites of nerve avulsion. CT scanning with contrast gives the best information on the extent of the damage and is superior to MRI scanning. In the last resort surgical exploration may be needed to localise the lesion definitively, especially in the first few days after injury when the prospect of successful repair is most favourable. The measurement of intra-operative nerve action potentials is valuable: when these are present distal to the lesion a substantial number of large fibres have survived the injury, so excision and grafting are unnecessary.

Treatment. For irrecoverable (preganglionic) lesions all that can be done is to make the best use of any function that remains. Tendon or muscle transfers, to replace the action of paralysed muscles, may be appropriate in selected cases, and arthrodesis of the shoulder may sometimes be indicated if strong scapular muscles and useful hand function are preserved.

If, however, it is confirmed at operation that the roots have been torn across rather than avulsed, repair by nerve grafting may be attempted with some hope of success. Nerve transfers that have been used include: redirection of the accessory nerve to the suprascapular nerve to improve shoulder function; and transfer of the third or fourth intercostal nerve to the musculocutaneous nerve to restore elbow flexion. Even limited recovery is well worth-while, and may reduce the level of severe causalgic pain; nevertheless the outlook for good recovery of motor and sensory function is always very doubtful, especially in the forearm and hand, and severe permanent disability is usually to be expected.

Part 3

In this part the features of the common disorders of the trunk and limbs will be outlined against the background of the systematic descriptions covered in Part 2. For each region emphasis will be placed on those diseases producing unique clinical features, or where the investigation and treatment of the condition is specific to the anatomical site. At the beginning of each chapter an outline of the important points in history taking and clinical examination is provided.

12 | Neck and cervical spine

The commonest orthopaedic cause of neck disorders is degeneration of a cervical intervertebral disc. This may lead to protrusion of part of the disc contents (prolapsed cervical disc) or, more often, it may give rise to secondary osteoarthritic changes in the intervertebral joints (cervical spondylosis). These conditions together make up a large proportion of the disabilities of the neck encountered in an orthopaedic out-patient department. Another major cause of prolonged pain and stiffness of the neck is the common post-traumatic musculo-ligamentous strain known generally as whiplash injury.

A disorder of the cervical spine often interferes with the roots of the brachial plexus, causing radiating pain, muscle weakness, or sensory impairment in the corresponding upper limb. Indeed, the clinical importance of a cervical disorder often lies in its neurological effects rather than in the local lesion itself.

SPECIAL POINTS IN THE INVESTIGATION OF NECK COMPLAINTS

HISTORY

It is important to ascertain the relationship of the present symptoms to any previous neck disorder. Has there been any previous injury to the neck? Or a sudden jerk of the head that might have jarred the cervical spine? Is there a history of 'stiff neck' – a common feature in the early stages of prolapsed cervical disc?

If pain in the upper limb is an associated symptom, it is important to determine its exact distribution. Pain caused by pressure upon a nerve root in the cervical region follows a clearly defined course which depends upon the particular nerve root involved, and it is usually severe. It commonly extends down the upper arm into the forearm and hand, radiating to one or more of the fingers. It is often accompanied by paraesthesiae, described as 'pins and needles' or 'numbness'. In contrast, pain referred down the limb from a lesion of the shoulder or humerus is more diffuse and ill defined, and it seldom extends below the elbow.

EXPOSURE

The patient must be stripped to the waist. Preferably he should stand, or he may sit upon a stool.

STEPS IN CLINICAL EXAMINATION

A suggested routine for clinical examination of the neck is summarised in Table 12.1.

Table 12.1 Routine clinical examination in suspected disorders of the neck

1. LOCAL EXAMINATION OF NECK, WITH NEUROLOGICAL AND VASCULAR SURVEY OF UPPER LIMBS

Inspection	**Movements**
Bone contours: ?deformity	Flexion–extension
Soft-tissue contours	Lateral flexion
Colour and texture of skin	Rotation
Scars or sinuses	? Pain on movement
Palpation	? Crepitation on movement
Skin temperature	**Neurological state of upper limb**
Bone contours	Muscular system
Soft-tissue contours	Sensory system
Local tenderness	Sweating
Vascular state of upper limb	Reflexes
Colour	
Temperature	
Pulses	

2. EXAMINATION OF POTENTIAL EXTRINSIC SOURCES OF NECK SYMPTOMS

Symptoms suggestive of a neck disorder may arise from the ears or throat. Symptoms in the upper limb suggesting a neck disorder with involvement of the brachial plexus may arise from shoulder, elbow, or nerve trunks in their peripheral course

3. GENERAL EXAMINATION

General survey of other parts of the body. Neck symptoms may be only one manifestation of a more widespread disease

DEFORMITY

The cervical spine normally has a slight anterior curvature (lordosis). Straightening of this curve, or an angulation in the reverse direction (kyphosis), is sometimes significant and may suggest an underlying abnormality. Any lateral or rotational deformity (torticollis) must also be noted.

MOVEMENTS

The movements to be examined are flexion, extension, lateral flexion to right and left, and rotation to right and left (Fig. 12.1). Flexion–extension movements occur mainly at the occipito-atlantoid joint but to some extent throughout the

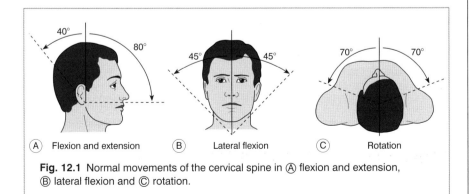

(A) Flexion and extension   (B) Lateral flexion   (C) Rotation

Fig. 12.1 Normal movements of the cervical spine in (A) flexion and extension, (B) lateral flexion and (C) rotation.

cervical spine. Lateral flexion takes place throughout the cervical spine. Rotation occurs largely at the atlanto-axial joint, with a small range of movement at the other joints. It is important to find out whether movement causes pain and, if so, whether the pain is felt locally in the neck or whether it is referred down the upper limbs. It should be noted also whether movement is accompanied by audible or palpable crepitation.

NEUROLOGICAL EXAMINATION OF UPPER LIMBS

This is an essential step in the investigation of the neck because cervical lesions so often interfere with the brachial plexus.

Muscular system. The muscles of the shoulder girdle, arm, forearm, and hand must be examined for wasting or fasciculation, a comparison being made on the two sides. The tone and power of each muscle group are then tested in turn and a comparison is made with the opposite limb. It is worth remembering the major root innervation for each muscle group when testing; C5 to deltoid, C6 biceps and wrist extensors, C7 triceps and wrist flexors, C8 finger flexors, and T1 to intrinsic muscles of hand.

Sensory system. Examine the patient's sensibility to touch and pin prick. In appropriate cases test also the sensibility to deep stimuli, joint position, vibration, and heat and cold. The nerve roots supplying the sensory dermatomes in the upper limb are shown in Fig. 12.2. In the assessment of sensory loss it should be remembered that the middle or long finger, representing the central axis of the limb, is innervated mainly from the seventh cervical nerve. The radial half of the hand is innervated by the proximal roots of the brachial plexus (C5, C6) whereas the ulnar half is innervated from the more distal roots (C8, T1).

Sweating. Feel whether the digits are moist or dry. Sweating is dependent upon intact sudomotor nerve fibres.

Reflexes. Compare on the two sides the biceps jerk (mainly C6), the triceps jerk (mainly C7), and the brachioradialis jerk (mainly C6).

From the findings elicited it should be possible to determine whether there is a neurological disturbance and, if so, whether it is of upper or lower motor neurone type, and the identity of the roots, trunks, or branches involved.

VASCULAR EXAMINATION OF THE UPPER LIMB

The subclavian artery is sometimes interfered with by a lesion of the neck. The efficiency of the circulatory system in each upper limb must therefore be determined. Judge and compare on the two sides the colour and warmth of the forearm, hand and fingers. Test and compare the radial pulses, first with the limb at rest, then with the shoulder depressed and the head rotated towards the side examined.

EXTRINSIC CAUSES OF NECK SYMPTOMS

Occasionally neck symptoms have their origin outside the neck itself. Thus pain may be referred to the neck from the ears or throat. These sites should be examined routinely for evidence of disease.

Symptoms in the upper limb that might suggest the possibility of a neck disorder involving the brachial plexus may in fact have their origin in the shoulder or elbow, or at any point along the peripheral distribution of the nerve trunks.

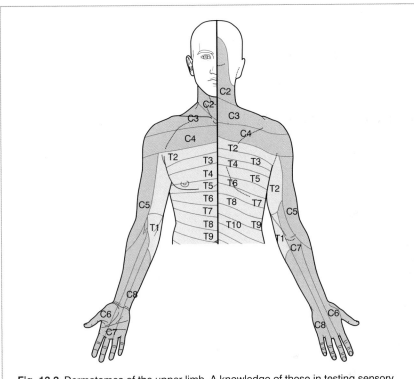

Fig. 12.2 Dermatomes of the upper limb. A knowledge of these in testing sensory impairment will assist in determining the level of root involvement in cervical spine disease.

DIAGNOSTIC IMAGING

Radiographic examination. Routine radiographs of the cervical spine include an antero-posterior and a lateral projection. Additional projections are often required when it is desired to show a particular structure more clearly. For a study of the dens (odontoid process) of the axis a special antero-posterior projection is made through the open mouth. Occasionally oblique projections are required for a proper investigation of the intervertebral foramina and the facet joints, and is also valuable in revealing the size and shape of a cervical rib.

Other techniques of imaging. Magnetic resonance imaging (MRI) is used increasingly to demonstrate the relationship between the bony and neurological structures in the cervical spine. Computerised tomography (CT scanning) and radioisotope scanning may sometimes be required to demonstrate pathological changes in the bony structures.

DEFORMITIES AND CERVICAL INSTABILITIES

INFANTILE TORTICOLLIS ('Congenital' torticollis; muscular torticollis)

In infantile torticollis (wry neck) the head is tilted and rotated by contracture of the sternomastoid muscle of one side. Strictly this is not a true congenital deformity because it arises after birth. With improvements in obstetrical practice it is now seen much less often than it was in the past.

Cause. This is uncertain. Probably there is interference with the blood supply of the sternomastoid muscle, caused by injury during birth.

Pathology. In the established condition, part of the affected muscle is replaced by contracted fibrous tissue. In some cases contracture is known to have been preceded, in early infancy, by a tumour-like thickening of the muscle ('sternomastoid tumour'), the histology being that of muscle infarction and replacement by fibrous tissue.

Clinical features. The child, often between 6 months and 3 years old when brought for consultation, is noticed to hold the head on one side. On examination, the contracted sternomastoid muscle is felt as a tight cord. The ear on the affected side is approximated to the corresponding shoulder. In long-established cases there is retarded development of the face on the affected side, with consequent asymmetry (Fig. 12.3).

Diagnosis. The condition has to be distinguished from other forms of wry neck, including structural deformities of the cervical spine, ocular torticollis, muscle spasm from a local inflammatory lesion such as infected glands, and psychogenic (hysterical) torticollis. The important diagnostic features are the history, the cord-like contracted sternomastoid muscle, and the facial asymmetry. Imaging of the spine with plain radiographs is important to exclude any underlying vertebral abnormalities or subluxations.

Treatment. If the condition is seen at the stage of 'sternomastoid tumour', repeated stretching of the muscle under the supervision of a physiotherapist is effective. In established cases the contracted muscle should be divided at its lower attachment. After operation corrective exercises should be encouraged.

CONGENITAL SHORT NECK (Klippel–Feil syndrome)

This is an uncommon non-familial congenital malformation of the cervical spine characterised clinically by short neck and limitation of head movements. The cause is unknown.

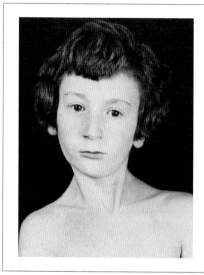

Fig. 12.3 Infantile torticollis. Note the tense cord-like left sternomastoid muscle and the facial asymmetry.

The degree of abnormality varies widely. The bony deformity consists in fusion of two or more of the cervical vertebrae. Clinically, the neck appears short or absent, and the hair-line is low. The neck may also be webbed to the shoulder. Movements of the head are restricted. Radiographs show the underlying bony abnormality, but operation is seldom indicated.

CONGENITAL HIGH SCAPULA (Sprengel's shoulder[1])

Congenital high scapula is an uncommon congenital deformity characterised by an abnormally high position and relative fixity of the scapula. The cause is unknown. The anomaly represents a failure of the scapula – originally a cervical appendage – to descend during development to its normal thoracic position. The scapular muscles are ill developed and may be represented only by tough fibrous bands.

Clinically, the scapula on one or both sides is abnormally high. Its attachments seem almost rigid and it does not rotate freely during abduction of the arm. The range of shoulder abduction is consequently impaired, but the functional disability is slight.

Treatment. The condition is often best left alone, but some cases are suitable for operation. The upper part of the scapula (above its spine) is excised after division of the contracted levator scapulae muscle and of tight fascial bands. The blade of the scapula is then divided vertically throughout its length near the vertebral border. This allows the main (lateral) part of the scapula to be displaced downwards relative to the medial strip, and the two parts are re-united with sutures through drill holes.

CERVICAL SUBLUXATION AND DISLOCATION (Spontaneous subluxation of the cervical spine; cervical spondylolisthesis)

Most displacements of the cervical spine are caused by injury, but in some circumstances there may be spontaneous displacement, usually forwards, of a cervical vertebra upon the one next below it.

Causes and pathology. There are three types, caused by:

1. congenital failure of fusion of the dens (odontoid process) with the axis vertebra
2. inflammatory softening of the transverse ligament of the atlas
3. instability from previous injury or from rheumatoid arthritis.

Congenital or acquired non-fusion of dens. Occasionally the dens fails to fuse with the body of the axis by bone, being attached only by fibrous tissue (os odontoideum). Under the constant stress of superimposed weight the fibrous bond slowly stretches, allowing the dens, and with it the atlas and skull, to slide gradually forwards upon the axis (Fig. 12.4A). A similar condition may exist after fracture of the dens, but this would be preceded by a history of trauma. Instability may also be present in patients with Down's syndrome and radiological screening may be indicated in patients with this condition.

[1]Otto Sprengel (1852–1915) Head surgeon at Children's Hospital in Dresden, Germany. Described the deformity in 1891.

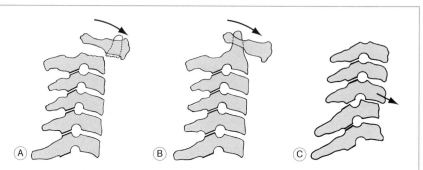

Fig. 12.4 Three types of cervical spondylolisthesis or spontaneous subluxation. Ⓐ Displacement of atlas with the dens permitted by congenital or post-traumatic non-fusion of the dens with the axis. Ⓑ Displacement of atlas on axis, from softening of the transverse ligament of the atlas. Ⓒ Subluxation of a cervical vertebra upon the one next below it from instability of the intervertebral joint after previous injury. Instability may also be caused by rheumatoid arthritis.

Inflammatory softening of the transverse ligament of the atlas. In this type the underlying cause is an inflammatory lesion in the upper part of the neck, such as rheumatoid arthritis or a severe local infection of the throat or glands. There is rarefaction of the atlas, with softening of the transverse ligament. In consequence the atlas is able to slide forwards upon the axis (Fig. 12.4B).

Instability from previous injury or from arthritis. A traumatic fracture-dislocation or subluxation at any level in the cervical spine may cause permanent instability, with a liability to slow redisplacement months or years after the initial injury (Fig. 12.4C).

In all types the upper segment is displaced forwards in relation to the lower. The spinal canal becomes progressively more flexed and narrowed, and there is always a grave risk of compression of the spinal cord.

Clinical features. In the inflammatory type there is complaint of 'stiff neck'. The head is held rigidly, the cervical muscles being in spasm. In subluxation from congenital or post-traumatic instability there are discomfort and stiffness in the neck, and flexion deformity is apparent. Radiographs will show the displacement, its level and its type (Fig. 12.5).

Complications. In all types the complication to be feared is compression of the spinal cord. The first symptoms appear in the upper limbs and consist of root pain, paraesthesiae, motor weakness, or sensory impairment. Eventually, increasing cord compression may lead to spastic paralysis below the level of the lesion, and to bladder and bowel dysfunction.

Treatment. This depends upon the underlying cause and upon whether or not neurological disturbance is present.

Inflammatory type. The displacement is reduced by head traction, which is continued for two weeks. Thereafter the neck is immobilised in extension in a plaster jacket for 2 months. Atlanto-axial fusion may be required.

Congenital or post-traumatic instability. If subluxation is not complicated by neurological disturbance, treatment may be expectant (observation only), by a plastic collar to give support, or by local fusion of the spine, according to the

Neck and cervical spine

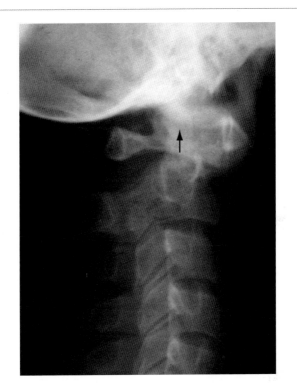

Fig. 12.5 Lateral radiograph of upper cervical spine in rheumatoid arthritis showing atlanto-axial subluxation. The anterior arch of the atlas has displaced anteriorly because of destruction by the rheumatoid inflammatory process of the transverse ligaments that normally hold it against the odontoid process of the axis. As a result the odontoid peg (arrow) will compress the anterior aspect of the spinal cord and medulla with severe neurological complications.

severity of the displacement and of the local symptoms. If neurological disturbance is present, treatment is by preliminary skull traction to reduce the displacement, followed by operative fusion of the affected segments of the spine.

TUBERCULOSIS OF THE CERVICAL SPINE
(Tuberculous cervical spondylitis)

Tuberculosis is far less common in the cervical spine than in the thoracic and lumbar regions. It is now seldom seen in Britain, but it still occurs commonly in Africa and in Eastern countries. The general features of tuberculosis of bone were described in Chapter 7 (p. 92).

Pathology. The infection begins in the front of a vertebral body, or in an inter-vertebral disc (Fig. 12.6A). Destruction of bone and intervertebral disc leads to anterior collapse with consequent cervical kyphosis (Fig. 12.6B). The degree of destruction varies widely, depending upon the virulence of the organism and the resistance of the patient. Formation of pus leads either to a retropharyngeal abscess (behind the prevertebral fascia), which may eventually point at the posterior margin of the sternomastoid muscle, or, if the pus tracks posteriorly,

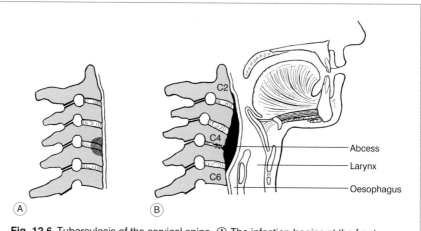

Fig. 12.6 Tuberculosis of the cervical spine. Ⓐ The infection begins at the front margin of a vertebral body close to the intervertebral disc, or possibly in the disc itself, as indicated by the shaded area. Ⓑ The opposing surfaces of the bodies of C4 and C5 have been eroded and the intervening disc is destroyed. Pus has collected behind the prevertebral fascia, forming a bulging retropharyngeal abscess.

to a suboccipital abscess. The spinal cord may be damaged by direct pressure of an abscess, or by secondary thrombosis of the vessels of the cord.

Clinical features. The disease occurs mainly in children and young adults. There is pain in the neck and occiput, aggravated by movement. In addition, one or more of the following symptoms may be present: difficulty in swallowing; abscess or sinus at the side or back of the neck; neurological symptoms from spinal cord dysfunction, the upper limbs being affected before the lower. On examination the head is held rigidly, often supported by the hands. The cervical muscles stand out in spasm. One or more of the spinous processes may appear prominent, due to cervical kyphosis. There is local tenderness on firm palpation over the spinous processes. All movements of the head and neck are restricted, and cause pain if forced. An abscess may be present in the suboccipital region, behind the sternomastoid muscle, or behind the pharynx (see below). Associated tuberculous lesions elsewhere are common.

Imaging. Radiographs always show diminution of disc space, usually some destruction of bone (Fig. 12.6B), and sometimes an abscess shadow. MRI scans will provide more detailed information on the extent of the soft tissue abscess and assist in planning surgical drainage.

Investigations. The erythrocyte sedimentation rate is raised in the active stage. The Mantoux test is positive. Pus obtained by aspiration of an abscess may yield tubercle bacilli.

Complications. Retropharyngeal abscess. This causes difficulty in swallowing (dysphagia), and the posterior wall of the pharynx is seen to bulge forwards in the midline. Eventually the abscess may point behind the sternomastoid muscle. If neglected, it may rupture into the pharynx.

Spinal cord dysfunction. If the spinal cord is affected there will be neurological signs (sensory, motor, and visceral) at and below the level of the lesion, which may progress to complete paralysis.

Diagnosis. Important diagnostic features are the history of tuberculous contact or disease, spasm of the neck muscles with restriction of all movements, abscess formation, and the radiographic findings.

Treatment. The principles of treatment are the same as for other forms of skeletal tuberculosis. Antibacterial therapy: combinations of antituberculous drugs were described on page 102. Local treatment is by support for the cervical spine by a halo splint or by a plastic collar until the disease is quiescent – often a matter of several months.

Operation is sometimes required and the following are the main indications:

1. to drain a retropharyngeal abscess that threatens to rupture or to cause asphyxia
2. in a florid case, to remove necrotic bone and debris and then to embed a bone graft in the cavity
3. to decompress a spinal cord damaged by pressure of abscess or granulation tissue
4. in the quiescent stage, to fuse the affected region of the spine if it is judged to be unstable.

PYOGENIC INFECTION OF THE CERVICAL SPINE (Pyogenic cervical spondylitis)

Infection of the cervical vertebrae or intervertebral discs with pyogenic organisms is uncommon. It is usually caused by the staphylococcus, streptococcus, or pneumococcus, and occasionally by other bacteria, including salmonella organisms or *Brucella abortus*.

Pathology. The organisms reach the spinal column by the general blood stream (from a septic focus elsewhere), by lymphatic channels (from a local infection, for instance in the pharynx), or possibly by the spinal venous plexus (from a focus in the pelvis). As in tuberculous spondylitis, there is destruction of bone and intervertebral disc, with or without abscess formation. The spinal cord may be damaged by direct pressure or by thrombosis.

Clinical features. The onset is usually acute or subacute, with pyrexia. The clinical features resemble those of tuberculous spondylitis (p. 192), but the course is more rapid. A suppurative process elsewhere in the body (for instance, in the pharynx or pelvis) is usually present. *Radiographs* show local osteoporosis or erosion of bone, diminution of disc space, and sometimes subligamentous new bone formation.

Investigations. The erythrocyte sedimentation rate and C-reactive protein level is raised and polymorphonuclear leucocytosis is to be expected.

Diagnosis. The condition must be distinguished from tuberculous spondylitis; the relatively rapid onset and course, with pyrexia and leucocytosis, and identification of the causal organism in pus, are the main diagnostic criteria.

Treatment. Appropriate antibiotic drugs (see p. 89) should be given systemically. The cervical spine must be immobilised in a rigid collar or brace; sometimes sustained head traction with a halo splint is required for relief of spasm. When there is an abscess it should be drained, especially if the spinal cord is threatened. Spontaneous fusion of the affected vertebrae usually makes operative fusion unnecessary.

Neck and cervical spine

RHEUMATOID ARTHRITIS (General description of rheumatoid arthritis, p. 134)

The cervical spine is the third most commonly affected in rheumatoid polyarthritis, after the hands and feet. In sero-positive disease up to 50% will show evidence of destructive synovitis in the vertebral joints. It is important that this be recognised, because there is a risk that destruction of the intervertebral joints may allow gradual forward subluxation of a cervical vertebra upon the one next below it, with danger to the integrity of the spinal cord. There is a particular risk of subluxation at the atlanto-axial joint due to softening of the transverse ligament of the atlas (see Fig. 12.5). Destructive changes may also occur at multiple levels below the axis vertebra and may result in subluxation causing progressive spinal cord or nerve root compression. It is important to remember that these destructive changes may occur insidiously without significant symptoms because of the involvement of the upper and lower limb joints; thus they may be overlooked until the onset of paralysis.

Warning symptoms that should alert the clinician to impending cord damage are sensory paraesthesia and sensations of 'electric shocks' in the hands with increased muscle tone and spasticity in the legs. Dizziness, tinnitus and vertigo may also occur and are indicative of vertebral artery insufficiency.

Treatment. If the patient experiences significant neck pain and erosion of the intervertebral joints or subluxation at any level are demonstrated radiologically, the neck should be splinted with a moulded soft plastic collar. In a few patients when neurological impairment becomes progressive MRI scanning is required to evaluate the extent of spinal cord compression. If this is present more active surgical treatment is indicated; initially with skull traction or a halo brace to correct the subluxation, followed by posterior spinal fusion or occipito-cervical fusion.

ANKYLOSING SPONDYLITIS

Ankylosing spondylitis is a disease that creeps up the spine from below having originated in the sacro-iliac joints and the lumbar spine. In a high proportion of cases – though by no means in all – it extends to involve the cervical region, with aching pain and permanent stiffness – sometimes total rigid ankylosis – of the intervertebral joints. Very occasionally the neck may become ankylosed in an extreme degree of flexion producing a 'chin on chest' deformity. When this interferes with swallowing and the ability to see ahead it may justify surgical correction by osteotomy and fusion. This is very high-risk surgery with a 20% mortality rate and should only be undertaken in specialised centres by surgeons with the necessary skills. The disease of ankylosing spondylitis as a whole will be described in Chapter 13 (p. 229).

CERVICAL SPONDYLOSIS (Cervical spondylarthritis; cervical spondylarthrosis; cervical osteoarthritis; cervical osteoarthrosis)

Degenerative changes are common in the cervical spine. Indeed, they are found almost universally in some degree in persons over 50 years of age. Beginning in the intervertebral discs, they affect the posterior intervertebral (facet) joints secondarily, causing pain and stiffness of the neck, sometimes with referred symptoms in an upper limb.

Cause. The primary degenerative changes may be initiated by injury, but usually the condition is simply a manifestation of normal ageing processes.

Pathology. Degenerative arthritis occurs most commonly in the lowest three cervical joints. The changes affect first the central intervertebral joints (between the vertebral bodies) and later the posterior intervertebral (facet) joints. In the central joints there is degenerative narrowing of the intervertebral disc, and bone reaction at the joint margins leads to the formation of osteophytes (Fig. 12.7A). In the posterior intervertebral joints the changes are those of osteoarthritis in any diarthrodial joint – namely, wearing away of the articular cartilage and the formation of osteophytes (spurs) at the joint margins (Fig. 12.7B).

Secondary effects. Osteophytes commonly encroach upon the intervertebral foramina, reducing the space for transmission of the cervical nerves (Fig. 12.7B). If the restricted space in a foramen is reduced still further by traumatic oedema of the contained soft tissues, manifestations of nerve pressure are likely to occur. Exceptionally, the spinal cord itself may suffer damage from encroachment of osteophytes within the spinal canal.

Clinical features. The symptoms are in the neck or in the upper limb, or both.

Neck symptoms consist chiefly of aching pain in the back of the neck or in the trapezius area, a feeling of stiffness, and 'grating' on movement. Usually slight, they are liable to periodic exacerbations, probably from unremembered strains or repetitive movements: exacerbations may be interspersed with periods of freedom from pain. Occipital headache may be a feature if the upper half of the cervical spine is affected.

In the upper limb there may be a vague, ill-defined and ill-localised 'referred' pain spreading over the shoulder region, or there may be more serious symptoms from interference with one or more of the cervical nerves in their foramina. The main feature of nerve root irritation is radiating pain along the course of the affected nerve or nerves, often reaching the digits. There may also be paraesthesiae in the hand, in the form of tingling or 'pins and needles'. Noticeable muscle weakness is uncommon.

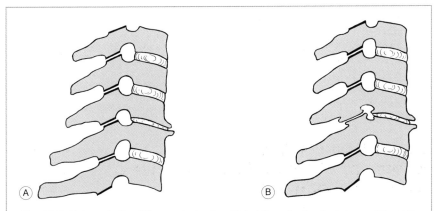

Fig. 12.7 Osteoarthritis of the cervical spine. At first there is simply degeneration and narrowing of the intervertebral disc, with the formation of osteophytes anteriorly Ⓐ. Later, the posterior or facet joints are affected: the articular cartilage is worn away and marginal osteophytes may encroach upon the intervertebral foramen Ⓑ.

On examination, the neck may be slightly kyphotic. The posterior cervical muscles may be somewhat tender but they are not in spasm. Movements are not markedly diminished except during acute exacerbations or when the degenerative changes are very advanced. Audible crepitation on movement is common. In the upper limb objective findings are usually slight or absent, for nerve pressure is seldom great enough to produce well-defined objective neurological signs (compare prolapsed intervertebral disc). Thus demonstrable motor weakness or sensory impairment is exceptional. Depression of one or more of the tendon reflexes is, however, fairly common.

Radiographic features. There is narrowing of the intervertebral disc space, with formation of osteophytes at the vertebral margins, especially anteriorly (Fig. 12.8A). A single vertebral level may be affected – often at the C5–C6 or C6–C7 level – or there may be changes at more than one level. Encroachment of osteophytes upon an intervertebral foramen is demonstrated best in oblique projections (Fig. 12.8B) or on CT scans. In a few patients with clinical evidence of neurological impairment MRI scanning may be indicated to identify nerve root or cord compression.

Diagnosis. Distinction has to be made from:

1. *Other causes of neck pain.* These include prolapsed cervical disc, tuberculous or pyogenic infection, tumours involving the vertebral column, and fibromyalgia.
2. *Other causes of upper limb pain* (Fig. 12.9). These are as follows: central lesions – tumours involving the spinal cord or its roots; cervical spondylolisthesis. Plexus lesions – tumours at the thoracic inlet (Pancoast); cervical rib; prolapsed intervertebral disc. Shoulder lesions with radiating pain in the upper arm. Skeletal lesions such as a tumour, infection, or Paget's disease of a bone of the upper extremity. Elbow lesions such as tennis elbow or arthritis. Distal nerve lesions such as friction neuritis of the ulnar nerve at the elbow or compression of the median nerve in the carpal tunnel.

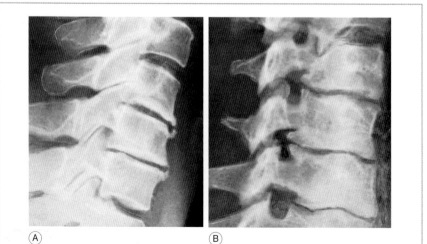

(A)   (B)

Fig. 12.8 Cervical spondylosis. Note in the lateral view Ⓐ the narrowed intervertebral space, with marginal osteophyte formation, at C5–C6 and at C6–C7. The oblique view Ⓑ shows severe encroachment of osteophytes upon an intervertebral foramen (compare with the normal foramen below).

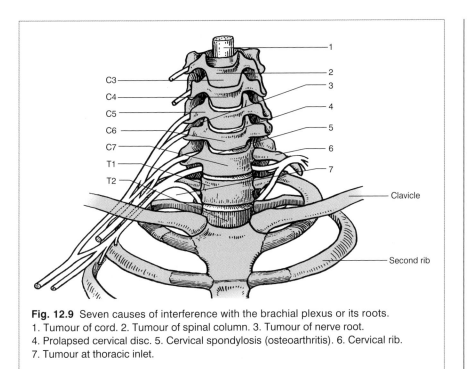

C3
C4
C5
C6
C7
T1
T2

1
2
3
4
5
6
7

Clavicle

Second rib

Fig. 12.9 Seven causes of interference with the brachial plexus or its roots. 1. Tumour of cord. 2. Tumour of spinal column. 3. Tumour of nerve root. 4. Prolapsed cervical disc. 5. Cervical spondylosis (osteoarthritis). 6. Cervical rib. 7. Tumour at thoracic inlet.

Treatment. There is a strong tendency for the symptoms of cervical spondylosis to subside spontaneously, though they may persist for many weeks and the structural changes are clearly permanent. Treatment is thus aimed towards assisting natural resolution of temporarily inflamed or oedematous soft tissues. In mild cases such measures include anti-inflammatory analgesic drugs and muscle relaxants as well as various forms of physiotherapy. Ultrasound, short-wave diathermy, massage, and intermittent traction have all been used, but none have been shown to be effective in large clinical trials. Some benefit has been shown for mobilisation and strengthening exercises. Manipulation is sometimes recommended, but in the presence of extensive osteophytes it is hazardous because it may damage the spinal cord; it should therefore be employed with extreme caution, and only by those familiar with a gentle technique. In the more severe cases it is wise to provide rest and support for the neck by a closely fitting protective cervical collar (Fig. 12.10A), but this should only be worn for a few weeks until the acute symptoms subside to prevent atrophy of the spinal muscles.

In the exceptional cases in which radiculopathy or myelopathy is progressive and bony impingement can be demonstrated by imaging, surgical decompression may be required. For nerve root compression this can be achieved by a foraminotomy procedure, but where cord compression is present the type of operation is dictated by the site of bone impingement. In the commoner anterior compression from osteophytes on the vertebral body, an anterior discectomy combined with an interbody fusion gives best results. When compression is posterior from thickening of the laminae, a posterior laminectomy is required with a lateral facet joint wiring and fusion.

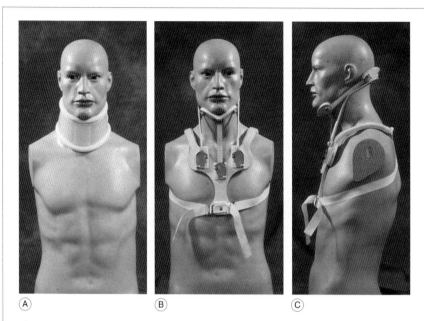

(A)   (B)   (C)

Fig. 12.10 Cervical collars used in the treatment of painful neck disorders. The simple polythene support Ⓐ gives only symptomatic relief and minimal support. The more rigid adjustable orthosis Ⓑ and Ⓒ can be fitted to limit flexion and extension of the spine and provides some stability in more severe disease.

PROLAPSED CERVICAL DISC

Displacement of intervertebral disc material in the cervical spine is much less common than it is in the lumbar region. It is characterised by pain and stiffness in the neck, often with neurological manifestations in the upper limb and occasionally with signs of spinal cord compression.

Cause. Sudden jarring injury may be a predisposing factor, though a history of injury cannot be obtained in every case. Probably an intrinsic degenerative change in the substance of the disc makes it prone to rupture and displacement.

Pathology. The disc between C5–C6 and that between C6–C7 are those most frequently affected. Part of the gelatinous nucleus pulposus protrudes through a rent in the annulus fibrosus at its weakest part, which is posterolateral; or part of the annulus itself may be displaced. If slight, the protrusion bulges against the pain-sensitive posterior longitudinal ligament, causing local pain in the neck. If large, the protrusion herniates through the ligament and may impinge upon the nerve leaving the spinal canal at that level (posterolateral prolapse) (Fig. 12.11A), or occasionally upon the spinal cord itself (central prolapse) (Fig. 12.11B). Healing is probably by shrinkage and fibrosis of the extruded material rather than by its reposition within the disc. *Secondary effects:* Prolapse of a disc accelerates its degeneration and predisposes to the development of osteoarthritis (cervical spondylosis) in later years.

Clinical features. Central protrusions. These lead to manifestations of spinal cord compression and may be confused with spinal cord tumours or other

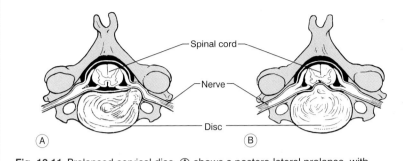

Fig. 12.11 Prolapsed cervical disc. Ⓐ shows a postero-lateral prolapse, with compression of the issuing nerve. Ⓑ shows the much less common central prolapse, with impingement upon the spinal cord.

central neurological disorders. They fall within the province of the neuro-surgeon rather than the orthopaedic surgeon.

Postero-lateral protrusions. A typical clinical picture is as follows. The patient sustains an injury to the neck – often a jarring or twisting strain – which may seem slight at the time and may cause no immediate effects. Hours or days later there is a rapid development of acute 'stiff neck' with severe pain made worse by coughing or similar strains. Later still, the pain begins to radiate over the shoulder and throughout the length of the upper limb; it is felt strictly in the course of a cervical nerve, and characteristically it is severe. Paraesthesiae are felt in the digits. On examination, there is limitation of certain neck movements by pain, but movement in at least one direction (often lateral flexion) is free. In the upper limb there is a full range of joint movements. There are slight muscle wasting and slight sensory impairment in the distribution of a cervical nerve. The corresponding tendon reflex (biceps jerk in C5–C6 lesions; triceps jerk in C6–C7 lesions) is depressed or absent.

Variations. The characteristic features described are not always present. Variations are common. Thus a history of injury is not always obtainable. The symptoms may be confined to the neck, the upper limb being spared; or they may be confined entirely to the upper limb. Motor changes (wasting and weakness) may be marked, sometimes amounting to almost complete paraly-sis of a muscle or a group of muscles; or on the other hand they may be absent. Similarly, wide variations in the degree of sensory impairment are noted.

Imaging. Radiographs characteristically show a normal appearance in the first attack, but narrowing of one of the disc spaces (usually C5–C6 or C6–C7), denoting long-standing disc degeneration, is often demonstrable. Magnetic res-onance imaging may show the displaced disc material and its relationship to the nerve roots and cord (Fig. 12.12).

Diagnosis. Prolapsed cervical disc has to be differentiated:

1. from other causes of neck pain
2. from other causes of upper limb pain (Fig. 12.9).

The main conditions that may be confused with it are the same as those listed in the differential diagnosis of cervical spondylosis (p. 196). A confident diag-nosis is justified only when a suggestive history is associated with the signs of a

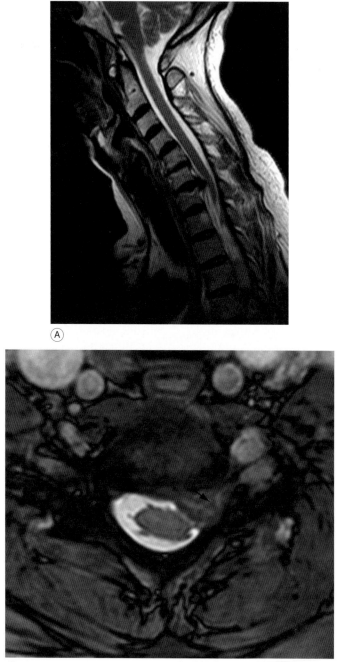

Fig 12.12 Ⓐ and Ⓑ Sagittal and axial MR scans showing a posterior cervical disc protrusion at the C6–C7 level. On the axial scan Ⓑ the disc material is seen lying on the left side of the canal extending into the exit foramen (arrow) and compressing the underlying C6 nerve root.

lesion of a single cervical nerve, and provided always that other possible causes have been excluded by careful investigation.

Relationship between prolapsed disc and cervical spondylosis

The clinical features of the two conditions are similar. Distinction is difficult if the radiographs show arthritic changes, because the arthritis may be only incidental and itself symptomless. Nerve pressure is probably greater in prolapsed disc than in osteoarthritis: consequently the symptoms tend to be more clearly defined and pain very severe; and the objective signs are more marked.

Course. There is a strong tendency to spontaneous recovery, but symptoms often persist with decreasing severity for as long as six months or more.

Treatment. This depends upon the nature and severity of the individual case. When the symptoms are slight no treatment other than perhaps a mild analgesic drug is required. In the more severe cases treatment is advisable, especially in the early acute stage. If the neck is 'stiff' and if movements aggravate the neck and limb pain, rest for a few weeks in a supportive collar made from heat-moulded reinforced plastic or a more rigid adjustable orthosis (Fig. 12.10) is the most satisfactory method. Pain is usually severe, necessitating fairly intensive analgesic therapy. As the acute symptoms gradually subside, physiotherapy in the form of graduated neck exercises to restore full mobility and muscle strength is often helpful.

In cases of intractable radicular pain or myelopathy surgical treatment may be required. Removal of the affected degenerative disc material can be achieved through an antero-lateral approach to the vertebral bodies (Fig. 12.13). This displaces the sterno-mastoid muscle and contents of the carotid sheath laterally, with the strap muscles, trachea and oesophagus moved medially to expose the pre-vertebral fascia. It is important to confirm the correct intervertebral space with intra-operative radiography before disc removal. Distraction of the vertebral bodies facilitates removal of the disc and the space created is then filled with a block of autogenous cortico-cancellous bone graft

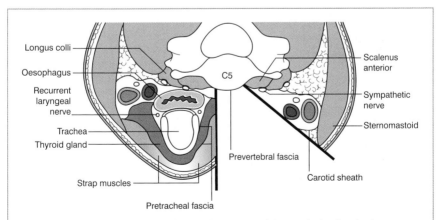

Fig 12.13 Surgical approach to the anterior aspect of the cervical spine. In the mid-cervical spine, dissection between the trachea and oesophagus medially and the carotid sheath laterally is relatively avascular compared with the posterior approach through thick muscle layers.

to produce an anterior interbody fusion. The technique can also be applied to disc degeneration at more than one level by the use of a longer strut graft (see Fig. 4.4A), usually reinforced with a plate and screws. Postoperatively the neck is immobilised in a light collar until there is radiological evidence of bone healing.

Because of the loss of movement that follows intervertebral fusion, attempts are now being made to replace the degenerate disc with an artificial prosthetic replacement, but as yet the procedure is experimental and no long-term results are available.

CERVICAL RIB

A cervical rib is a congenital over-development, bony or fibrous, of the costal process of the seventh cervical vertebra. It often exists without causing symptoms, especially in the young, but in adult life the tendency to gradual dropping of the shoulder girdle may lead to its causing neurological or vascular disturbance in the upper limb.

Pathology. The over-developed costal process may be unilateral or bilateral. It may be of any size from a small bony protrusion, often with a fibrous extension, to a complete supernumerary rib. The subclavian artery and the lowest trunk of the brachial plexus arch over the rib. In a proportion of cases the nerve trunk suffers damage at the site of pressure against the rib; this accounts for the neurological manifestations. The vascular changes are probably similarly accounted for by local damage to the subclavian artery, from which thrombotic emboli may be repeatedly discharged into the peripheral vessels of the upper limb.

Clinical features. Cervical rib is often symptomless. When symptoms occur, they usually begin during early adult life. They may be neurological, vascular, or combined.

Neurological manifestations. The sensory symptoms are pain and paraesthesiae in the forearm and hand, most marked towards the medial (ulnar) side, and often relieved temporarily by changing the position of the arm. The motor symptoms include increasing weakness of the hand, with difficulty in carrying out the finer movements.

On examination, there is usually an area of sensory impairment – sometimes complete anaesthesia – in the forearm or hand. The affected area does not correspond in distribution to any of the peripheral nerves, but may be related to the lowest trunk of the brachial plexus. There may be wasting of the muscles of the thenar eminence or of the interosseous and hypothenar muscles.

Vascular manifestations. The changes that have been observed range from dusky cyanosis of the forearm and hand to gangrene of the fingers. The radial pulse may be weak or absent.

Radiographic features. Radiographs show the abnormal rib: if small, it is seen best in oblique projections (Fig. 12.14). In cases of suspected vascular obstruction arteriography is required.

Diagnosis. Radiographic demonstration of a cervical rib does not prove that it is the cause of symptoms. The condition has to be distinguished:

1. from other causes of pain and paraesthesiae in the forearm and hand (Fig. 12.9)
2. from other causes of muscle wasting in the hand, including neurological disorders and muscular dystrophy
3. from other causes of peripheral vascular changes in the upper limb including Raynaud's disease.

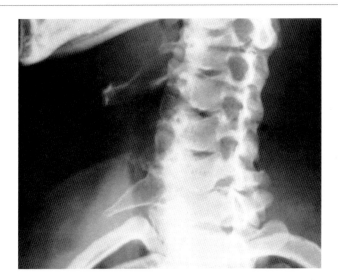

Fig. 12.14 Cervical rib. Typical appearance of a small supernumerary rib. This one caused severe neurological symptoms and signs. A cervical rib is shown best in an oblique radiograph such as this.

The diagnosis of symptomatic cervical rib depends upon the detection of the characteristic neurological signs or vascular disturbance in association with a demonstrable supernumerary rib. Prolapsed intervertebral disc at C7–T1 gives a similar clinical picture neurologically, and indeed it may often be the true cause of symptoms ascribed to a cervical rib; but in prolapsed disc there is a strong tendency to natural recovery, which is not the case with cervical rib. Arteriography may be conclusive by revealing obstruction of the subclavian artery.

Treatment. This depends upon the severity of the subjective and objective manifestations. In mild cases physiotherapy in the form of 'shrugging' exercises, to improve the tone of the elevator muscles of the shoulder girdle, is adequate. But if the neurological or vascular signs are well marked, and especially if they are increasing, operation is advisable. First the scalenus anterior muscle is divided. If this does not demonstrably release the lowest nerve trunk from constricting pressure the scalenus medius should be divided and the abnormal rib removed.

Occlusion of the subclavian artery may be amenable to reconstruction by vein grafting if the diagnosis is made before irreversible changes in the limb have occurred.

SCALENUS SYNDROME (First rib syndrome; thoracic outlet syndrome)

Occasionally the neurological manifestations characteristic of cervical rib occur in the absence of a demonstrable skeletal abnormality. They have been ascribed to trapping of nerves between the first rib and the clavicle (costo-clavicular compression), or between the first rib and the scalenus anterior muscle; and to stretching of the lowest trunk of the brachial plexus over the normal first rib. More often, they are caused by a tough fibrous band in the scalenus medius muscle, which may lead to kinking of the lowest trunk of the brachial plexus, demonstrable at operation. The symptoms are easily confused with those from a prolapsed intervertebral disc between C7 and T1. Treatment should be conservative at first, as for prolapsed disc. Gradual improvement would support the diagnosis of disc prolapse. But if the symptoms persist with undiminished intensity for a long time a true scalenus syndrome is probably the cause. In that event it may be justifiable to explore the plexus, to divide the scalenus anterior and the scalenus medius, and if necessary to excise the first rib.

SOFT-TISSUE STRAIN OF THE NECK ('Whiplash' injury)

Soft-tissue strain of the neck – commonly termed whiplash injury – is a common cause of persistent pain and stiffness in the neck. It occurs frequently in occupants of cars struck violently from behind by other vehicles ('rear-end shunts'). Similar strains may also occur in head-on collisions.

Mechanism of injury and pathology. At the moment of impact the head is first thrown backwards as the vehicle in which the victim is seated is suddenly jolted forwards, often without any warning. This is followed by rebound flexion of the neck, often so extreme that the chin abuts against the manubrium of the sternum, and by a second extension movement. It is assumed that there is strain of the deep muscles and ligaments of the cervical spine. In the great majority of cases in which the patient attends at a hospital, radiographs do not show any structural damage in the spinal column.

Clinical features. At impact the patient usually feels jolting or 'wrenching' of the neck or of one or other shoulder; but often there is no severe pain initially and the patient may think at first that he has escaped significant injury. However, within hours of the accident – occasionally as late as a day or more afterwards – there is increasing pain and 'stiffness' in the back of the neck, often with extension of the pain to the top and back of one or other shoulder. The neck pain is usually accompanied by severe headache, which may be persistent. *Examination* shows restriction of the range of movement of the cervical spine, usually in all directions at first, but later more localised.

Symptoms from whiplash injury of the neck are often very slow to subside, and whereas some patients show full recovery in a matter of weeks, it is common for patients to complain of lingering neck and shoulder pain, with or without recurrent headaches, for as long as one or two years, and sometimes even longer. In long protracted cases it is often found that the patient has become demoralised, and consequent psychological upset may delay recovery.

Treatment. Whiplash strain does not respond well or regularly to any particular form of treatment: as is so often the case with soft-tissue strains, time is the best healer. In general, the principles of treatment should be to provide support and rest for the neck in the initial stages, in the form of a protective cervical collar. But after a week or so the emphasis should be rather on the restoration of mobility by regular exercises within the limits imposed by pain, preferably under the supervision of a physiotherapist.

TUMOURS IN RELATION TO THE CERVICAL SPINE AND EMERGING NERVES

Tumours involving the cervical spine or the related nerves may arise:

1. in the spinal column itself
2. in the meninges or, rarely, the spinal cord
3. in the fibrous components of a peripheral nerve (neurofibroma)
4. in adjacent soft tissues.

Tumours of the spinal column are more often malignant than benign, and predominantly metastatic rather than primary tumours. A meningeal tumour (meningioma) is an uncommon cause of compression of the spinal cord. A tumour arising in nerve (neurofibroma) occurs occasionally within an intervertebral foramen, where it may grow inwards to compress the spinal cord and outwards towards the surface ('dumb-bell' tumour). A tumour at the apex of the lung (Pancoast's tumour) is a well-recognised cause of severe pain from invasion of the brachial plexus.

Clinical features. The effects of these tumours vary according to their site and nature. Broadly, there may be:

1. local destruction and collapse of cervical vertebrae
2. spinal cord compression
3. interference with the brachial plexus.

Destruction and collapse of cervical vertebrae. The commonest cause is a metastatic carcinoma (Fig. 12.15). The clinical features are local pain and, usually, flexion deformity. The spinal cord or the issuing cervical nerves may be involved, with corresponding signs of spinal cord compression or peripheral nerve defect.

Spinal cord compression. Interference with the function of the spinal cord may be caused by tumours of the cord itself or of its meninges, by tumours of nerves (neurofibroma), or by tumours of the bony spinal column. The clinical

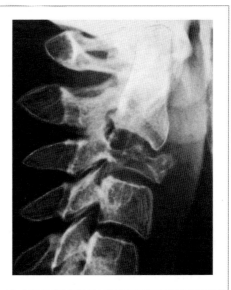

Fig. 12.15 Partial destruction of the body of the third cervical vertebra by a metastasis from a renal carcinoma.

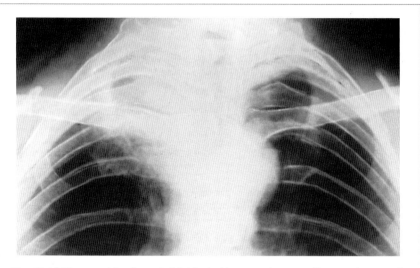

Fig. 12.16 Tumour at the thoracic inlet (apical lung carcinoma or Pancoast's tumour) causing well-marked opacity at the apex of the right lung. This tumour should always be borne in mind in the differential diagnosis of pain in the upper limb.

manifestations depend upon the location of the tumour. Typically, root pain at the level of the lesion is followed by lower motor neurone changes at the same level and by progressive upper motor neurone paralysis and visceral dysfunction below the lesion.

Interference with the brachial plexus. Nerves forming the brachial plexus may be involved by tumours of the nerves themselves (neurofibroma), by bone tumours, or by tumours at the thoracic inlet (Fig. 12.16). The predominant features are severe pain along the course of the nerve or nerves affected (neck or upper limb) and increasing motor and sensory impairment in the distribution of the nerves.

Imaging. Plain radiographs will usually help in discovering a tumour arising in the bones of the spinal column or eroding the bones from outside (Fig. 12.15). They may also reveal a tumour at the thoracic inlet (Fig. 12.16). Computerised tomography or magnetic resonance imaging may give more precise information. Radiographs of the chest may reveal an apical lung tumour or pulmonary metastases.

13 | Trunk and spine

Pain in the back is the commonest symptom encountered in orthopaedic practice. Indeed, if accident cases are excluded, it probably accounts for nearly a third of all orthopaedic out-patient attendances.

When this huge mass of material is sifted and categorised it is found that the cases fall into two broad groups. In the first group clear-cut physical signs, with or without distinctive radiographic changes or other abnormal findings, allow a precise determination of the nature of the lesion and of its site. The diagnosis is positive, and rational treatment can be applied. In the second group, almost as large as the first, there are few or no abnormal findings on clinical examination or from imaging investigations; so the pathology is unclear. Diagnosis is largely a matter of conjecture, and treatment is empirical. For want of more accurate knowledge these rather vague and unsatisfactory cases are generally classed as 'chronic ligamentous strain' or 'postural back pain'.

Lumbar back pain is often accompanied by radiating pain in the buttock, thigh, or leg, usually on one side but occasionally on both sides. This pain is generally referred to as sciatica, though the term should strictly be reserved for pain in the distribution of the sciatic nerve. It should be noted that sciatica is often a much more disturbing and persistent symptom of back disorders than the back pain itself, which indeed may be slight or transient.

SPECIAL POINTS IN THE INVESTIGATION OF BACK AND SCIATIC SYMPTOMS

History

Special attention should be paid to the mode of onset of the symptoms, whether they are periodic or constant, whether they are getting worse or better, and what relieves them or aggravates them. The precise location of the back pain and its character should be determined. The patient should be asked to what he or she attributes the symptoms: a history of a jarring strain, a fall, or an unaccustomed lifting job may be pertinent. Exacerbation of the pain on coughing or sneezing, which raises intracranial pressure, is indicative of an organic lesion.

Significance of sciatica. If pain radiates into the lower limb its character and exact distribution must be ascertained. Two distinct types of sciatica can be recognised. If the pain is severe and radiates in a well-defined course that can be outlined on the skin surface, and especially if it is accompanied by motor, sensory, or reflex impairment, it suggests mechanical interference with nerve fibres of the lumbar or sacral plexus, as for instance by a prolapsed disc or a tumour. On the other hand, if it takes the form of a vague diffuse ache, ill defined in its distribution, it is more likely to be a 'referred' pain originating in a disordered joint or ligament.

Exposure

The patient should be stripped completely, except for undergarments and, in women, a brassière.

Steps in routine examination

A suggested plan for the routine clinical examination of the back is summarised in Table 13.1.

Assessment of deformity

Any visible or palpable alteration of shape or posture of the spinal column should be noted. Deformity may occur in the sagittal plane, in the form of kyphosis (excessive forward curve or stoop) or lordosis (hollow back); or it may occur in the coronal plane as a lateral curvature (scoliosis). Combined curves and rotational deformity may also occur.

Table 13.1 Routine clinical examination in suspected disorders of the back

1. LOCAL EXAMINATION OF THE BACK, WITH NEUROLOGICAL SURVEY OF THE LOWER LIMBS

(Patient standing)	*Costo-vertebral joints*
Inspection	Range indicated by chest expansion
Bone contours and alignment:	*Sacro-iliac joints*
(?visible deformity)	(Impracticable to assess range)
Soft-tissue contours	? Pain on movement imparted by
Colour and texture of skin	lateral compression of pelvis
Scars or sinuses	*(Patient recumbent)*
Palpation	**Palpation of iliac fossae**
Skin temperature	Examine specifically for abscess
Bone contours	or mass
Soft-tissue contours	
Local tenderness	**Neurological state of lower limbs**
Movements	Straight leg raising test
Spinal joints	Muscular system
Flexion	Sensory system
Extension	Reflexes
Lateral flexion	
Rotation	
? Pain on movement	
? Muscle spasm	

2. EXAMINATION OF POTENTIAL EXTRINSIC SOURCES OF BACK PAIN AND SCIATICA

This is important if a satisfactory explanation for the symptoms is not found on local examination. The investigation should include:
1. the abdomen
2. the pelvis, including rectal examination
3. the lower limbs
4. the peripheral vascular system

3. GENERAL EXAMINATION

General survey of other parts of the body. The local symptoms may be only one manifestation of a widespread disease

Movements of the spinal column and related joints

The spinal column. The joints of the spinal column must necessarily be considered as a group, for it is impracticable to study the movement of each joint independently. The movements to be examined are flexion, extension, lateral flexion to right and left, and rotation to right and left. It should be noted particularly whether the spinal muscles go into protective spasm when movement is attempted. *Flexion*: Instruct the patient to stretch the fingers towards the toes, keeping the knees straight. It is important to judge what proportion of the movement occurs at the spine and how much is contributed by hip flexion (Fig. 13.1). Some patients can almost reach their toes, despite a stiff back, simply by flexing unusually far at the hips. (Normally the hamstrings limit hip flexion to about 90° when the knees are straight.) The range may be expressed roughly as a percentage of the normal, or as the distance by which the fingers fail to reach the floor. A more accurate assessment is made by measuring the linear widening of the interspinous spaces as indicated by a tape measure laid along the line of the spinous processes, which may be marked with a pen. The excursion of the spinous processes between full extension and fullest flexion may thus be measured on the tape. An excursion of four centimetres between the twelfth thoracic spinous process and the first sacral prominence between full extension and fullest flexion indicates good lumbar mobility. *Extension*: Instruct the patient to arch the spine backwards, looking up at the ceiling. Judge the range and express approximately as a percentage of the normal; or measure the excursion as described above. *Lateral flexion*: Instruct the patient to slide each hand in turn down the lateral side of the corresponding thigh. Observe the range. *Rotation*: With the feet fixed, the patient rotates the shoulders towards each side in turn. Hold the pelvis steady, and note the range of spinal rotation as distinct from that which occurs at the knees and hips.

Related joints. *The costo-vertebral joints*: The mobility of the costo-vertebral joints is judged from the range of chest expansion. The normal difference in chest girth between full inspiration and full expiration is about 7 or 8 cm.

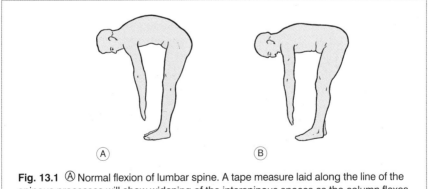

Ⓐ   Ⓑ

Fig. 13.1 Ⓐ Normal flexion of lumbar spine. A tape measure laid along the line of the spinous processes will show widening of the interspinous spaces as the column flexes. Ⓑ Apparent or false flexion due entirely to movement at the hips, the hamstrings being unusually lax. A tape measure laid along the line of the spinous processes shows little excursion of their tips. In assessing trunk flexion it is important to judge in this way how much of the movement occurs at the spinal joints and how much at the hips.

A marked reduction of chest expansion is of particular significance when ankylosing spondylitis is suspected. *The sacro-iliac joints*: It is not practicable to measure the range of sacro-iliac movement. But the joints should be moved passively to determine whether pain is produced, as it will be in arthritic conditions of the joints. A simple method is to grip each iliac crest and compress the pelvis strongly from side to side.

Palpation of iliac fossae and groins

Palpation of the iliac fossae and groins is an essential step in the examination of the back. Its specific purpose is to determine whether or not there is a soft-tissue thickening or abscess. It should be remembered that a 'psoas' abscess originating from a tuberculous lesion of the lumbar spine first becomes palpable deep in the iliac fossa. Such an abscess is felt most easily by pressing the flat palmar surface of the hand and fingers against the flat inner aspect of the iliac bone. To do this the surgeon must stand at the side of the couch corresponding to the side being examined – that is, he must stand on the right of the patient to examine the right iliac fossa and on the left to examine the left iliac fossa (Fig. 13.2).

Neurological examination of the lower limbs

Disorders of the back are so frequently accompanied by radiating pain, paraesthesiae, or other manifestations in the lower limb that a neurological survey should be carried out as a routine.

Straight leg raising test. Holding the knee straight, lift each lower limb in turn to determine the range of pain-free movement (normal = 90°; often more in women) (Fig. 13.3). When associated with clearly defined sciatica (and in the absence of gross disease of the hip), marked impairment of straight leg raising by pain suggests mechanical interference with one or more of the roots of the sciatic nerve. The pain is easily explained. Even a normal sciatic nerve is tautened by straight leg raising, though not to the point of causing pain by dragging on the meningeal sheath that encloses the nerve root. If a nerve is already stretched or anchored, as by a protruded piece of an intervertebral disc or a tumour, the further tautening entailed in lifting the limb is sufficient to cause pain.

When a nerve is tensely stretched, raising the straight leg on the unaffected side may cause pain on the affected side. This sign, termed the crossed sciatic

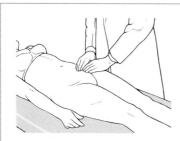

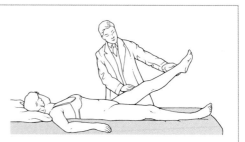

Fig. 13.2 Palpating the iliac fossae for abscess. This is an essential step in the routine examination of the spine.

Fig. 13.3 The straight leg raising test, an important part of the neurological examination of the lower limbs.

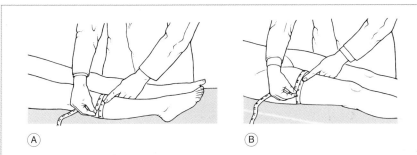

Fig. 13.4   Ⓐ Girth measurement at the widest part is a reliable method of comparing the bulk of the calf muscles on the two sides. Ⓑ Measurement is less reliable in comparing the bulk of the thigh muscles because of the conical shape of the thigh and the difficulty of taking the measurement at an exactly comparable level on each side.

reflex, is a well-recognised feature of prolapsed lumbar intervertebral disc with nerve pressure.

Muscular system. Examine the muscles for wasting, hypertrophy, and fasciculation. Note the tone and test the power of each muscle group, comparing it with its counterpart in the opposite limb. Circumferential measurement is a reliable method of comparing the bulk of the calf muscles, the girth being measured at the widest part or 'equator' (Fig. 13.4A). Circumferential measurement of the thighs, on the other hand, tends to be inaccurate, and may be misleading, on account of the conical shape of the thigh (Fig. 13.4B). Often a more accurate assessment of the relative volume of the two thighs is obtained from inspection and palpation. If the thighs are measured, the girth should be taken on each side at an equal distance above the knee – 12 or 15 cm above the upper margin of the patella is usually a convenient level.

Power of the muscles is estimated in comparison with the opposite side. Not only the major muscle groups should be tested: significant information may emerge from assessing the power of the toe muscles, and in particular of the extensor hallucis longus, which characteristically is weakened by lesions (such as prolapsed intervertebral disc) involving the fifth lumbar nerve.

Sensory system. Examine the patient's sensibility to touch and pin prick, paying particular attention to the sites of any impairment. A knowledge of the innervation of the dermatomes (Fig. 13.5) is essential as this may give an indication of the level of any nerve roots affected. When indicated, test also the sensibility to deep stimuli, joint position, vibration, and heat and cold.

Reflexes. Compare on the two sides the knee jerk (dependent mainly on the L4 nerve) and the ankle jerk (mainly S1). It is important to note not only the presence or absence of the response, but also any difference of intensity (Fig. 13.6). Test the plantar reflex.

Electromyography. Electromyographic examination of selected muscles in the lower leg may have an occasional place in helping to establish whether or not there is degeneration in the innervating lumbar or sacral nerve, as indicated by abnormal potentials in the resting muscle. For instance, abnormal potentials in the lateral half of the gastrocnemius muscle or in the extensor digitorum brevis suggest degeneration of the fifth lumbar nerve, whereas abnormal potentials in the medial half of the gastrocnemius or in the soleus indicate the first sacral nerve.

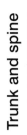
Trunk and spine

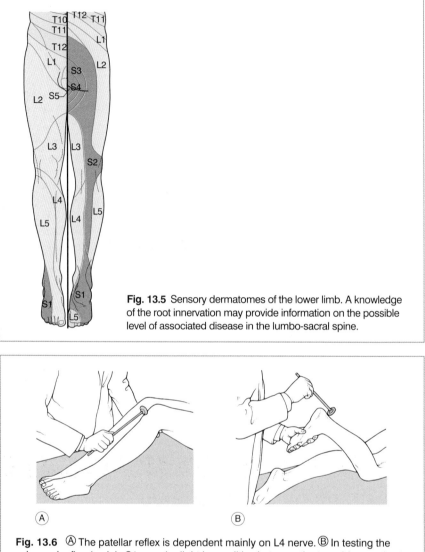

Fig. 13.5 Sensory dermatomes of the lower limb. A knowledge of the root innervation may provide information on the possible level of associated disease in the lumbo-sacral spine.

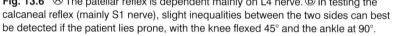

(A)   (B)

Fig. 13.6 Ⓐ The patellar reflex is dependent mainly on L4 nerve. Ⓑ In testing the calcaneal reflex (mainly S1 nerve), slight inequalities between the two sides can best be detected if the patient lies prone, with the knee flexed 45° and the ankle at 90°.

Imaging

Radiographic examination. If the complaint is clearly localised to the thoracic spine, antero-posterior and lateral radiographs of that area alone will usually suffice. If the lumbar spine is the part complained of, radiographs should include not only antero-posterior and lateral views of the lumbar spine but also at least one view of the sacro-iliac joints, pelvis, and hip joints. In cases of doubt additional projections may be required. Oblique projections – from half right and half left – are essential for the proper study of the sacro-iliac joints and the posterior intervertebral (facet) joints of the lumbar region. If a spinal tumour is suspected further imaging with magnetic resonance scanning is required.

Other methods of imaging. *Radioisotope bone scanning* (p. 21) is of particular value in examination of the spinal column, especially in the early detection of metastatic deposits.

Computerised tomography (CT scanning) (p. 12) is valuable in selected cases. It gives cross-sectional images of the trunk that reveal bony abnormalities very clearly.

Magnetic resonance imaging (MRI) is even more informative in demonstrating the intervertebral disc substance, the nerve roots, other soft tissues, and their relationship to the bony structures.

Discography (radiography after injection of radio-opaque fluid into the nucleus pulposus) indicates the integrity or otherwise of the disc, but the technique has been largely superseded by magnetic resonance imaging.

Extrinsic sources of back pain and sciatica

The back offers many pitfalls in diagnosis. Sometimes there are no local symptoms to indicate that the spine is the seat of the disorder, pain being referred entirely to the buttock or to the lower limb. Thus patients often complain only of pain 'in the hip' or 'in the leg' when the true source of the trouble is the lumbar spine. Conversely, the symptoms may suggest a spinal lesion when in fact they arise from an affection of the abdomen, pelvis, or lower limb, or from occlusion of a major artery or a leaking aortic aneurysm. Finally, it should always be remembered that back symptoms may be no more than a local manifestation of a generalised skeletal disease.

Thus the investigation of back or sciatic symptoms must extend further than a study of the spine itself; it must include an examination of the abdomen, pelvis, lower limbs, and vascular system, and a general survey of the rest of the body.

CONGENITAL ABNORMALITIES AND DEFORMITIES

LUMBAR AND SACRAL VARIATIONS

Minor variations of the bony anatomy are common, especially in the lumbar and sacral regions. Most are of little practical importance. They include: deficient or rudimentary lowest ribs; incomplete or complete incorporation of the fifth lumbar vertebral body in the sacrum (sacralisation of the fifth lumbar vertebra); persistence of the first sacral segment as a separate vertebra (lumbarisation of the first sacral vertebra); and over-development of the fifth lumbar transverse process on one or both sides with, in marked cases, a false joint between the hypertrophied process and the ilium (Fig. 13.7A). In the last-mentioned condition the false joint is sometimes a source of pain.

HEMIVERTEBRA

In this anomaly a vertebra is formed in one lateral half only. The defect may occur at any level. The body of the half-vertebra is wedge-shaped, and the spine is angled laterally at the site of the defect (Fig. 13.7B). This anomaly is a rare cause of scoliosis.

Trunk and spine

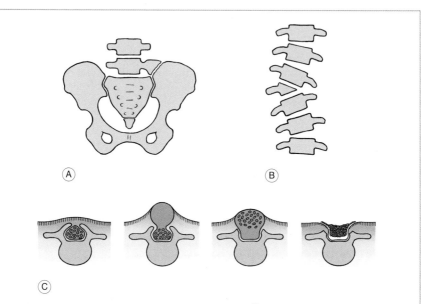

Fig. 13.7 Three congenital anomalies of the spine. Ⓐ Hypertrophied transverse process forming false joint with ilium. Ⓑ Hemivertebra, an occasional cause of scoliosis. Ⓒ Four examples of spina bifida. In all, the neural arch of the vertebra is deficient posteriorly. In the first diagram, representing spina bifida occulta, there is no other deficiency; the skin and soft tissues are intact. In the second diagram overlying soft tissues are also deficient and the spinal theca bulges backwards to form a meningocele. In the third diagram nerve elements are also displaced backwards within the bulging sac (myelomeningocele). In the final diagram skin is deficient as well, and nerve elements are exposed on the surface (rachischisis).

SPINA BIFIDA (Spinal dysraphism)

The basic fault in spina bifida is a failure of the embryonic neural plate to fold over to form a closed neural tube, or of mesodermal tissue fully to invest the neural tube as it does in the normal embryo to form the vertebral arch with its spinous process and the surrounding muscles and ligaments. Different grades of the anomaly are shown in Figure 13.7C.

In most cases spina bifida is of minor degree and not a cause of disability. Indeed it is often found incidentally during radiography for some other reason. The importance of spina bifida lies in the fact that in the more severe forms there is a co-existing lesion of the nerve elements. The subject of spina bifida with neurological involvement was discussed in Chapter 11 (p. 171).

SCOLIOSIS

The term *scoliosis* denotes lateral curvature of the spine. The deformity may be 'structural', implying a permanent change in the bones or soft tissues, or it may be no more than a temporary disturbance produced by reflex or postural activity of the spinal muscles. Five types can be recognised:

1. infantile scoliosis, a type seen in very young children which may either resolve to normal or become progressively worse
2. primary or 'idiopathic' structural scoliosis, a well-defined group of unknown cause arising in children
3. secondary structural scoliosis, a miscellaneous group in which the curvature is secondary to a demonstrable underlying disorder
4. compensatory scoliosis
5. sciatic scoliosis, a temporary deformity.

Infantile scoliosis

Infantile scoliosis begins in the first year of life as a simple curve, usually convex to the left, without known cause. There are two subgroups – resolving and progressive – and it is usually possible to distinguish them by the radiographic appearance.

Idiopathic structural scoliosis

Idiopathic scoliosis is the commonest and the most important type of structural scoliosis. It begins in childhood or adolescence and tends to increase progressively until the cessation of skeletal growth. It sometimes leads to severe and ugly deformity, especially when the thoracic region is the part affected. The exact cause of the growth disturbance is unknown: the children are otherwise healthy. The condition is much commoner in girls than in boys. This fact, together with its frequent onset at puberty, suggests a possible link with the hormonal control of bone growth. Recent evidence has suggested a genetic link with the disorder and several candidate genes are currently under investigation.

Pathology. Any part of the thoraco-lumbar spine may be affected. There is a primary structural curve, with secondary compensatory curves above and below. The pattern of curve and its natural evolution are fairly constant for each site, and the following types are recognised: lumbar scoliosis, thoraco-lumbar scoliosis, and thoracic scoliosis (Fig. 13.8A). The lateral curvature is constantly accompanied by rotation of the vertebrae on a vertical axis, the body of the vertebra rotating towards the convexity of the curve and the spinous process away from the convexity. By thrusting the ribs backwards on the convex side this rotation increases the ugliness of the deformity (Fig. 13.8).

Clinical features. The onset is usually in middle childhood – often between the ages of 10 and 12 years, at the time of the adolescent growth spurt.

In children deformity is usually the only symptom. Pain is occasionally a feature in adults with long-standing deformity, particularly with structural curves in the lumbar region of the spine.

Course and prognosis. The outlook depends upon the age at onset and upon the site of the primary curve. The ultimate visible deformity tends to be worst in thoracic scoliosis and least in lumbar scoliosis. The curvature tends to increase until the end of the period of spinal growth, but not significantly thereafter. In general, therefore, the earlier the onset the worse the prognosis.

Treatment. The first essential is to assess the prognosis for progression of the deformity from a consideration of the age of onset and the site and severity of the curve. This requires the identification of the first and last vertebrae in the primary curve and the measurement of the Cobb angle between them on an erect AP radiograph of the spine (Fig. 13.9). When the prognosis is good (for instance, in most cases of lumbar scoliosis) expectant treatment, with regular

Trunk and spine

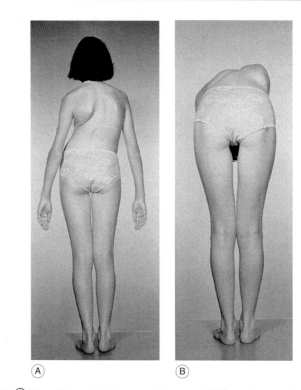

(A)   (B)

Fig. 13.8 (A) Idiopathic scoliosis in an adolescent girl. The main curve is in the thoracic region. There is marked rotation of the vertebrae, causing posterior prominence of the ribs on the side of the convexity. In lumbar scoliosis the deformity is much less noticeable. (B) In forward flexion the ugliness of the deformity caused by the backward rotation of the ribs on the convex side of the curve becomes more apparent.

clinical and radiological reviews every six months, may be all that is required. But when the prognosis is poor (as in thoracic scoliosis with early onset or a curve in excess of 45–50°) active treatment is advised. This usually necessitates operation, and much surgical endeavour has been spent in the quest for an effective and safe method of correcting the deformity and maintaining the correction while fusion occurs. Surgical treatment is usually deferred until early adolescence to minimise the loss of height which may result from fusion of a significant length of the growing spine. To prevent further deterioration in the curvature during this waiting period, conservative management with various types of orthotic bracing has been used.

For many years the brace most commonly employed was the Milwaukee brace. This used the principle of three-point correction by distracting the spine between a pelvic band and an occipito-cervical support, with additional lateral pressure from a pad applied to the chest wall at the apex of the curvature. Recently doubt has been cast on the effectiveness of this type of bracing, and because of frequent problems of acceptance by the patient, an alternative

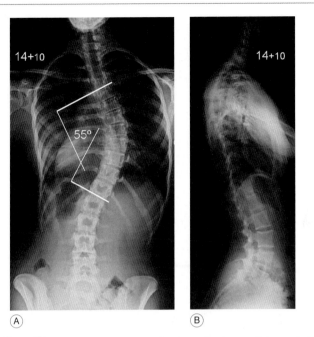

Fig. 13.9 Ⓐ and Ⓑ Radiographs of thoraco-lumbar spine in an adolescent girl with an idiopathic scoliois. The measurement of the Cobb angle on the AP film shows a severe curve of 55° that would justify surgical treatment.

under-arm thoraco-lumbar jacket, or Boston brace (Fig. 13.10), has been used. This provides only two-point correction and it acts by flattening the lumbar lordosis; thus it is most suitable for lower curvatures with an apex below the ninth thoracic vertebra.

The principle of surgical treatment is to fuse the joints of all the vertebrae within the primary curve, after having first achieved the greatest possible correction of the curvature. When surgical treatment was first introduced correction was obtained by pre-operative traction or corrective plaster casts. It is now routinely gained at the time of operation by the use of an internal corrective implant. For many years the device used for this purpose was the Harrington distraction rod. This was inserted posteriorly in the concavity of the curve between two hooks placed under the laminae of the top and bottom vertebrae and then forcibly elongated to produce straightening. The results from this technique were encouraging, with up to 50% correction of the lateral curvature, though this was not reflected in improvement of the cosmetic deformity, which largely results from vertebral rotation. This led to a search for other methods of correction including the use of anterior interbody fixation devices, though these necessitated thoracotomy with its associated morbidity in terms of decreased lung function. Currently most specialist surgeons favour posterior correction with multiple-level segmental pedicle screw fixation devices (Cotrel-Dubousset instrumentation) (Fig. 13.11). This was an advance over the Harrington instrumentation because it improved correction in both the sagittal and coronal planes.

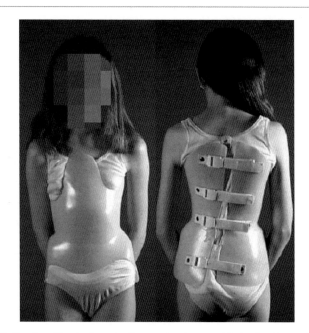

Fig. 13.10 Front and back view of a thoraco-lumbar moulded orthosis used for the conservative treatment of scoliois. The brace does not correct the deformity, but may prevent further deterioration of minor curves until skeletal maturity is reached.

Other methods of fixation and correction may be required for more severe curvatures, or when abnormal vertebral pathology exists, as in congenital curvatures which may include a kyphotic component.

The place of these various specialised techniques has not yet been finally established: they all carry a risk of neurological complications and require intraoperative spinal cord monitoring, which is only available in specialist centres.

It must be emphasised that it is impossible to prevent the increase of a progressive scoliotic deformity by exercises alone, though these are an important adjunct to bracing, and useful in preserving mobility. The aim of all treatment must be to minimise progression, or to correct the deformity to an acceptable level at skeletal maturity. It is difficult and often impracticable to correct long-standing deformity in adults by any method.

Secondary structural scoliosis

In this group the spinal curvature is secondary to a demonstrable underlying abnormality.

Causes. The three commonest underlying causes are congenital abnormalities (especially hemivertebra), poliomyelitis with residual weakness of the spinal muscles (paralytic scoliosis), and neurofibromatosis.

Pathology. In *congenital hemivertebra* there is a sharp angulation at the site of the anomaly, with compensatory curves above and below (Fig. 13.7B). Scoliosis following *poliomyelitis* is explained by unequal pull of the muscles on the two

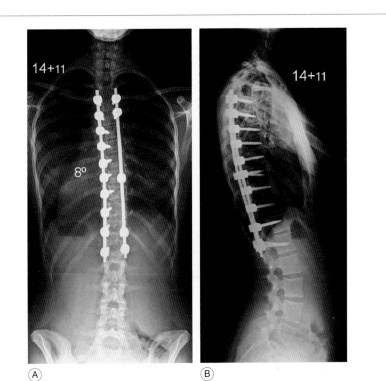

Fig. 13.11 Ⓐand ⒷRadiographs of the same patient shown in Figure 13.9 after surgical correction and fusion with segmental pedicle fixation which has reduced the curve to 8°.

sides. The mechanism of scoliosis complicating *neurofibromatosis* is not clear; in this type the deformity may be very severe.

Clinical features. In most cases the visible deformity is the only symptom. The age of onset, site, nature, and severity of the curve vary with the underlying cause.

Complications. In exceptional cases of severe long-standing scoliosis the sharp angulation of the spinal cord over the apex of the deformity may cause interference with cord function, with consequent neurological manifestations leading in the worst cases to total paralysis below the level of the obstruction.

Treatment. In most cases treatment is along the lines suggested for idiopathic scoliosis.

Compensatory scoliosis

Lumbar scoliosis is seen as a compensatory device when the pelvis is tilted laterally – as, for instance, when the lower limbs are unequal in length, or when there is a fixed abduction or adduction deformity at one or other hip. In such a case it is only by curving the lumbar spine through an angle equal to the pelvic tilt that the trunk can be held vertical. Usually there is no intrinsic abnormality of the spine itself, and the scoliosis disappears automatically when the pelvic tilt is corrected. In cases of many years' duration, however, the lumbar scoliosis may become fixed by adaptive shortening of the tissues on the concave side.

Sciatic scoliosis

Sciatic scoliosis is a temporary deformity produced by the protective action of muscles in certain painful conditions of the spine.

Cause. In many cases the underlying cause is a prolapsed intervertebral disc impinging upon a lumbar or sacral nerve. But the deformity may also be observed in some cases of acute low back pain (p. 241), the pathogenesis of which is not entirely clear.

Pathology. The curve is in the lumbar region. The abnormal posture is assumed involuntarily in an attempt to reduce as far as possible the painful pressure upon the affected nerve or joint, usually from a lumbar disc protrusion.

Clinical features. The predominant feature is severe back pain or sciatica, aggravated by movements of the spine (see prolapsed lumbar intervertebral disc, p. 236). The onset is usually sudden. The scoliosis is poorly compensated; so the trunk may be tilted over markedly to one side (see Fig. 13.27, p. 238). The curvature is not associated with rotation of the vertebrae.

Treatment. The treatment is that of the underlying condition.

KYPHOSIS

Kyphosis is the general term used to define excessive posterior curvature of the spinal column. The deformity may take the form of a long rounded curve ('round back'), or there may be a localised sharp posterior angulation ('hump back').

In the thoracic region there is normally a considerable posterior curvature: thoracic kyphosis exists only if this curve is excessive. In the cervical and lumbar regions there is normally an anterior curvature (lordosis): any reversal of this constitutes cervical or lumbar kyphosis.

Causes. Kyphosis is a manifestation of an underlying disorder of the spine. The causes are numerous. The following are the most important:

1. tuberculosis of the spinal column
2. wedge compression fracture of a vertebral body
3. Scheuermann's kyphosis
4. ankylosing spondylitis
5. osteoporosis
6. destructive tumours of the spinal column (especially metastatic carcinoma).

Treatment. The treatment is that of the underlying condition. Often the deformity is best accepted unless it is unduly severe.

LORDOSIS

Lordosis is the opposite deformity to kyphosis. The term denotes excessive anterior curvature of the spinal column ('hollow back'). In practice, lordosis is seen only in the lumbar region, where a slight anterior curve is normal. Strictly, the term lordosis should be used only when this normal curve is exaggerated.

Causes. Spinal disorders tend to cause kyphosis or scoliosis rather than lordosis. In many cases lordosis is simply a postural deformity, predisposed to by lax muscles and heavy abdomen. Sometimes it is compensatory, balancing a kyphotic deformity above or below, or a fixed flexion deformity of a hip.

TUBERCULOSIS OF THE THORACIC OR LUMBAR SPINE (TUBERCULOUS SPONDYLITIS; POTT'S DISEASE[1])

Tuberculosis of thoracic or lumbar vertebral bodies was formerly one of the commonest forms of skeletal tuberculosis, and it is still prevalent in some Eastern countries, though now seen only rarely in the West.

Pathology. The infection begins at the anterior margin of a vertebral body, near the intervertebral disc (Fig. 13.12A). The disc itself is usually involved at an early stage. The extent of the destruction varies widely from case to case. Commonly there is complete destruction of one intervertebral disc with partial destruction of the two adjacent vertebrae, most marked anteriorly (Fig. 13.12B). But the changes may extend over several spinal segments; or, on the other hand, they may be confined to a single intervertebral disc, without evident bone involvement (Fig. 13.13A). Anterior collapse of the affected vertebrae leads to an angular kyphosis (Figs 13.12B, 13.13B and 13.14).

Abscess formation is usual. In the thoracic region pus collects around the spinal column, forming a fusiform paraspinal abscess (Fig. 13.14); or it may track towards the surface between ribs. From the lower thoracic or lumbar region pus tracks downwards behind the fascial sheath of the psoas muscle and generally bursts into the compartment behind the iliacus fascia to form a palpable abscess in the iliac fossa (psoas abscess). An abscess occasionally points posteriorly, or in the thigh. As in most instances of skeletal tuberculosis, the inflammation is low-grade and chronic rather than acute: hence the term 'cold abscess' for the quiet suppuration that is a common feature.

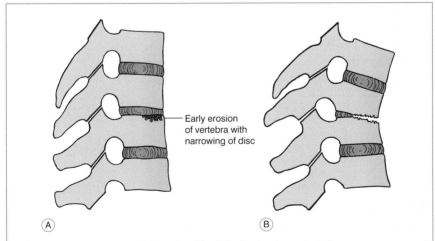

Early erosion
of vertebra with
narrowing of disc

Ⓐ   Ⓑ

Fig. 13.12 Tuberculosis of the spine. The infection begins anteriorly near an intervertebral disc, which is soon destroyed Ⓐ. It may spread to adjacent vertebrae, which collapse in front, with consequent angular kyphosis Ⓑ.

[1]Percivall Pott (1714–1788) London surgeon who worked at St. Bartholomew's Hospital and described the paraplegia from spinal disease in 1779 as well as the ankle fracture that bears his name.

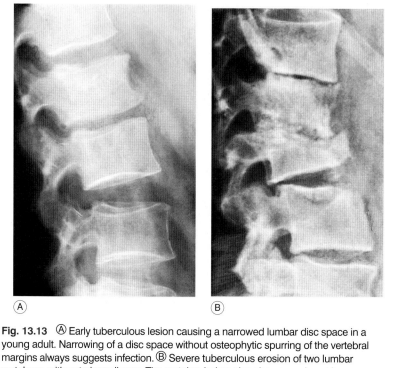

(A)   (B)

Fig. 13.13 Ⓐ Early tuberculous lesion causing a narrowed lumbar disc space in a young adult. Narrowing of a disc space without osteophytic spurring of the vertebral margins always suggests infection. Ⓑ Severe tuberculous erosion of two lumbar vertebrae, with anterior collapse. The vertebra below also shows erosion at its upper anterior corner. One intervertebral disc is destroyed and the one above is much narrowed.

Secondary effects. An abscess or mass of granulation tissue encroaching upon the spinal canal may interfere with the spinal cord or with a spinal nerve. In cases of long-standing severe kyphosis the spinal cord is occasionally damaged by the bony ridge at the site of deformity.

Clinical features. The disease is commonest in young adults. One or more of the following symptoms may be present:

1. pain in the back
2. stiffness of the back
3. visible deformity of the back (kyphosis)
4. localised swelling (abscess)
5. weakness of legs or visceral dysfunction from involvement of the spinal cord.

On examination, the patient often looks ill. There may be visible or palpable angular kyphosis. There is local tenderness on firm palpation or percussion over the affected vertebrae. All spinal movements are greatly restricted and when they are attempted the spinal muscles go into protective spasm. An abscess may be detected over the thoracic wall or in the flank, iliac fossa, or upper thigh. Signs of spinal cord compression ('Pott's paraplegia') or of a nerve root lesion may be present. Tuberculous lesions are often manifest elsewhere.

Imaging. On *radiographic examination* the earliest signs are narrowing of an intervertebral space (Fig. 13.13A) and local vertebral osteoporosis. Later, there is

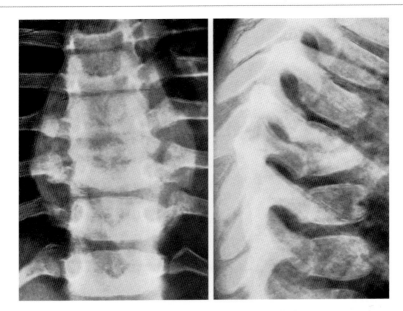

Fig. 13.14 Tuberculosis of the thoracic spine in a child. Note in the antero-posterior view the typical fusiform appearance of a paraspinal abscess, an almost constant feature of thoracic spinal tuberculosis. In the lateral view two vertebral bodies are seen partly collapsed in a wedge-shaped mass; the disc between them has been destroyed.

usually destruction of bone at the anterior margin of one or more of the vertebral bodies, leading to anterior collapse and wedge-shaped deformity of the affected vertebrae (Figs 13.13B and 13.14). An abscess shadow is nearly always visible: in the thoracic region it is seen as a fusiform paraspinal shadow (Fig. 13.14); in the lumbar region it is indicated by lateral bulging of the psoas outline, usually on one side. In the healing stage the bone outline in the area of destruction becomes sharper, and normal density is regained. Abscesses may become calcified. *Magnetic resonance imaging (MRI)* is useful in defining the extent of the soft-tissue abscess more clearly, especially if there are signs of spinal cord dysfunction (Fig. 13.15). *Ultrasound scanning* is useful in defining the extent of an abscess.

Investigations. The erythrocyte sedimentation rate is raised in the active stage. The Mantoux test is positive. Tubercle bacilli can sometimes be isolated from aspirated pus.

Complications. These include:

1. chronic discharging sinus
2. tuberculous infection of other organs, such as meninges, kidneys, or lungs
3. interference with the spinal cord, causing weakness or paralysis in the lower limbs with or without sensory impairment or disturbance of bladder and bowel function ('Pott's paraplegia').

Paraplegia may arise early – that is, during the active stage of the disease – when it is caused by the pressure of pus or granulation tissue; or it may arise many years after healing has occurred, from mechanical impedance of the spinal cord where it is sharply angled at the apex of a severe kyphos ('late onset paraplegia').

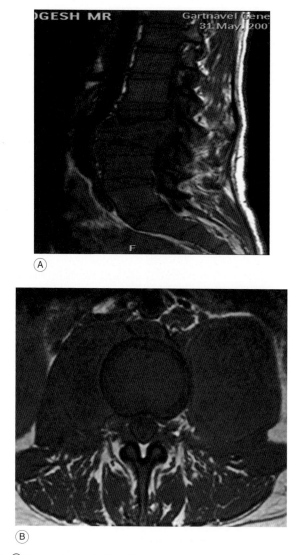

Fig. 13.15 Ⓐ Tuberculous infection of the lumbar spine shown on sagittal MR scan. The L2 disc is destroyed as are the adjacent end vertebral endplates and a soft-tissue mass is seen anterior to the spine with some abnormal soft tissue also extending into the spinal canal. Ⓑ An axial T2 scan demonstrates large fluid-filled para-spinal masses, which are the 'cold' psoas abscesses typical of tuberculous infections.

Prognosis. The prognosis is worse in certain Asian and African countries where the disease tends to be more florid, than in Britain, North America and the Antipodes where it is usually mild and responsive to treatment.

Treatment. Treatment of spinal tuberculosis is now much more often ambulatory than it was in the past, largely because of the efficacy of antituberculous drugs. Nowadays treatment may entail only a brief stay in hospital – or indeed it may often be carried out entirely on an out-patient basis.

Conservative treatment. Conservative management relies almost entirely upon antibacterial agents. Results from long-term controlled trials have now shown that short-course regimens based on isoniazid, rifampicin and pyrazin-amide for six to nine months are as effective as longer-term treatment for up to 18 months with the addition of streptomycin. In more severe disease local treatment for the spine may be required by a short period of bed rest or immobilisation by a plaster jacket for relief of pain, but in most cases antibiotic treatment can be continued on an ambulant outpatient basis. Adjuvant operation may be required in certain circumstances, mainly for the drainage of an abscess.

1. An abscess that is superficial should be either aspirated or drained by simple incision followed by immediate suture of the wound
2. A paraspinal abscess in the thoracic region may be drained from the back by removing the head and neck of a rib and the adjacent transverse process (costo-transversectomy).

With this regimen, satisfactory healing may be expected in a high proportion of patients, though often with some residual kyphosis.

Operative treatment. The alternative management is by radical operation as developed by Hodgson in Hong Kong. This may promote more rapid healing. The affected part of the spinal column is approached anteriorly and all diseased bone is excised. Thereafter the gap is bridged by bone grafts. Adjuvant antibacterial agents are given. By this method the duration of treatment is shortened and kyphosis may often be prevented or corrected.

Relief of paraplegia. If paraplegia from compression of the spinal cord does not show rapid improvement after the commencement of antibacterial therapy the spinal canal should be decompressed by operation. Occasionally this may be achieved by costo-transversectomy alone (see above), particularly if a paraspinal abscess is the chief factor responsible for the compression. More reliably, it may be done by clearance of pus, necrotic tissue and diseased bone from the region of the spinal theca, either through an anterior approach or through a lateral route by unilateral excision of the pedicles of three or four vertebrae (lateral rhachotomy; antero-lateral decompression).

Assessment of cure. Signs of quiescence are: good general health; diminishing blood sedimentation rate; and arrest of the destructive process with hardening of the bony outlines as seen radiographically.

PYOGENIC INFECTION OF THE THORACIC OR LUMBAR SPINE (Pyogenic spondylitis; osteomyelitis of the spined; discitis)

Pyogenic infection of the spine is uncommon. It has often been confused with tuberculous spondylitis, which it may resemble clinically and radiographically, though it tends to run a more acute course.

Cause. It is caused by infection with the staphylococcus, streptococcus, pneumococcus, or occasionally with other bacteria such as the typhoid bacillus or other salmonella organisms, or *Brucella abortus*.

Pathology. Organisms usually reach the spinal column through the general blood stream, from a septic focus elsewhere. Other possible routes are through the spinal venous plexus from a focus in the pelvis, or through lymphatic channels from a neighbouring focus. As in tuberculous spondylitis, there is destruction of an intervertebral disc and erosion of the adjacent bone, with or without abscess formation. The spinal cord may be damaged by pressure, or by thrombosis of its vessels.

Clinical features. The clinical picture is inconstant: there are remarkable variations in the severity of the symptoms from case to case. The onset is often acute or subacute, and may be accompanied by pyrexia, with local pain and restriction of all movements by muscle spasm. A suppurative process elsewhere in the body is usually present or has recently subsided; or infection may follow operation for removal of displaced disc material, with consequent 'discitis'.

Imaging. Radiographs show local rarefaction or erosion of bone, diminution of disc space, and sometimes sub-ligamentous new bone formation. MRI scanning may also reveal the extent of soft tissue and bone involvement by the infective abscess (Fig. 13.16). After healing, spontaneous bony fusion of affected vertebrae is often observed.

Investigations. The erythrocyte sedimentation rate is raised. Polymorphonuclear leucocytosis is to be expected. Serological studies can occasionally incriminate a particular organism, such as one of the salmonella group.

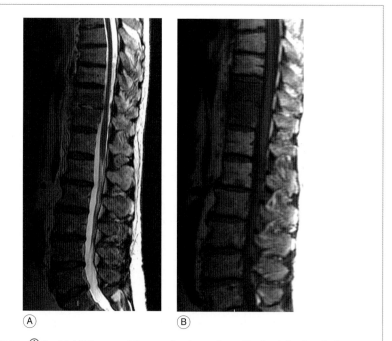

Fig. 13.16 Ⓐ Sagittal MR scan of thoraco-lumbar spine with disc infection. In the lower thoracic region there is a narrowed disc space (arrow) which shows high signal on T2 indicating the presence of fluid. The discs above and below this level appear normal. Ⓑ Sagittal T1 image of the same patient showing that the vertebrae on either side of the disc are of much lower signal. This indicates the presence of marked bone oedema and combined with the fluid in the narrowed disc allows a diagnosis of infective discitis to be made.

Treatment. Appropriate antibacterial drugs are given. The spine is rested, at first in bed, but later with a suitable brace, until healing occurs. An abscess may require early drainage, especially if the spinal cord is threatened.

RHEUMATOID ARTHRITIS OF THE SPINAL JOINTS (General description of rheumatoid arthritis, p. 134)

It has been noted above that rheumatoid arthritis often affects the cervical spine. Joints of the thoracic and lumbar spine may likewise be affected, but clinical manifestations are relatively uncommon. They consist in aching pain of a rather diffuse type, with impairment of spinal movements. The symptoms develop insidiously, without preceding injury. Examination of the limbs will usually reveal typical rheumatoid changes in several joints.

OSTEOARTHRITIS OF THE THORACIC AND LUMBAR SPINE (Spondylarthritis; spondylarthrosis; spondylosis)

Osteoarthritis of the thoracic or lumbar intervertebral joints is found very commonly in those used to heavy work, but it is not necessarily accompanied by symptoms.

Cause. Predisposing factors are:

1. previous injury to the spinal joints
2. previous disease involving the joints (for example, Scheuermann's kyphosis or an intervertebral disc lesion).

As in other joints the cause of degeneration is unknown, but may be the manifestation of an ageing process in the cartilage tissue.

Pathology. The changes affect the central intervertebral (body-to-body) joints and the posterior intervertebral (facet) joints. One segment or several segments may be affected. In the central joints, which are affected first, there is degeneration with consequent narrowing of the intervertebral disc, and hypertrophy of bone at the joint margins leads to the formation of osteophytes (Fig. 13.17). In the posterior intervertebral (facet) joints the changes are those of osteoarthritis in any diarthrodial joint – namely, attrition of the articular cartilage and osteophyte formation (spurring) at the joint margins. These changes in the facet joints are probably the more important from a clinical point of view.

Secondary effects. Rarely, osteophytes encroach upon an intervertebral foramen sufficiently to interfere with the function of the issuing nerve. Thinning of the articular cartilage of the posterior intervertebral (facet) joints reduces the stability of the affected segment and predisposes to one type of spondylolisthesis (p. 242). In severe cases the osteophytes around the facet joints may encroach on the spinal canal resulting in the syndrome of spinal stenosis (p. 245).

Clinical features. Spinal osteoarthritis can exist in quite marked degree without causing symptoms. But there is often a complaint of aching pain in the affected area, worse on activity or after prolonged standing or sitting in one position, and especially after stooping or lifting. Pain is often worse first thing in the morning, and there may be a feeling of stiffness when rising from a sitting position. In the lumbar region there is a tendency to acute exacerbations of pain, usually arising suddenly and lasting a few weeks. These are possibly explained by strain or momentary subluxation of an unstable degenerate joint. Interference with a nerve

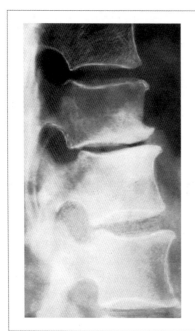

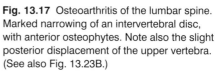

Fig. 13.17 Osteoarthritis of the lumbar spine. Marked narrowing of an intervertebral disc, with anterior osteophytes. Note also the slight posterior displacement of the upper vertebra. (See also Fig. 13.23B.)

in a narrowed intervertebral foramen leads to radiating pain in the distribution of the affected nerve (girdle pain or sciatica according to the level affected).

On examination in the quiet phase, the objective findings are slight. Spinal movements may be moderately restricted, especially flexion; but there is no muscle spasm. If there is interference with a lumbar nerve root straight leg raising on the affected side is likely to be restricted. Apart from this, objective neurological signs are exceptional. During an acute exacerbation of pain there may be marked impairment of spinal movements, with muscle spasm.

Radiographic features. The changes are most obvious in the central (body-to-body) intervertebral joints, which show narrowing of the intervertebral space and osteophyte formation (spurring) at the joint margins (Fig. 13.17). Later the posterior intervertebral (facet) joints also show changes: there is narrowing of the joint space with sharpening of the margins of the facets. These changes are seen clearly only in oblique projections or on CT scans.

Diagnosis. Osteoarthritis has to be distinguished from other causes of back pain and from other causes of radiating nerve pain (girdle pain or sciatica) (see Fig. 13.29, p. 240). It should be remembered that the demonstration of osteoarthritic changes in the radiographs does not necessarily mean that the arthritis is the cause of a patient's symptoms, for spinal osteoarthritis is common and often painless. The diagnosis is always presumptive rather than proved, and it is justified only when other possible causes have been excluded by careful consideration of the history, clinical examination, and radiographs.

Treatment. This depends upon the severity of the disability. In mild cases treatment is unnecessary: explanation and reassurance suffice.

Thoracic spine. In osteoarthritis of the thoracic spine the symptoms are seldom severe, and if treatment is required a course of active spinal exercises to strengthen the posterior muscles is usually sufficient.

Lumbar spine. In lumbar osteoarthritis with moderate disability a well-fitted surgical corset (orthotic brace) will usually afford adequate relief. Physiotherapy, mainly by exercises and passive mobilisation, may also be helpful. Heavy lifting and similar strains to the back should be strictly avoided. Rarely, if the pain from a localised lesion is bad enough to cause serious hardship, operative fusion of the affected segments of the spine may be required.

ANKYLOSING SPONDYLITIS

In ankylosing spondylitis there is chronic inflammation, progressing slowly to bony ankylosis, of the joints of the spinal column and occasionally of the proximal limb joints.

Cause. This is unknown, but may represent an auto-immune response to an infecting organism. The condition is distinct from rheumatoid arthritis, although it has sometimes been loosely termed 'rheumatoid spine'. There is a strong hereditary link to the HLA-B27 gene, which is present in 80–90% of patients. There is also a relationship with certain types of sero-negative chronic juvenile arthritis in members of the family.

Pathology. The disease usually begins in the sacro-iliac joints, whence it usually extends upwards to involve the lumbar, thoracic, and often the cervical spine. In the worst cases the hips or shoulders are also affected. The articular cartilage, synovium, and ligaments show chronic inflammatory changes and eventually they become ossified. After several years the inflammatory process becomes quiescent.

Clinical features. The disease has a strong male preponderance (M:F = 3:1) and it nearly always begins between the ages of 16 and 25. The early symptoms are aching pain in the lower back and increasing stiffness. Later, the pain migrates upwards. Diffuse radiating pain down one or both lower limbs is also common. *On examination* the predominant finding is marked limitation of all movements in the affected area of the spine ('poker back'). When the thoracic region is involved chest expansion is markedly reduced – often to less than 2.5 cm (normal = 7.5 cm) – from ankylosis of the costo-vertebral joints: this is an important diagnostic feature. In a few cases the hips or shoulders are affected, with pain and limitation of movement.

Imaging. Radiographs in the early stage show fuzziness and widening of both the sacro-iliac joints, so that the joint outline is no longer clearly defined (Fig. 13.18). MRI scanning is far more sensitive in detecting these early changes in the sacro-iliac joints (Fig. 13.19). Later, the sacro-iliac joints are completely obliterated and, if the disease progresses, the intervertebral joints in the lumbar, thoracic, and sometimes even the cervical region undergo bony ankylosis, with prominent anterior bridging of the vertebral bodies producing the so-called 'bamboo spine' (Fig. 13.20).

Investigations. The erythrocyte sedimentation rate and C-reactive protein levels are raised while the disease is active. In 90% of cases the test for HLA-B27 antigen is positive.

Diagnosis. In the early stages ankylosing spondylitis has to be distinguished from other causes of back pain and sciatica (see Fig. 13.29, p. 240). The marked limitation of spinal movement, the reduced chest expansion, the typical radiographic features, and the raised erythrocyte sedimentation rate are diagnostic.

Trunk and spine

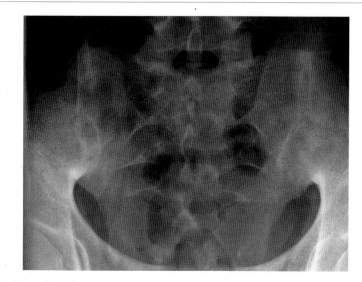

Fig. 13.18 AP radiograph of sacroiliac joints. The joints are completely fused showing the typical appearances of advanced sacroiliitis seen in ankylosing spondylitis.

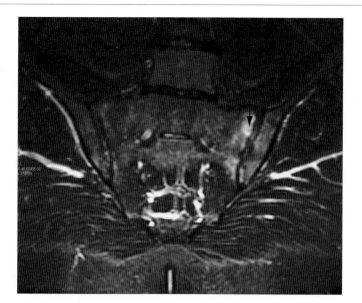

Fig. 13.19 Coronal T2 weighted MR scan of sacroiliac joints in ankylosing spondylitis. There is oedema seen as high signal on either side of the left SI joint (arrow), which indicates an active sacroiliitis. The MR scan is much more sensitive than plain radiographs at detecting early changes in the disease.

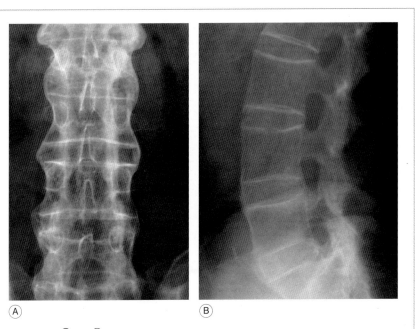

(A)   (B)

Fig. 13.20 Ⓐ and Ⓑ Radiographs of a fused lumbar spine in advanced ankylosing spondylitis. There is ossification of the anterior longitudinal ligament and of the annulus of the discs at all levels giving the so-called 'bamboo spine' appearance typical of the disease.

Course and complications. The disease usually ceases to progress after ten or fifteen years, leaving permanent stiffness, the extent of which varies widely from case to case. Complications include fixed flexion deformity of the spine (Fig. 13.21A), intercurrent respiratory infections, and iridocyclitis, which in severe cases may lead to blindness. There is also a relationship with Crohn's disease (regional ileitis), which may co-exist.

Treatment. Treatment is rather unsatisfactory, in that no method is known by which the disease process can be halted and spinal mobility preserved. In most cases the mainstay of treatment is a non-steroidal anti-inflammatory agent in the first instance. Steroid drugs are inappropriate except for ophthalmic complications. The advent of new biological drugs based on monoclonal antibodies has allowed anti-tumour necrosis factor alpha (antiTNF-α) to be used in the early stages of the disease with moderate success, but the long-term results are not yet available.

Apart from these measures, treatment should be directed towards preserving function and preventing spinal deformity. Activity rather than rest should be prescribed. Special exercises should be practised to make the most of such movement as remains. The patient should adopt the habit of sleeping flat on a firm mattress, ideally in the supine position with a single pillow, to maintain normal spinal alignment.

If a severe flexion deformity of the spine occurs through neglect of these precautions it can result in severe functional disability. This is particularly the case when the hips are involved and develop flexion contractures in addition to the spinal deformity. Relief may be obtained by replacement arthroplasty of both

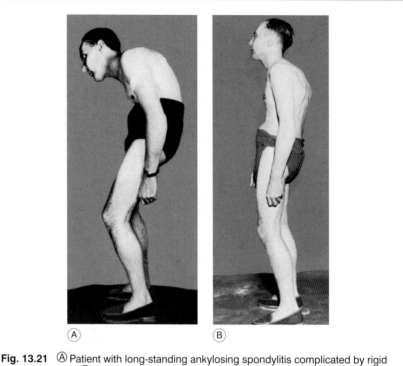

Fig. 13.21 Ⓐ Patient with long-standing ankylosing spondylitis complicated by rigid flexion deformity. Ⓑ After corrective osteotomy in the lumbar region.

hips to restore an upright stance. In a few patients where this fails it may be necessary to undertake a corrective wedge osteotomy of the spine in the lumbar region followed by internal fixation (Fig. 13.21). This is high-risk surgery and should only be performed by surgeons experienced in the procedure.

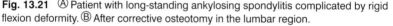

SCHEUERMANN'S KYPHOSIS (Adolescent vertebral osteochondritis; adolescent kyphosis)

Formerly termed *osteochondritis*, Scheuermann's disease[1] is now regarded as unrelated to osteochondritis juvenilis (p. 130) and should no longer be so called. Basically, it seems to be an intrusion of part of the intervertebral disc into the vertebral end plate at multiple levels, mostly in the thoracic region. This leads to a rounded kyphosis. The cause and precise nature of the affection are uncertain. It is uncommon.

Pathology. The vertebral bodies ossify from three centres – a primary centre for the middle of the body, and secondary centres for the upper and lower surfaces. These secondary centres, known as the ring epiphyses, appear at about the time of puberty in the cartilaginous end plates that separate the vertebral

[1]Holger Scheuermann (1877–1960) a famous Danish radiologist who worked at the Cripples Hospital in Copenhagen and described the deformity and its cause in 1921.

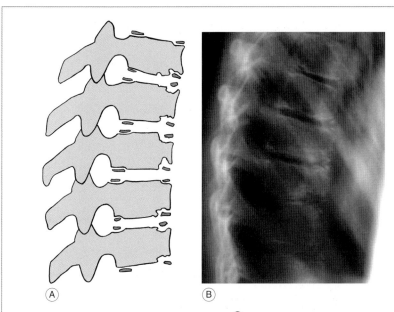

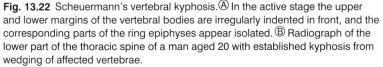

Fig. 13.22 Scheuermann's vertebral kyphosis.Ⓐ In the active stage the upper and lower margins of the vertebral bodies are irregularly indented in front, and the corresponding parts of the ring epiphyses appear isolated. Ⓑ Radiograph of the lower part of the thoracic spine of a man aged 20 with established kyphosis from wedging of affected vertebrae.

bodies from the adjacent intervertebral discs. In Scheuermann's disease there is a disturbance of the normal development of the cartilage plates and ring epiphyses, possibly because they are damaged by bursting of the disc contents through the cartilage into the subjacent vertebral body (Fig. 13.22A). The changes occur predominantly near the anterior margins of the vertebrae, where the greatest weight-thrust is borne. In consequence the disc is somewhat narrowed anteriorly, and through deficient growth of the affected part of the ring epiphysis the vertebral body becomes slightly wedge-shaped (Fig. 13.22B). The deformity predisposes to the later development of osteoarthritis.

Characteristically Scheuermann's disease affects several vertebrae in the thoracic region. Occasionally similar changes are confined to a single vertebra, and this localised form of the disease is as common in the lumbar as in the thoracic region.

Clinical features. The patient is usually 13 to 16 years old, and more often a boy than a girl. In the active stage there is pain in the thoracic spine, with 'round' back. After some months the pain subsides, leaving a rounded kyphosis of varying severity (Fig. 13.23A). In later life there may be renewed pain from the development of osteoarthritis. *On examination* there is a slight or moderate rounded kyphosis in the thoracic region. In the active stage there is tenderness on firm palpation over the affected vertebrae.

Radiographic features. In the active stage of the disease the affected vertebral bodies show deep notched defects at their anterior corners, and the corresponding parts of the ring epiphyses may be irregular in shape and size

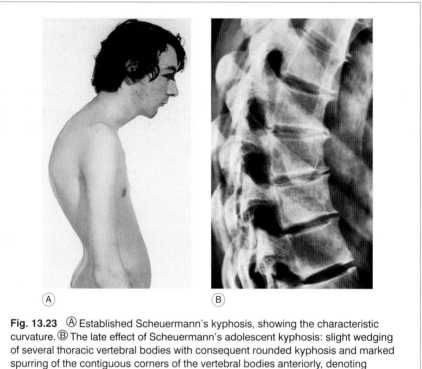

Fig. 13.23 Ⓐ Established Scheuermann's kyphosis, showing the characteristic curvature. Ⓑ The late effect of Scheuermann's adolescent kyphosis: slight wedging of several thoracic vertebral bodies with consequent rounded kyphosis and marked spurring of the contiguous corners of the vertebral bodies anteriorly, denoting osteoarthritis.

(Fig. 13.23B). The disc spaces are slightly narrowed but never totally destroyed. After healing, there is slight antero-posterior wedging of the affected vertebral bodies. Years later, osteoarthritic spurring of the anterior vertebral margins is observed, probably as a result of the vertebral malalignment (Fig. 13.23B).

Diagnosis. In its characteristic form the affection is easily diagnosed from the history, clinical appearance, and radiographs. If localised to a single vertebra it may easily be confused with tuberculous spondylitis. Radiologically, the chief points of distinction are that in osteochondritis the margins of the notched defect in the vertebral body tend to be sclerotic rather than rarefied, and a paraspinal abscess shadow (almost a constant feature of thoracic spinal tuberculosis) is never seen. Furthermore, the erythrocyte sedimentation rate is not raised in Scheuermann's kyphosis.

Course and prognosis. The affection is self-limiting, the active stage lasting for one or two years. If the epiphyses become deformed, permanent wedging of the affected vertebrae, with consequent slight or moderate kyphosis, remains as a cosmetic blemish. Osteoarthritis often supervenes in later life but it is not of major significance clinically.

Treatment. In a mild case treatment is often unnecessary. If pain is troublesome, support for the spine in extension, by a brace or plaster jacket, may be advisable. Bracing may have to be continued for up to six months, according to progress. Meanwhile active exercises to strengthen the posterior spinal muscles are encouraged. In the worst cases – a small minority – operative correction may be considered. Operation entails excision of intervertebral discs, with inter-body grafting, in the affected region of the spine, and it usually entails posterior instrumentation to provide correction and stability. It is a major procedure and clearly must not be undertaken without very careful assessment of every facet of the problem, since at best only 40% of the deformity can be corrected.

CALVÉ'S[1] VERTEBRAL COMPRESSION (Vertebra plana; vertebral osteochondritis)

Whereas in Scheuermann's disease it is the vertebral ring epiphyses that are affected, Calvé's disease affects the central bony nucleus of a vertebral body. It is generally confined to a single vertebra. It is uncommon.

Pathology. From its radiological features and benign course, Calvé's disease was regarded as an osteochondritis. Histological studies have shown that the majority of cases are in fact caused by an *eosinophilic granuloma* (p. 72).

In a typical case the bony nucleus of one of the vertebral bodies, usually in the thoracic region, becomes soft and is condensed into a thin wafer. Later, this may re-develop to a more normal size though it is doubtful if it is ever restored to full height. The intervertebral discs above and below are intact and unaffected.

Clinical features. The affection occurs in children of 2 to 10 years of age. The complaint is of pain, usually in the thoracic region of the spine. *On examination*, there may be slight localised kyphosis. Percussion of the spinal column reveals deep tenderness in the affected region. Movements of the spine as a whole are impaired little, if at all.

Radiographic features. Radiographs show the characteristic extreme flattening of the affected vertebral body, which appears greatly increased in density (Fig. 13.24): it has been likened to a coin seen end on.

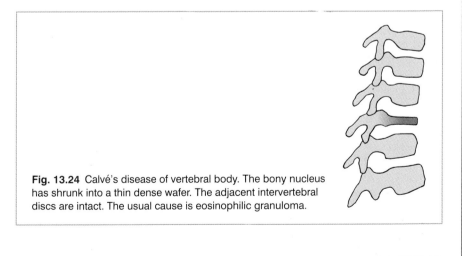

Fig. 13.24 Calvé's disease of vertebral body. The bony nucleus has shrunk into a thin dense wafer. The adjacent intervertebral discs are intact. The usual cause is eosinophilic granuloma.

[1]Jacques Calvé (1875–1954) French orthopaedic surgeon; worked in TB Hospital at Berck Plage and described the vertebral condition thought to be an osteochondritis, in 1925.

Treatment. Calvé's disease is non-progressive, and in practice treatment is required only for as long as the symptoms last. If pain is severe the child should be kept recumbent in bed, but in most cases he may safely resume an active life without external support within a few weeks.

PROLAPSED LUMBAR INTERVERTEBRAL DISC

Herniation of part of a lumbar intervertebral disc is a common cause of combined back pain and sciatica.

Cause. Prolapse of a disc is often precipitated by injury, but it may also occur in the absence of any remembered injury. Spontaneous age-degeneration of the disc is probably an important predisposing factor.

Pathology. The discs between L5 and S1 and between L4 and L5 are those most often affected. Part of the gelatinous nucleus pulposus protrudes through a rent in the annulus fibrosus at its weakest part, which is postero-lateral (Figs 13.25 and 13.26); or sometimes the torn annulus itself protrudes backwards. If it is small, the protrusion bulges the pain-sensitive posterior longitudinal ligament, causing pain in the back. If it is large, the protrusion herniates through the posterior ligament and may impinge upon an issuing nerve to cause sciatic pain. The nerve affected is that which leaves the spinal canal at the interspace next below the site of the disc lesion. Thus the first sacral nerve is impinged upon by a prolapse between L5 and S1, the fifth lumbar nerve by a prolapse between L4 and L5, and so on. Natural healing is by shrinkage and fibrosis of the extruded disc material; not by its reposition within the disc.

Secondary effects. Progressive degeneration of the disc leads, after months or years, to altered joint mechanics, with ultimate involvement of the posterior intervertebral (facet) joints as well as the central (body-to-body) joints.

Clinical features. In a typical case of disc prolapse at the L4–L5 or L5–S1 level the clinical picture is clearly defined. The patient is aged between 18 and 60. A few hours or days after jarring or straining the back he or she is seized, while twisting, stooping, or coughing, with agonising pain in the lumbar region. Any

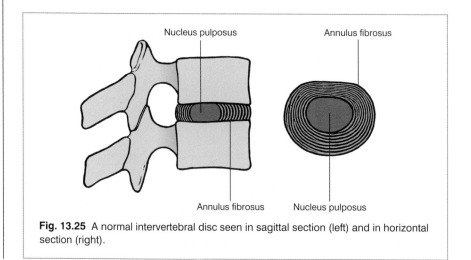

Fig. 13.25 A normal intervertebral disc seen in sagittal section (left) and in horizontal section (right).

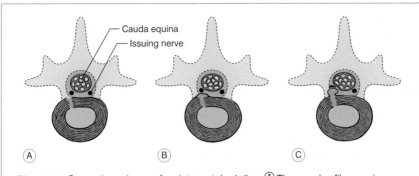

Fig. 13.26 Stages in prolapse of an intervertebral disc. Ⓐ The annulus fibrosus is torn but there has been no extrusion of the nucleus pulposus. Ⓑ Extrusion of nuclear material through the rent. The posterior longitudinal ligament is stretched but the protrusion has not reached the nerve. Ⓒ The protrusion is larger and the nerve is stretched over it. Sometimes a fragment of the torn annulus itself protrudes backwards.

movement of the back is impossible. The acute pain gradually lessens in severity, but after a few days a radiating pain is felt in one or other buttock and down the back or side of the thigh to the calf and foot. Tingling or numbness is felt in the calf or foot. The pain is aggravated by coughing or sneezing.

On examination the patient with a fully developed acute attack stands either with a lumbar scoliosis (sciatic scoliosis) (Fig. 13.27) or with the normal anterior lumbar curve obliterated. Forward flexion is greatly restricted, as also may be extension. Lateral flexion, on the other hand, is usually free and painless – certainly to one side if not to both. Straight leg raising is restricted on the affected side, usually markedly – an important clinical sign. Careful tests may reveal slight muscle wasting or weakness in the distribution of the affected nerve, and the corresponding tendon jerk (knee jerk in L3–L4 lesions; ankle jerk in L5–S1 lesions) is impaired or absent.

Variations. Atypical cases are common. Thus a definite history of injury or strain is often lacking. The pain may begin gradually rather than suddenly. The symptoms may be confined to the back and never radiate to the lower limb (acute lumbago). On the other hand, the pain is sometimes felt predominantly in the limb and is relatively mild in the back. The severity of the pain varies greatly from case to case, and its exact distribution depends upon the level of the disc prolapse: for instance, in the relatively uncommon cases of mid-lumbar (L3–L4) prolapse the pain radiates towards the groin and the front of the thigh rather than to the back of the thigh and leg.

In a severe case in which the prolapse is almost central there may be pressure upon the cauda equina, with consequent loss of bladder sensibility and retention of urine. This is the dangerous *cauda equina syndrome*, which must be regarded as an acute surgical emergency, for in the absence of immediate effective treatment serious permanent disability is likely to ensue (see below, p. 241).

Imaging. *Radiographic features.* In a case of acute prolapsed disc plain radiographs do not show any abnormality, and the purpose of radiography is mainly to exclude other causes of back pain and sciatica. It is only when a disc has

Trunk and spine

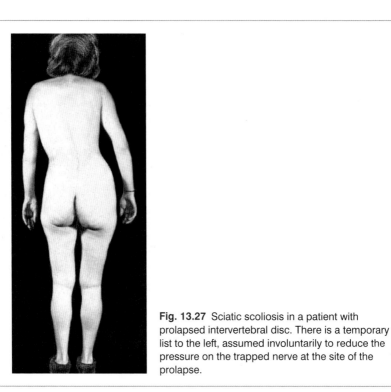

Fig. 13.27 Sciatic scoliosis in a patient with prolapsed intervertebral disc. There is a temporary list to the left, assumed involuntarily to reduce the pressure on the trapped nerve at the site of the prolapse.

been deranged for many months or years that appreciable narrowing of the disc space and spurring of the joint margins, denoting secondary degenerative arthritis (osteoarthritis), are observed.

Magnetic resonance imaging (MRI scanning) can show the intervertebral disc substance and the nerve roots: the bulging disc material can thus be visualised directly, particularly on sagittal projection (Fig. 13.28). *Discography* has only an occasional place as a diagnostic tool to confirm the level of symptomatic disc disease.

Correlation of pathology with clinical features. The initial injury or strain marks the time when the annulus fibrosus is torn or damaged. The nucleus pulposus is very gelatinous and an interval elapses before it becomes extruded. Bulging of the extruded material beneath the posterior longitudinal ligament corresponds to the stage of acute back pain. Herniation through the ligament with impingement against the adjacent nerve is responsible for the radiating limb pain and, in low lumbar lesions, the restriction of straight leg raising.

Diagnosis. Prolapsed intervertebral disc must be differentiated from other causes of pain in the back or leg (Fig. 13.29). A dramatically sudden onset is always suggestive of a mechanical derangement and especially of a prolapsed disc, whereas pain that increases relentlessly without intermission suggests a progressive lesion, inflammatory or neoplastic. Although the clinical features are often highly suggestive, definitive diagnosis rests upon appropriate imaging, preferably by magnetic resonance scans.

Treatment. *Conservative treatment* is successful in relieving the symptoms in a high proportion of cases – probably at least nine out of ten, though most of this improvement may be the result of natural healing. Prolonged bed rest,

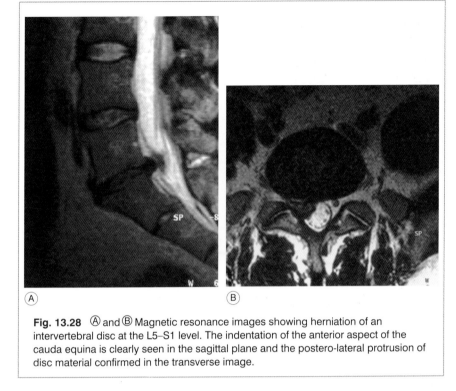

Fig. 13.28 Ⓐ and Ⓑ Magnetic resonance images showing herniation of an intervertebral disc at the L5–S1 level. The indentation of the anterior aspect of the cauda equina is clearly seen in the sagittal plane and the postero-lateral protrusion of disc material confirmed in the transverse image.

other than for a few days when symptoms are most acute, should be avoided. The patient should be encouraged to mobilise but the lumbar spine may be supported with a moulded plastic jacket or a well-fitted spinal orthosis (Fig. 13.30). The patient should be encouraged to discard the support as soon as the severe pain has subsided and mobilise the spine with physiotherapy supervision.

Intradiscal injection of chymopapain. Chymopapain is an enzyme with the property of dissolving fibrocartilaginous tissue. Injected into the disc substance, it causes partial dissolution of the nucleus pulposus and, in a favourable case, of protruding disc material. This treatment was popular for a few years but has now been discarded because of the risk of nerve damage due to leakage of the enzyme into the spinal canal. In the long term there is marked narrowing of the disc space as seen radiologically. Intradiscal injection of chymopapain is a method of treatment that has been slow in gaining acceptance, largely because the potential dangers were not at first fully assessed. It may be used in selected cases as a possible alternative to excision of the disc, with the advantage that operation is avoided. In most reported series the success rate in cases that would otherwise entail operation is in the order of 80%. Rarely, inadvertent leakage of the enzyme into the spinal canal has led to nerve damage and even death, but when the method is used with proper skill and with due precautions the risks are probably no greater than those of operation.

Trunk and spine

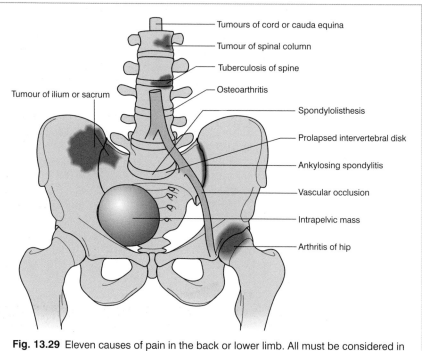

Fig. 13.29 Eleven causes of pain in the back or lower limb. All must be considered in differential diagnosis of prolapsed intervertebral disc.

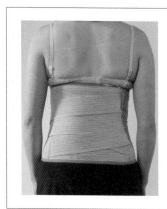

Fig. 13.30 Reinforced surgical corset used for mild cases of prolapsed intervertebral disc and for certain types of chronic low back pain.

Operative treatment. Excision of the displaced disc material, or discectomy, is indicated in the following circumstances:

1. when the sciatic pain is so excruciating from the beginning that it prevents sleep and leads to deterioration of the general health
2. when severe sciatic pain is unrelieved by appropriate conservative treatment continued for at least 8 weeks

3. when sciatic pain is accompanied by progressive signs of neurological impairment from root compression
4. when severe neurological disturbance suggests massive prolapse with compression of the cauda (cauda equina syndrome). In this last condition operation must be carried out as an emergency procedure because the attendant impairment of bladder, bowel, and sexual function quickly becomes irreversible.

At operation the disc is exposed from behind by retraction of the posterior spinal muscles away from the midline, excision of the ligamentum flavum and perhaps part of a lamina at the appropriate level, and gentle retraction of the theca. The protruded part of the disc forms an obvious rounded bulge, over which the emerging spinal nerve may be seen tightly stretched. The extruded material is removed, together with as much of the remaining nuclear tissue as can be pulled out from between the vertebral bodies. Many surgeons now favour excision by a magnification technique, the so-called 'microdiscectomy', utilising the operating microscope through a limited interlaminar approach using a small 'stab' incision. This obviates the need for extensive stripping of muscles from the back of the spinal column and reduces the associated post-operative morbidity, allowing the patient a more rapid return to normal activity.

ACUTE LOW BACK PAIN (LUMBAGO)

Back pain is a symptom rather than a disease. In a typical acute attack the patient is suddenly seized with agonising pain in the lumbar region of the spine, usually while stooping, lifting, turning, or coughing. The pain is often so severe that any movement is difficult and the patient is 'stuck'. With rest, the pain gradually subsides, but in some cases the acute back pain is accompanied by sciatica, suggesting irritation of a lumbar or sacral nerve.

The pathogenesis of acute low back pain is not entirely clear. Indeed there may be more than one cause. Probably in many cases the underlying lesion is a prolapsed disc that has not yet been retropulsed far enough to interfere with a nerve root (Fig. 13.26B). It is in these cases that sciatica may develop later, as the size of the prolapse increases. But other examples of acute back pain are more convincingly ascribed to some other mechanical fault, such as sudden nipping of synovial membrane in one of the facet joints, or momentary subluxation at an intervertebral joint that is unstable on account of disc degeneration or degenerative arthritis. Nerve irritation may also be the result of leakage of inflammatory cytokines from the degenerative lumbar disc. In most cases acute attacks of pain may recur at intervals of months or years, with intervals of relative freedom between the attacks.

Treatment should be conservative and similar to that used for prolapsed lumbar intervertebral disc. Mobility should be maintained and prolonged bed rest discouraged. Mobilisation and postural retraining under physiotherapy supervision has been shown to be beneficial.

SPONDYLOLYSIS

In spondylolysis there is a defect in the neural arch of the fifth (rarely the fourth) lumbar vertebra. There is loss of bony continuity between the superior and the inferior articular processes, the deficiency being bridged by fibrous tissue

Trunk and spine

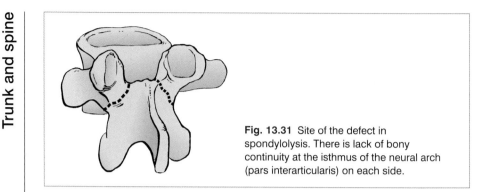

Fig. 13.31 Site of the defect in spondylolysis. There is lack of bony continuity at the isthmus of the neural arch (pars interarticularis) on each side.

(Fig. 13.31). If this stretches or gives way, the consequent vertebral displacement constitutes one variety of spondylolisthesis (see below).

Though the defect was formerly regarded as congenital it is now widely believed that it may be caused by injury; or, more specifically, it may be the result of a stress fracture in childhood or adolescence.

Clinically, spondylolysis (the defect without displacement) is often symptomless, but it is sometimes a cause of deep lumbar back pain. *Radiographically,* the defect is usually best shown in oblique projections or on a CT scan.

Treatment. This is often unnecessary. Aching may be relieved by a surgical corset or belt. If pain is unusually troublesome an attempt may be made to close the defect in the pars interarticularis on each side by transfixing it with a screw and laying in slender bone grafts ; or alternatively, local fusion of the spine may be undertaken (see p. 245).

SPONDYLOLISTHESIS (Lumbar spondylolisthesis)

Spondylolisthesis is the term applied to spontaneous displacement of a lumbar vertebral body upon the segment next below it. Displacement is usually forwards: only rarely does backward displacement occur (retrospondylolisthesis).

Cause. There are three predisposing factors leading to spondylolisthesis of three distinct types:

1. congenital malformation of the articular processes (rare)
2. spondylolysis (a defect in the pars interarticularis of the neural arch which may be developmental or the result of stress fracture) (p. 241)
3. osteoarthritis of the posterior (facet) joints.

Pathology. In the normal spine forward displacement of a vertebral body is prevented by engagement of its articular processes with those of the segment next below it. In spondylolisthesis there is a failure of this check mechanism, and the attachments of the intervertebral disc alone are not strong enough to hold the vertebral bodies in alignment.

In the first type of spondylolisthesis, the least common, there is a congenital basis for the displacement. The posterior intervertebral joints are unstable because the articular processes are congenitally malformed or even rudimentary: thus they form no bar to forward displacement of the spinal column (Fig. 13.32).

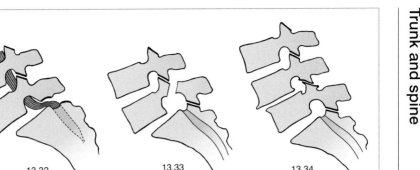

Fig. 13.32 (Left) Spondylolisthesis secondary to congenital malformation of the articular processes at the lumbo-sacral joint. The cauda equina is trapped between the body of the sacrum and the lamina of the displaced fifth lumbar vertebra. In this type of spondylolisthesis neurological signs are to be expected.

Fig. 13.33 (Middle) Spondylolisthesis due to defect of the neural arch of a vertebra, in this case affecting the fifth lumbar vertebra. The body and superior articular processes have slipped forwards, leaving the spinous process and inferior articular processes in normal relationship with the sacrum. (Radiographically the defect is seen best in oblique projections.)

Fig. 13.34 (Right) Spondylolisthesis secondary to osteoarthritis. Wearing down of the cartilage of the posterior intervertebral (facet) joints has permitted slight forward displacement of the fourth lumbar vertebra on the fifth. The condition may occur at any level in the lumbar spine.

This defect occurs most often at the lumbo-sacral joint. Displacement may be severe and, since the whole vertebra is displaced complete with its neural arch, the cauda equina may be trapped, with consequent severe neurological disturbance (Fig. 13.32).

In the second type, which is the best recognised, a defect in the neural arch of a vertebra allows separation of its two halves (see spondylolysis, and Fig. 13.33). The body, with the pedicles and superior articular processes (and the whole of the spinal column above it), slips forwards, leaving behind the laminae and inferior articular processes (Fig. 13.33). The fifth lumbar is the vertebra usually affected, the fourth occasionally. Displacement may gradually increase, especially during adolescence, and it sometimes reaches a severe degree. There may be minor irritation of one of the issuing nerves, with consequent sciatica; but despite severe bony displacement serious interference with the nerves of the cauda equina is exceptional in this type of spondylolisthesis.

In the third type of spondylolisthesis (sometimes termed pseudospondylolisthesis), seen fairly commonly, the arthritic posterior intervertebral facet joints become unstable with degeneration of the articular cartilage and osteophyte formation displacing the joint surfaces (Fig. 13.34). It may occur at any level in the lumbar spine — most commonly between the fourth and fifth lumbar vertebrae. In this type the vertebral displacement is occasionally backwards rather than forwards (see Fig. 13.17), but in either case displacement is never severe, and neurological disturbance is unusual.

The intervertebral disc at the site of vertebral slipping is inevitably damaged, and disc prolapse may occur.

Clinical features. The clinical features of spondylolisthesis are inconstant: they depend to some extent upon the nature of the causative lesion and upon the degree of displacement. Thus in spondylolisthesis from under-development of the articular processes (Fig. 13.32), and in that from a defect of the pars interarticularis (Fig. 13.33), the patient is usually a young adult, whereas displacement from degeneration of the facet joints in osteoarthritis (Fig. 13.34) is seen characteristically in patients beyond middle age. In some cases the deformity is entirely symptomless. When symptoms occur they take the form of chronic backache, with or without sciatica. The back pain is worse on standing.

On examination there is often a visible or palpable 'step' above the sacral crest, due to the forward displacement of the spinal column; but this is obvious only when the displacement is severe. Spinal movements are restricted only slightly, if at all. *Abdomen*: When displacement is severe the spinal column is projected forwards and the lumbar vertebral bodies may be palpable through the abdominal wall. *Lower limbs*: Minor irritation of a sciatic root is often evidenced by impairment of straight leg raising; but severe neurological disturbance is seldom observed except in the rare cases in which congenital malformation of the articular processes allows dislocation of the whole vertebra complete with its neural arch (Fig. 13.32).

Radiographic features. Lateral and oblique views will sometimes demonstrate a defect of the neural arch (Fig. 13.35), but CT scans will show this more clearly (Fig. 13.36).

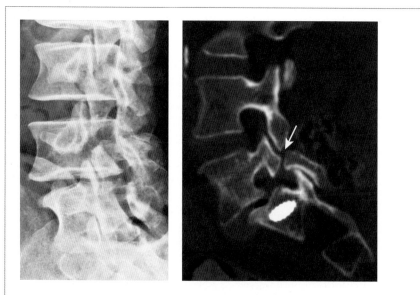

Fig. 13.35 Oblique radiograph of the lower lumbar region of a patient with spondylolisthesis, showing a defect of the pars interarticularis of the neural arch of the fourth lumbar vertebra (centre of illustration). Oblique radiographs such as this are important in the differentiation of spondylolisthesis caused by a neural arch defect from the other two types of spondylolisthesis.

Fig. 13.36 Sagittal CT scan of lumbar spine to show a defect in the pars interarticularis of the L5 vertebra (arrow). This has led to a forward slip of the L5 vertebra on the sacrum.

Treatment. When spondylolisthesis is symptomless treatment is not required.

Non-operative treatment. Moderate symptoms are often adequately relieved by a well-fitted surgical corset and this should be tried before operation is considered.

Operation. This is justified only when the disability (from back pain or neurological disturbance) is severe. The operation entails the release of stretched or compressed nerves, followed by fusion of the affected segments of the spinal column. Fusion of the spine is normally achieved by bridging the vertebrae with bone grafts, usually obtained from the ilium, though sometimes allograft bone may be used. In *posterior fusion* the grafts are fitted between or alongside the spinous processes, superficial to the laminae. In *anterior fusion* blocks of bone are inlayed in deep slots cut in the vertebral bodies after excision of most of the intervertebral disc from the front. In *lateral fusion* bone grafts are wedged between the transverse processes or, in the case of the lumbo-sacral joint, between transverse processes above and the lateral masses of the sacrum below. Each method has its special application, but the choice also depends largely on the nature of the pathology to be treated and the surgeon's individual preference.

SPINAL STENOSIS (Claudication of the cauda equina)

In the syndrome of spinal stenosis standing and walking beyond a certain duration are associated with increasingly severe pain in the gluteal region and lower limb on one or both sides, ascribed to cramping of nerves and their blood vessels in a constricted spinal canal.

Pathology. The dimensions of the spinal canal in the lumbar region show considerable variation between individuals. The cross-sectional shape of the canal also varies, it being sometimes rounded and sometimes almost triangular. Thus in some persons there is a congenital narrowing or constriction of the canal which, though providing adequate room for the cauda equina in the absence of other pathology, nevertheless allows little or no margin of safety, so that if the canal becomes further narrowed from secondary causes such as the formation of osteophytes about the facet joints, or bulging of an intervertebral disc, the normal functioning of nerves of the cauda equina will be impaired by lack of room and constriction of their blood supply. To some extent the constriction seems to be selective rather than uniform throughout the cauda equina, the nerves lying in the narrow lateral recesses of a triangular canal being particularly vulnerable. For a long time the impairment of nerve function is intermittent rather than permanent, being rapidly reversible when the patient assumes a sitting posture.

Clinical features. The clinical history is characteristic. The patient, often an elderly man, complains that after walking for a matter of 10–15 minutes, he develops a heavy aching sensation in one or both lower limbs, and that this steadily increases to such an extent that eventually he is forced to sit down. In most cases similar symptoms develop when the patient stands for a while, even without walking. Relief is obtained only by sitting or by lying with the hips and knees drawn up in a sitting posture: it is not sufficient just to stop walking. Sitting relieves the symptoms within a few minutes because on flexion of the spine the canal is widened, and the patient can then resume walking or standing for a further period.

Examination may reveal little abnormality, though frequently there are features to suggest degenerative change in the lumbar spine – for instance impairment of spinal mobility.

Imaging. *Plain radiographs* may give the impression that the spinal canal is narrower than usual and they may show further constriction of the canal by posterior osteophytes upon the margins of the vertebral bodies or in relation to the facet joints. *Magnetic resonance imaging (MRI)* shows very clearly the shape of the spinal canal, and may also show bony or soft-tissue outgrowths encroaching upon either a normal or a congenitally constricted canal (Fig. 13.37).

Diagnosis. The spinal stenosis syndrome bears superficial resemblance to intermittent claudication from vascular disease. Confusion should be avoided, however, because of the important distinction that pain in spinal stenosis, unlike that from arterial disease, comes on not only with walking but also with standing, and is relieved only by sitting or by flexing the spine. Moreover, examination of the vascular system shows no abnormality.

Treatment. Mild symptoms may be controlled by appropriate modification of activities – for instance by using a bicycle instead of walking, and by the avoidance of prolonged standing. In the fully established case with severe intractable symptoms, treatment should be by operation to decompress the

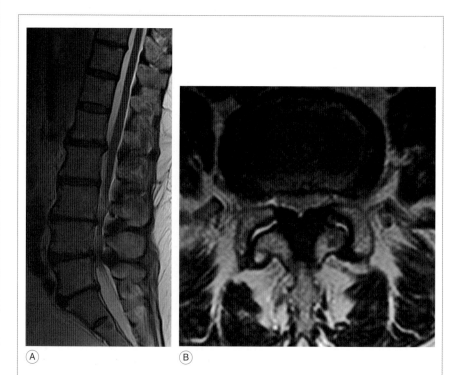

Ⓐ　　　　　　　　　Ⓑ

Fig. 13.37 Ⓐ Sagittal and Ⓑ axial MR scans of lumbar spine in spinal stenosis. There is marked narrowing of the spinal canal at the L4–L5 level, in part due to the bulging disc, though much of the compromise is from the posterior aspect by the ligament flavum which is buckled and hence appears thickened.

spinal canal by removal of intruding osteophytes and enlargement of the lateral recesses at the level of the constriction. Decompression may have to be carried out over a number of segments, depending upon the longitudinal extent of the constriction as shown by appropriate imaging.

TUMOURS OF THE TRUNK AND SPINE

TUMOURS IN RELATION TO THE SPINAL COLUMN, SPINAL CORD, OR EMERGING NERVES

Classification and pathology. As in the cervical region, tumours involving the spine or related nerves may arise:

1. in the bony spinal column itself
2. in the meninges or, rarely, the spinal cord
3. in the fibrous component of a peripheral nerve (neurofibroma)
4. in adjacent soft tissues.

Tumours of the spinal column may be benign (for instance chondroma, giant-cell tumour, haemangioma, osteoblastoma) but are more often malignant. Such tumours may be primary (sarcoma, multiple myeloma, chordoma), but metastatic tumours predominate. A meningeal tumour (meningioma) is an occasional cause of compression of the spinal cord or cauda equina. Nerve compression may also be a consequence of a neurofibroma growing within the spinal canal.

Clinical features. The effects of these tumours vary according to their site and character. Broadly, the effects may be placed in three groups:

Local destruction of the skeleton. The commonest cause is a malignant tumour of the bones of the spinal column (Fig. 13.38) – usually a metastatic carcinoma. The predominant symptom is pain, which is constant and increases relentlessly in its severity. Frequently there are associated neurological manifestations from involvement of the spinal cord or nerve roots. Sometimes deformity, from collapse of the bony structure, is evident clinically; or there may be marked restriction of spinal movement, with protective muscle spasm.

Compression of the spinal cord. This may occur from tumours of the spinal cord itself or of its meninges, from tumours of nerves (neurofibroma), or from tumours of the bony spinal column. The clinical manifestations depend upon the exact location of the tumour. Typically, when the spinal cord is slowly compressed, initial root pain (girdle pain in thoracic involvement, lower limb pain in lumbar involvement) is followed by lower motor neurone paresis at the segmental level corresponding to the site of the tumour, by progressive sensory and upper motor neurone paralysis below the lesion, and often by bladder or bowel dysfunction.

Interference with peripheral nerves. Peripheral nerves – especially the nerves of the cauda equina – may be involved by tumours of the nerves themselves (neurofibroma), by tumours of the spinal column (benign or malignant), or by tumours in the peripheral course of the nerves (for example, a tumour of a rib, or a tumour arising from or within the pelvis). The clinical features depend upon the particular nerve or nerves affected and upon the extent of the involvement. Typically, there will be constant, progressive, and ultimately severe pain along the course of the affected nerve, with sensory impairment, increasing

Trunk and spine

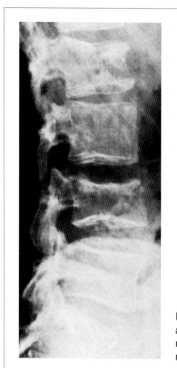

Fig. 13.38 Partial collapse of the second and fourth lumbar vertebrae in a patient with myelomatosis. Note that the intervertebral discs are not destroyed.

motor weakness, and depression of reflexes in the distribution of the nerve. Retention of urine is usually a prominent feature of a tumour interfering with the cauda equina.

Imaging. *Plain radiographs* will usually help in discovering a tumour arising in the bones of the spinal column (Fig. 13.38), or eroding the bone from outside. In cases of vertebral destruction by a tumour the adjacent intervertebral discs are typically preserved. This point helps in the distinction from erosion and collapse due to infection, in which the discs are destroyed at an early stage (compare Figs 13.13A and 13.38).

Radiographs of the chest may reveal a primary lung tumour or a metastasis; and radiographs of the rest of the skeleton may be helpful in the diagnosis of disseminated tumours. *Magnetic resonance imaging* is indispensable in showing the full extent of the tumour and the extent to which the adjacent tissues have been infiltrated (Fig. 13.39).

Radioisotope scanning may show evidence of a lesion before it is evident radiographically. CT scanning is capable of showing even quite small tumours within the vertebrae.

Diagnosis. The possibility of a tumour has to be borne in mind constantly in the differential diagnosis of back pain and lower limb pain, especially when associated with radiological signs of vertebral erosion or collapse or with neurological disturbance affecting the trunk, lower limbs, or viscera (Fig. 13.29).

A history of insidious onset, with relentless increase of symptoms without remission, always suggests the possibility of tumour. Careful search should always be made for a primary tumour elsewhere in the body.

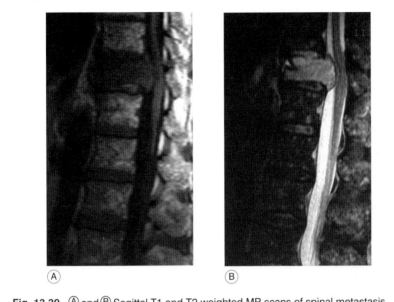

Fig. 13.39 Ⓐ and Ⓑ Sagittal T1 and T2 weighted MR scans of spinal metastasis. The T12 vertebra is replaced by abnormal marrow signal and there is some collapse with retropulsion of tissue into the spinal canal, features typical of a metastatic deposit in the spine.

Treatment. This is dependent on the site and nature of the tumour, but it should be remembered that many of these patients will survive for a considerable period of time and may require more active treatment than analgesic therapy alone for their increasing pain. Radiotherapy to the bone lesions and sometimes operative spinal decompression and fusion may be required in selected cases.

OTHER TUMOURS OF THE TRUNK

Tumours of the sternum and ribs

The sternum and ribs contain abundant red marrow, favourable to the development of blood-borne metastatic tumours or of deposits in myelomatosis or the lymphomas. Histological examination of the sternal marrow (obtained by sternal puncture) is often of diagnostic importance in suspected metastasising tumours, for the material will often show tumour cells even in the absence of clinically evident metastases.

Tumours of the scapula

The commonest tumour of the scapula is a chondroma. It grows outwards from the flat body of the bone and is therefore classed as an ecchondroma. It may attain a large size. Although it is often benign at first, there is a risk of malignant change, with the development of a chondrosarcoma. For that reason

Trunk and spine

a chondroma that appears to be enlarging should always be excised with an adequate margin of healthy bone. A large part of the scapula can be removed without causing serious disability.

Tumours of the pelvic girdle

The pelvic bones, like the scapula, are sometimes the seat of a chondroma (ecchondroma). It may reach a large size, and there is risk of malignant change to chondrosarcoma.

The considerable content of red marrow also renders the pelvic bones liable to carcinomatous metastatic deposits, and they are also a common site of tumour deposits in myelomatosis.

CHRONIC LOWER LUMBAR LIGAMENTOUS STRAIN (Postural back pain)

The terms *chronic ligamentous strain* and *postural back pain* are used to cover an ill-defined group of affections characterised by persistent backache without demonstrable pathology. These conditions are common – in fact they form a considerable proportion of the cases of back pain seen in orthopaedic practice.

Cause. It is assumed that the spinal muscles fail in their function of protecting the deep ligaments in maintaining posture. Predisposing causes include childbirth, overweight, general flabbiness of muscle, and debilitating illness.

Pathology. No precise lesion is demonstrable.

Clinical features. The pain is characteristically in the lumbar or lumbo-sacral region. It tends to be worse on activities such as stooping, or after prolonged standing or sitting in one position. *On examination* there may be no abnormal physical signs but in many cases there is some restriction of spinal movement. *Radiographs* are normal.

Diagnosis. This depends upon the exclusion of demonstrable pathological lesions by careful clinical and radiographic examination. A history of long-continued lumbar backache, with a total lack of clinical or radiological abnormalities, should always suggest this group of affections.

Course and prognosis. Aching often persists intermittently for many years despite treatment. Nevertheless in most cases the condition is a source of nagging discomfort rather than a serious handicap to most ordinary day-to-day activities.

Treatment. Often reassurance alone is required. Treatment may be required for short-term exacerbations, but should be focused on activity modification, weight loss, active exercises to strengthen the spinal muscles and postural correction under physiotherapy supervision. Other more invasive treatments such as local injections of anaesthetic solution or hydrocortisone should be avoided if possible.

COCCYDYNIA

In its widest sense, coccydynia includes any painful condition in the region of the coccyx. In practice, the term is restricted to the clinical entity in which persistent pain continues for many weeks or months after a local injury, despite the absence of demonstrable pathology. Eventually it is a self-limiting affection, but it may cause severe discomfort while it lasts – often for many months.

Cause. Typically coccydynia develops after an injury – usually a fall on the 'tail'. Occasionally a history of injury is lacking.

Pathology. In some cases there is probably a strain of the sacro-coccygeal joint; in others the lesion is thought to be simply a contusion of the periosteum over the lower sacrum or coccyx. Rarely, a crack fracture of the coccyx or sacrum is demonstrated.

Clinical features. There is pain localised to the sacro-coccygeal area, worse when sitting. In severe cases there is also pain on defaecation. Usually the patient is free from pain when standing or lying. *On examination* there is localised tenderness over the sacro-coccygeal region. In some cases the pain can be reproduced by moving the coccyx. In the absence of a fracture, *radiographs* do not show any alteration from the normal.

Diagnosis. It is important to consider other causes of pain in this area, especially infections of the sacro-coccygeal joint and tumours of the sacrum or coccyx. Investigation should include rectal examination, and radiographs must always be obtained.

Treatment. In most cases treatment is not required. All that is necessary is to exclude serious organic disease, and then to reassure the patient that the condition is harmless and that it may be expected to resolve spontaneously if left alone. In resistant cases manipulation and local injection of steroids have been used but none of these methods is uniformly successful. In unusually severe and persistent pain surgical excision of the coccyx may be required.

OSTEOPOROSIS

The vertebrae of the thoracic and lumbar spine are one of the commonest sites affected by osteoporosis, or so-called 'brittle bone' disease. This is a general affection of the skeleton and is described in more detail on page 81. It is commonest in postmenopausal women, but it can also affect men in the same age group. Its onset is insidious, but crush fracture of the vertebral body is the commonest of the fragility fractures associated with this condition. Its onset may be associated with an episode of minor trauma, but there is often no significant injury and only minor local pain. More commonly, the patient presents with progressive loss of height and an increasing kyphotic deformity of the thoracic spine. This results from collapse of the thoracic vertebrae at several levels with anterior wedging of the bodies (Fig. 13.40). In advanced cases the radiographs show little difference between the density of the bone and the intervertebral discs.

Treatment. Greater awareness of the morbidity of this condition in a rapidly increasing elderly population has led to more active medical and surgical interventions. All patients should be investigated to determine the cause and extent of their bone loss and, where appropriate, medical treatment instituted to prevent further progression. In selected cases where local pain is more severe and of recent onset, a new minimally invasive surgical treatment of balloon kyphoplasty may be considered. Using radiographic screening a percutaneous probe is inserted into the centre of the collapsed vertebral body and is then replaced with a balloon-like device which is inflated with contrast medium until the vertebral body height is restored. Finally the space is injected with semi-liquid polymethylmethacrylate cement which once solidified will restore the vertebral bone stability.

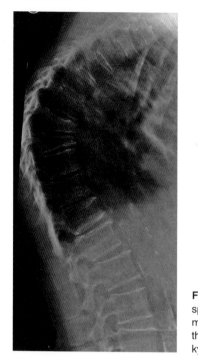

Fig. 13.40 Lateral radiograph of osteoporotic spine in an elderly female patient. There are multiple vertebral fractures with collapse in the mid thoracic region resulting in a rounded kyphotic deformity.

Disorders of the sacro-iliac joint

Sacro-iliac lesions are a rather uncommon but nervertheless important cause of back symptoms or of referred pain in the lower limb. Of the various types of arthritis, ankylosing spondylitis is the best recognised. Tuberculous arthritis is seen occasionally, but mainly in developing countries.

EXTRINSIC DISORDERS SIMULATING SPINAL DISEASE

ABDOMINAL DISORDERS

Peptic ulcer, renal and perirenal infections, renal calculus, and biliary calculus and cholecystitis may all produce retroperitoneal pain which may be felt in the back as well as the abdomen. Consideration of the other associated symptoms and abdominal signs should lead to the correct diagnosis.

PELVIC DISORDERS

Intrapelvic tumours interfering with the sacral plexus or its branches, may cause pain in the sciatic distribution simulating sciatica from a spinal cause. A full pelvic examination should form part of the routine investigation of lower limb pain and in cases of doubt magnetic resonance imaging may be helpful in diagnosis.

LOWER LIMB DISORDERS

Pain from an arthritic hip may sometimes simulate sciatic pain from a spinal lesion, but characteristically is referred from the groin down to the front of the thigh rather than on its posterior aspect. A full examination of the hip and if necessary radiology should establish the true diagnosis.

VASCULAR DISORDERS

Arterial occlusion in the lower limb and more rarely aortic aneurysm may present with muscle pain on exercise which may be confused with sciatica from a spinal cause. For this reason a full examination of the vascularity of the limb is essential to establish the true diagnosis.

14 | The shoulder region

The mechanics of the shoulder are rather complex. The shoulder 'joint' in fact comprises three components – the gleno-humeral joint or shoulder joint proper, the acromio-clavicular joint, and the sterno-clavicular joint. The gleno-humeral joint allows a free range of abduction, flexion, and rotation, under the control of the scapulo-humeral and pectoral muscles. The other two joints together allow 90° of rotation of the scapula upon the thorax and a moderate range of antero-posterior gliding of the scapula, under the control of the cervico-scapular and thoraco-scapular muscles.

Disorders of the shoulder include most varieties of arthritis; but it is notable that osteoarthritis – common in most joints – is less common in the gleno-humeral joint. As if to make up for this, the shoulder exhibits several affections peculiar to itself – notably tears of the musculo-tendinous cuff, the painful arc syndrome, and 'frozen' shoulder. Together these form a large proportion of shoulder disabilities.

The recent developments in soft tissue imaging and arthroscopy have revolutionised the diagnosis and treatment of many of these disorders. Open operative procedures have now been replaced in specialist centres by minimally invasive arthroscopic techniques with equally successful outcomes.

Pain in the shoulder and arm is notoriously prone to misinterpretation, and special care is required to differentiate intrinsic pain arising in the shoulder from extrinsic pain referred from the cervical spine, the thorax, or the abdomen.

SPECIAL POINTS IN THE INVESTIGATION OF SHOULDER SYMPTOMS

History

Characteristics of shoulder pain. It is important to find out the precise location and distribution of the pain. True shoulder pain is seldom confined to the shoulder itself. Typically, it radiates from a point near the tip of the acromion down the lateral side of the upper arm to about the level of the deltoid insertion. It is unusual for true shoulder pain to extend below the elbow.

Pain arising in the acromio-clavicular joint or sterno-clavicular joint is localised to the joint itself and does not radiate down the limb.

Referred pain in the shoulder region. The pain referred from an irritative lesion of the brachial plexus often extends from the base of the neck, over the top of the shoulder, and thence into the arm. Unlike true shoulder pain, it frequently radiates below the elbow into the forearm or hand, and it may be accompanied by paraesthesiae – often described as 'pins and needles' or 'a numb feeling'. Pain may also be referred to the shoulder from a lesion in the thorax or upper abdomen.

Exposure

The patient must be stripped to the waist. The examination is conducted most easily with the patient standing; alternatively he may sit upon a high stool. For the greater part of the examination the surgeon stands behind the patient, so that he may observe more easily the position of the scapula.

Steps in routine examination

A suggested plan for the routine examination of the shoulder is summarised in Table 14.1.

Movements at the shoulder

In examining shoulder movements it is important to determine how much of the movement occurs at the gleno-humeral joint and how much is contributed by rotation of the scapula. An accurate distinction between the two types of movement can be made only by grasping the lower half of the scapula so that its movements can be detected (Fig. 14.1). In the normal shoulder about half the range of abduction occurs at the gleno-humeral joint and half by scapular rotation. Disorders of the shoulder generally cause restriction of gleno-humeral movement rather than of scapular movement. If the shoulder joint proper (the

Table 14.1 Routine clinical examination in suspected disorders of the shoulder

1. LOCAL EXAMINATION OF THE SHOULDER REGION	
Inspection Bone contours alignment Soft-tissue contours Colour and texture of skin Scars or sinuses	**Power** *Cervico-scapular and thoraco-scapular muscles* (controlling scapular movement)—Test elevation of scapula, retraction of scapula, abduction-rotation of scapula
Palpation Skin temperature Bone contours Soft-tissue contours Local tenderness	*Scapulo-humeral muscles* (controlling movement at gleno-humeral joint)—Abduction, adduction, flexion, extension, lateral rotation, medial rotation
Movements Distinguish between true gleno-humeral movement and scapular movement during abduction, flexion, extension, lateral rotation, and medial rotation ? Pain on movement ? Muscle spasm ? Crepitation on movement	**Acromio-clavicular joint** Examine for swelling, increased warmth, tenderness, pain on movement, and stability **Sterno-clavicular joint** Examine for swelling, increased warmth, tenderness, pain on movement, and stability

2. EXAMINATION OF POTENTIAL EXTRINSIC SOURCES OF SHOULDER SYMPTOMS
This is important if a satisfactory explanation for the symptoms is not found on local examination. The investigation should include: 1. the neck, with the brachial plexus 2. the thorax, with special reference to the heart and pleura 3. the abdomen, for subdiaphragmatic lesions

3. GENERAL EXAMINATION
General survey of other parts of the body

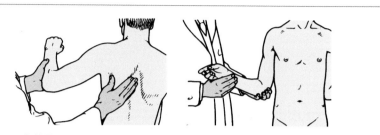

Fig. 14.1 (left) Examining shoulder abduction. One hand grasps the scapula while the other steadies the elbow. In this way the proportion of the total range contributed by gleno-humeral movement and by scapular rotation can be assessed.

Fig. 14.2 (right) Examining shoulder rotation. The elbow is supported by the examiner's hand and flexed to the right angle to eliminate forearm rotation. The forearm thus serves as a pointer to indicate the range of rotation at the shoulder.

gleno-humeral joint) is fused, either naturally or by operation, a range of abduction of up to 60 or 80° is possible by scapular movement alone.

Stand behind the patient. *Abduction*: Instruct the patient to try to raise both arms sideways from the body so that the palms of the hands meet above the head. Measure the range, and observe what proportion of the movement takes place at the gleno-humeral joint and how much is contributed by rotation of the scapula upon the thorax. *Flexion*: Instruct the patient to raise the arms forwards towards the vertical. Again observe (by means of the hand upon the scapula) what proportion of the movement occurs at the gleno-humeral joint and how much is contributed by rotation of the scapula on the chest wall. *Extension*: Ask the patient to raise the elbows backwards. *Lateral (external) rotation*: The elbows are held in to the sides and are flexed 90° (Fig. 14.2): the forearms then serve as convenient pointers to indicate the angle of rotation (normal range = 80°). *Medial (internal) rotation*: Instruct the patient to place the back of his hand in contact with his lumbar region and to carry the elbow forwards, bringing the finger tips up as high as possible between the shoulder blades (normal range = 110°).

Estimation of muscle power

In estimating the power of the shoulder muscles two groups must be distinguished:

1. the cervico-scapular and thoraco-scapular muscles
2. the scapulo-humeral muscles.

The cervico-scapular and thoraco-scapular muscles. These control movements of the scapula. Estimate the power of each group in turn and compare on the two sides. *Elevators of the scapula* (levator scapulae, upper fibres of trapezius): Instruct the patient to shrug the shoulders against the resistance of the examiner's hands. *Retractors of the scapula* (rhomboids and middle fibres of trapezius): Instruct the patient to brace the shoulders back. *Abductor-rotators of the scapula* (serratus anterior, with middle and lower fibres of trapezius): Instruct the patient to push horizontally forwards with the hand against a wall (Fig. 14.3) or simply to raise the

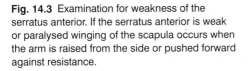

Fig. 14.3 Examination for weakness of the serratus anterior. If the serratus anterior is weak or paralysed winging of the scapula occurs when the arm is raised from the side or pushed forward against resistance.

arm from the side. If the serratus anterior is weak, winging of the scapula (backward projection of its vertebral border) will be observed (Fig. 14.3).

The scapulo-humeral muscles. These control movements of the gleno-humeral joint. Estimate the power of each muscle group, testing in turn the abductors, adductors, flexors, extensors, lateral rotators, and medial rotators. If the patient has lost the power to initiate active gleno-humeral movement from the dependent position, determine whether he can maintain abduction when the limb has been raised with assistance to 90°. Ability to *sustain* abduction but not to *initiate* it is characteristic of isolated rupture of the supraspinatus tendon (see Fig. 14.12, p. 267).

The acromio-clavicular and sterno-clavicular joints

The clavicle may be regarded as a link, jointed at each end, connecting the scapula to the sternum (Fig. 14.4). Movement of the scapula must occur about a fulcrum at one or both ends of this link. In the normal shoulder movement of the scapula, with consequent movement at the acromio-clavicular and sterno-clavicular joints, occurs mainly:

1. during elevation of the arm above 90°
2. when the shoulders are braced backwards or drawn forwards.

To examine the acromio-clavicular and sterno-clavicular joints stand in front of the patient. Examine the joints on each side for deformity, swelling, increase of local temperature, local tenderness, and pain on movement – especially at the extremes of elevation of the arm and backward bracing of the shoulders. Observe whether there is any tendency to subluxation or dislocation of the joint on movement.

Radiographic examination

Gleno-humeral joint. The routine shoulder film is a plain antero-posterior projection with the limb in the anatomical position. When additional information is required a special axillary projection with the arm abducted 90° (giving a lateral view of the humerus) should be obtained. Further films showing the

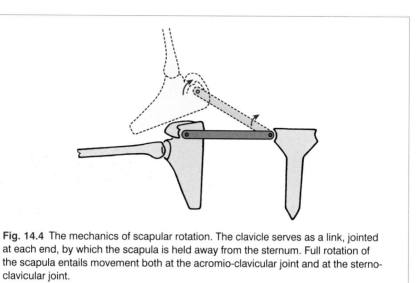

Fig. 14.4 The mechanics of scapular rotation. The clavicle serves as a link, jointed at each end, by which the scapula is held away from the sternum. Full rotation of the scapula entails movement both at the acromio-clavicular joint and at the sterno-clavicular joint.

upper end of the humerus in varying degrees of rotation are sometimes informative. *Arthrography*, after injection of radio-opaque fluid into the joint, will show whether or not the capsule is intact.

Acromio-clavicular joint and sterno-clavicular joint. Special projections are used to show each of these joints.

Other imaging techniques

Radioisotope scanning, computerised tomography, ultrasonography, and *magnetic resonance imaging* must each be considered in appropriate circumstances. Double contrast arthrography combined with computerised tomography or magnetic resonance imaging may be particularly valuable in demonstrating the extent of soft tissue damage in recurrent dislocation of the shoulder (see Fig. 14.10).

Arthroscopy

Arthroscopy has become a well-established method of investigation for difficult shoulder problems, as well as being used increasingly for closed operative treatment. The use of both anterior and posterior portals allows direct access to the glenoid fossa, the capsule, and the articular surfaces, as well as the rotator cuff musculature and sub-acromial space.

Extrinsic sources of shoulder and arm pain

In many cases in which the main complaint is of pain in the shoulder or arm there is no local abnormality, the symptoms being referred from a lesion elsewhere. Thus pain over the shoulder is a common symptom in affections of the neck, especially when the brachial plexus or its roots are involved. Shoulder pain is also a feature of irritative lesions in contact with the diaphragm, either in the thorax or in the abdomen. The possibility of such extrinsic lesions must always be considered in the investigation of shoulder pain.

Fortunately, with careful interrogation and clinical examination there is little difficulty in distinguishing intrinsic from extrinsic lesions. The important point is that intrinsic lesions of the shoulder always give rise to local physical signs that are readily demonstrable on examination. If the shoulder is clinically normal it is improbable that it is the seat of disease, and attention should be directed towards possible sources of referred pain.

DISORDERS OF THE SHOULDER (GLENO-HUMERAL) JOINT

PYOGENIC ARTHRITIS OF THE SHOULDER (General description of arthritis, p. 96)

Pyogenic arthritis of the shoulder is uncommon. It may complicate a penetrating wound, or it may be a haematogenous (blood borne) infection. In children infection may spread to the shoulder from a focus of osteomyelitis in the upper metaphysis of the humerus (p. 279).

The clinical features resemble those of pyogenic arthritis of other joints. The onset is rapid and is accompanied by pyrexia. The shoulder is swollen and abnormally warm, and all movements are greatly restricted. Treatment follows the lines suggested on page 98.

TUBERCULOUS ARTHRITIS OF THE SHOULDER (General description of tuberculous arthritis, p. 98)

Tuberculous arthritis of the shoulder has become a rare disease in Western countries. It occurs much less commonly than tuberculosis of the spine, hip, and knee. As with tuberculosis elsewhere, it occurs more commonly in African countries and in the East than in most countries of Europe and in North America.

The pathological and clinical features correspond to those of tuberculous arthritis in any major joint. Treatment with antituberculous drugs follows the general principles outlined on page 102. In early cases good recovery of function may occur, but in more advanced cases of bone and joint destruction surgical intervention with arthrodesis of the joint may be required.

RHEUMATOID ARTHRITIS OF THE SHOULDER (General description of rheumatoid arthritis, p. 134)

The shoulder is commonly affected by rheumatoid arthritis, though less commonly than the more peripheral joints such as hands, wrists and feet. Often both shoulders are affected simultaneously with other upper limb joints, with consequent serious impairment of function.

As in other superficial joints, the main clinical features are local pain and stiffness, increased warmth, swelling from synovial thickening, and marked restriction of movement. There is wasting of the deltoid muscle, with consequent flattening of the shoulder contour (Fig. 14.5A). Radiographs show rarefaction of bone, narrowing of the cartilage space, and eventually erosion of bone at the joint margins (Fig. 14.5B).

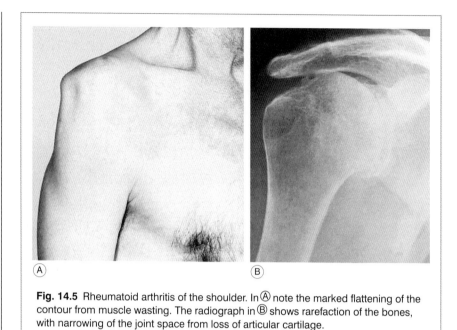

Fig. 14.5 Rheumatoid arthritis of the shoulder. In Ⓐ note the marked flattening of the contour from muscle wasting. The radiograph in Ⓑ shows rarefaction of the bones, with narrowing of the joint space from loss of articular cartilage.

Treatment. This is mainly that for rheumatoid arthritis in general, as described on page 137. Exercises are important in maintaining a useful range of movement.

Operative treatment. Severe disability often results from the bone and cartilage destruction produced by the inflammatory rheumatoid synovitis. When this occurs replacement arthroplasty of the joint may be indicated to restore mobility and relieve pain. Early designs used a metal humeral head prosthesis with a stem cemented into the shaft of the bone (Fig. 14.6). This articulated with a small concave polyethylene prosthesis to resurface the glenoid socket. Pain relief following this surgery is usually good, but full active movement, particularly in abduction, is never restored. The main problems that compromise the result are loosening of the glenoid prosthesis because of inadequate bone support and the degeneration of the scapulo-humeral muscles. Newer prosthetic designs to address these problems, including surface replacements and reversed prostheses are under trial, but no long-term results are yet available.

OSTEOARTHRITIS OF THE SHOULDER (General description of osteoarthritis, p. 140)

Unlike most other joints, the shoulder is seldom affected by osteoarthritis. When it is affected there is usually a clear predisposing factor, such as previous injury or disease, avascular necrosis of the humeral head, or senility. The rarity of osteoarthritis of the shoulder is explained by its freedom from pressure stresses.

Pathology. The articular cartilage is worn away. The underlying bone becomes eburnated and at the joint margins it hypertrophies to form osteophytes.

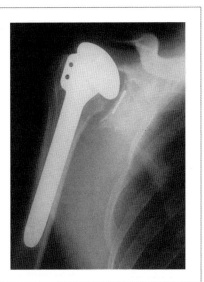

Fig. 14.6 Replacement arthroplasty of the gleno-humeral joint for rheumatoid arthritis of the shoulder, using a two-piece Neer prosthesis.

Clinical features. The patient is usually elderly: osteoarthritis is exceptional in the shoulders of younger patients. The main complaint is of pain in the shoulder and down the upper arm.

On examination there is no increase of local skin temperature and no synovial thickening. But a soft swelling due to effusion of fluid into the joint is common. Movements are restricted.

Radiographs show narrowing of the cartilage space: the joint outlines are clear-cut and often show some sclerosis; there is 'spurring' from osteophyte formation at the joint margins (Fig. 14.7).

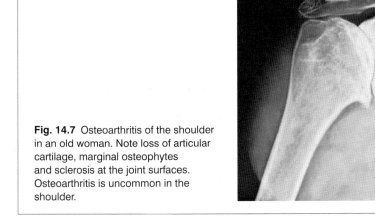

Fig. 14.7 Osteoarthritis of the shoulder in an old woman. Note loss of articular cartilage, marginal osteophytes and sclerosis at the joint surfaces. Osteoarthritis is uncommon in the shoulder.

Treatment. In most cases active treatment is unnecessary once the nature of the affection has been explained. If treatment is called for, conservative measures should usually be relied upon and gentle exercises are often helpful. If there is a large effusion it should be aspirated. Only exceptionally would operation be justified: if it were, replacement arthroplasty (see under rheumatoid arthritis, p. 260) would usually be advised, but arthrodesis might occasionally be appropriate.

'FROZEN' SHOULDER (Adhesive capsulitis; periarthritis)

'Frozen' shoulder is a common but ill-understood affection of the gleno-humeral joint, characterised by pain and uniform limitation of all movements but without radiographic change, and with a tendency to slow spontaneous recovery under appropriate treatment.

Cause. This is unknown. There is no evidence of infection. Injury is an inconstant factor and its significance is doubtful. Nevertheless it is accepted that symptoms of 'frozen' shoulder do often begin a few weeks after some form of injury.

Pathology. This is not fully understood, though the intense fibroblastic response may represent an auto-immune reaction similar to that seen with Dupuytren's contracture of the hand. There is a loss of resilience of the joint capsule, with adhesions between the synovial folds. Whatever their nature, the changes are reversible, and in most cases the range of joint movement is eventually restored to near normal.

Clinical features. The patient complains of severe aching pain in the shoulder and upper arm, of gradual and spontaneous onset. Pain is often severe enough to disturb sleep. *On examination* the only finding is uniform impairment of all gleno-humeral movements – abduction, flexion, extension, rotation – which are often reduced to about a quarter or half of their normal range. In a severe case much of the shoulder movement that remains is contributed by scapular movement, which is unimpaired. *Radiographs* do not show any abnormality.

Diagnosis. The characteristic feature of 'frozen' shoulder is the uniform limitation of all gleno-humeral movements without evidence of inflammatory or destructive changes.

Course. There is a tendency towards spontaneous recovery, usually within 6–12 months. The pain subsides first, leaving gleno-humeral joint stiffness, which thereafter gradually resolves with active use of the limb. If movements are not practised deliberately some permanent restriction of movement may remain.

Treatment. In the early, acutely painful stage the arm is rested in a sling, which is removed for short periods each day to permit gentle assisted shoulder exercises. Generally, non-steroidal anti-inflammatory drugs should be prescribed in addition to conventional analgesics. Steroid injections into the gleno-humeral joint may be of value in some patients with persistent severe pain. When the pain lessens, active exercises are intensified and continued for weeks or months until full movement is regained. If mobilisation is very slow after the pain has abated the shoulder may be manipulated gently under anaesthesia to break down residual adhesions. Manipulation may be required at some stage in up to a third of all cases, or arthroscopic distension with saline may be used as an alternative method.

It is important to warn the patient at the beginning that recovery may take many months, but at the same time to give assurance that eventually recovery is likely to be complete.

RECURRENT ANTERIOR DISLOCATION OF THE SHOULDER

Traumatic dislocation of the shoulder is liable to cause structural changes in the gleno-humeral joint which predispose to repeated dislocations. Rarely, dislocation may occur repeatedly in a patient with unduly lax ligaments, in the absence of trauma.

Pathology. This is twofold (Figs 14.8 and 14.9A):

1. The capsule, and with it the glenoid labrum, is stripped from the anterior margin of the glenoid rim (Bankart lesion) but retains an attachment farther down the neck of the scapula, where it becomes continuous with the periosteum. Thus there is created an intra-capsular 'pocket' in front of the glenoid margin, into which the humeral head may be displaced (Fig. 14.8).
2. The articular surface of the humeral head is dented postero-laterally (Hill-Sach), as if it were a table tennis ball, probably by impact against the sharp anterior corner of the glenoid fossa at the initial dislocation (Figs 14.8, 14.9 and 14.10).

The consequent defect in the contour of the articular surface allows the head to slip over the front of the glenoid when the arm is in lateral rotation, abduction, and extension. The dislocation is anterior, and it must be emphasised that the humeral head always remains within the capsule, in contradistinction to non-recurrent dislocation, in which the humeral head is displaced through a rent in the capsule.

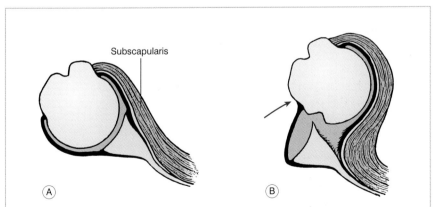

Fig. 14.8 Horizontal section of left shoulder showing the pathology of recurrent dislocation. The diagram on the left shows the normal condition. In the right-hand diagram the humeral head is shown dislocated forwards. It has stripped the capsule from the margin of the glenoid, creating a pocket in front of the neck of the scapula into which the humeral head is displaced. Note that the humeral head has been dented by the sharp glenoid margin, producing the typical defect of the articular surface.

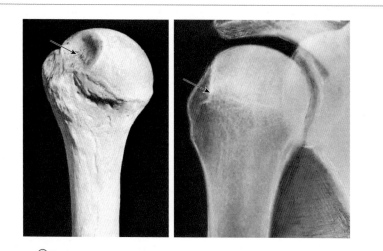

Fig. 14.9 Ⓐ Typical defect of articular surface of humeral head (arrow), found in most cases of recurrent dislocation of the shoulder. Ⓑ Radiographic appearance with the arm in 80° of medial rotation. The defect (arrow) is seen in profile at the upper and outer quadrant of the humeral head.

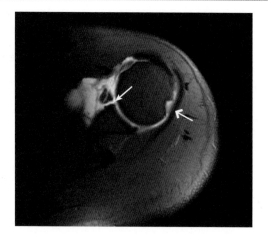

Fig. 14.10 Axial MR arthrogram of a patient with recurrent anterior shoulder dislocation. The large arrow indicates the presence of a bony defect (Hill-Sachs lesion) in the humeral head posteriorly. The smaller arrow points to a defect in the anterior cartilaginous labrum of the glenoid (the Bankart lesion). This has allowed the escape of contrast medium beneath the lax anterior capsule and predisposes the patient to further episodes of anterior dislocation.

Clinical features. The patient is usually a fit young adult, accustomed to sporting activities. Nearly always, recurrent dislocation follows an initial violent dislocation, often in a heavy fall. Thereafter dislocation recurs with trivial violence, characteristically during combined abduction, lateral rotation, and extension (for example, in putting on a coat).

On examination no clinical abnormality is apparent, but it may be found that the patient becomes apprehensive when the arm is placed in a position of abduction, extension, and lateral rotation – the position often adopted when putting on a coat.

Imaging. Routine radiographs with the limb in the anatomical position do not show any abnormality, but special profile views taken with the arm in 60–80° of medial rotation show the characteristic bony defect of the humeral head (Fig. 14.9B). The defect is not seen in any other projection, but it can be shown more clearly by computerised tomographic (CT) imaging or by magnetic resonance imaging (MRI). An MRI scan combined with arthrography provides the most detailed information on the bone and soft-tissue pathology (Fig. 14.10).

Treatment. Conservative treatment is not effective and if dislocation recurs frequently operation is justified. The two treatment principles used to prevent further dislocation are to either repair the defect in the glenoid labrum (Bankart[1] operation), or to create an overlapping buttress of muscle or bone on the anterior margin of the glenoid (Putti–Platt[2] or Bristow operations). Traditionally this required an open procedure through an anterior incision but increasingly this has been replaced by closed arthroscopic techniques for repair. However, it must be emphasised that the results in terms of functional outcome are identical with open or closed methods. Arthroscopic surgery, though more convenient for the patient, should only be undertaken by surgeons trained in the necessary specialist skills and equipped with the sophisticated equipment required.

Recurrent anterior dislocation from ligamentous laxity

There is a separate small group of patients in which the defects in the anterior capsule are not present. Instead, there is general laxity of the ligaments about the shoulder, with a voluminous capsule that allows subluxation or even full dislocation of the humeral head to occur without preceding injury. Such patients can often displace the humerus voluntarily and with increasing ease, and displacement may often be either anterior or posterior. The humeral head always remains within the lax capsule, and there is no capsular rupture.

Treatment. These patients should be dissuaded from repeatedly demonstrating their ability to subluxate or dislocate the joint, which can sometimes become an obsessive neurosis or at least a 'party trick'. If operation is called for, a bone-block operation, by which the area and depth of the glenoid fossa are increased by a suitably shaped bone graft, is generally to be recommended.

RECURRENT POSTERIOR DISLOCATION

Posterior dislocation of the shoulder is much less common than anterior dislocation. Often – indeed usually – the cause is an electric shock or an epileptiform

[1]Blundell Bankart, a technically brilliant English orthopaedic surgeon working in London, described the shoulder lesion in recurrent dislocation and the operation for its repair in 1923.
[2]Vittorio Putti, Professor of Orthopaedics in Bologna, and Sir Harry Platt of Manchester, later President of the Royal College of Surgeons of England, were jointly credited with developing this operation in 1923.

convulsion, and it is not uncommon for both shoulders to be dislocated together. The dislocation is prone to become recurrent. The pathology is analogous to that of recurrent anterior dislocation:

1. the capsule, glenoid labrum and periosteum are stripped from the back of the neck of the scapula
2. the humeral head is dented supero-medially rather than postero-laterally as in recurrent anterior dislocation.

Dislocation occurs on abduction and medial rotation.

Operative repair may be effected by reefing the infraspinatus tendon in a similar way to that used on the subscapularis for anterior dislocation. An alternative method is to deepen and widen the glenoid socket by screwing a suitably shaped block of iliac bone to the back of the neck of the scapula (bone-block operation).

Like recurrent anterior dislocation, recurrent posterior dislocation may sometimes occur spontaneously, without previous injury, in a patient with ligamentous laxity.

COMPLETE TEAR OF ROTATOR (TENDINOUS) CUFF (Torn supraspinatus)

It is important to distinguish complete tears of the rotator tendinous cuff from incomplete tears. The clinical effects are different. Whereas an incomplete tear is one cause of the 'painful arc syndrome' (p. 268), without obvious loss of power, a complete tear impairs seriously the ability to abduct the shoulder.

Cause. The tendon gives way under a sudden strain, usually caused by a fall. The injury is not necessarily a severe one; indeed it often seems to be mild. Age-degeneration of the tendon is a constant predisposing factor.

Pathology. The tear is mainly of the supraspinatus tendon, but it may extend into the adjacent subscapularis or infraspinatus tendons. The tear is close to the insertion of the tendons and usually involves the capsule of the joint, with which the tendons are blended. The edges of the rent retract, leaving a gaping eliptical hole which establishes a communication between the shoulder joint and the subacromial bursa (Fig. 14.11). In general, it may be said that a tendon that ruptures is usually already degenerate: thus rupture occurs mainly in the elderly.

Clinical features. The patient is usually a man over 60: only occasionally is a younger patient affected. After a strain or fall he complains of pain at the tip of the shoulder and down the upper arm, and of inability to raise the arm.

On examination there is local tenderness below the lateral margin of the acromion. When the patient attempts to abduct the arm no movement occurs at the gleno-humeral joint but a range of about 45–60° of abduction can be achieved, entirely by scapular movement (Fig. 14.12A). There is, however, a full range of passive movement; and if the arm is abducted with assistance beyond 90° the patient can sustain the abduction by deltoid action (Fig. 14.12B). Thus the essential and characteristic feature in cases of torn supraspinatus tendon is inability to initiate gleno-humeral abduction. The usual explanation is that the early stages of abduction demand the combined action of the deltoid muscle, which supplies the main motive force, and the supraspinatus, which stabilises the humeral head in the glenoid fossa (like the workman's foot against a ladder that is being raised from the ground).

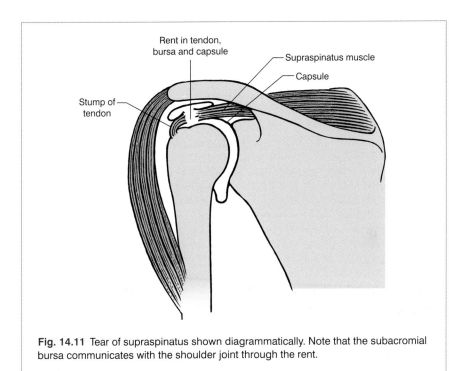

Fig. 14.11 Tear of supraspinatus shown diagrammatically. Note that the subacromial bursa communicates with the shoulder joint through the rent.

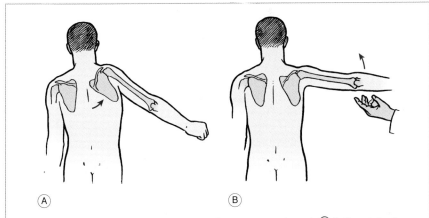

Fig. 14.12 Complete tear of tendinous cuff (torn supraspinatus). Ⓐ Active abduction from the resting position is possible only by scapular rotation, the deltoid being unable to initiate gleno-humeral abduction without the help of the supraspinatus. Ⓑ When the limb is raised passively beyond the horizontal abduction can be sustained actively by the deltoid.

Diagnosis. Complete tear of the rotator cuff must be distinguished from other causes of impaired gleno-humeral abduction, especially the painful arc syndrome and paralysis of the abductor muscles (as from poliomyelitis or nerve injury). Inability to initiate gleno-humeral abduction, with power to sustain abduction once the limb has been raised passively, is characteristic of a widely torn supraspinatus. In the painful arc syndrome the power of abduction is retained but the movement is painful.

Imaging. Examination by ultrasound scanning can identify a complete tear of the rotator cuff, but MR scans provide more detailed information on associated pathology in the surrounding structures (Fig. 14.13).

Treatment. In older patients operation should usually be avoided, because the degenerate state of the tendon makes satisfactory repair impracticable: the disability tends to become gradually less noticeable, and indeed the power of active abduction (by deltoid action alone) may sometimes be regained despite the persistence of a large tear.

In younger patients operation should be undertaken to repair both partial-thickness and full-thickness tears. As with other shoulder surgery this can be carried out as an open or an arthroscopic procedure depending on the experience of the surgeon. At the same operation it may be necessary to perform an acromioplasty to reduce impingement on the rotator cuff and to prevent repeat rupture. Thereafter passive movements may be begun within a few days but attempts to lift the arm actively should be deferred for 4 weeks, when provisional healing of the tendon may be expected to have occurred. The results of operation are not uniformly satisfactory, probably because of the poor quality of the degenerate tendon.

PAINFUL ARC SYNDROME (Supraspinatus syndrome)

This is a clinical syndrome characterised by pain in the shoulder and upper arm during the mid-range of gleno-humeral abduction, with freedom from pain at the extremes of the range. The syndrome is common to five distinct shoulder lesions.

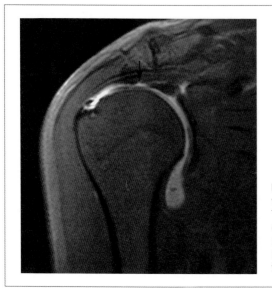

Fig. 14.13 Coronal T2 weighted MR scan of shoulder. There is a defect in the rotator cuff indicating a cuff tear (arrow). Most commonly this involves the supraspinatus tendon.

The shoulder region

Cause. The pain is produced mechanically by nipping of a tender structure between the tuberosity of the humerus and the acromion process and coraco-acromial ligament.

Pathology. Even in the normal shoulder, the clearance between the upper end of the humerus and the acromion process is small in the range of abduction between 45 and 160°. If a swollen and tender structure is present beneath the acromion it is liable to get nipped during the arc of movement in which the clearance is small (Fig. 14.14A), with consequent pain. In the neutral position and in full abduction the clearance is greater and pain is less marked or absent (Figs 14.14B and 14.14C).

Five primary lesions can give rise to the syndrome (Fig. 14.15). In general, though, these labels only represent variations of a process of degeneration which is the underlying defect.

1. *Minor tear of supraspinatus tendon*. Tearing or strain of a few degenerate tendon fibres causes an inflammatory reaction with local swelling, but power is not significantly impaired as it is after a complete tear of the tendinous cuff.
2. *Supraspinatus tendinitis*. In this condition there is believed to be an inflammatory reaction provoked by degeneration of the tendon fibres.
3. *Calcified deposit in supraspinatus tendon*. A white chalky deposit forms within the degenerate tendon, and the lesion is surrounded by an inflammatory reaction. As the chalky 'cyst' becomes increasingly tense, local pain becomes agonisingly acute.
4. *Subacromial bursitis*. The bursal walls are inflamed and thickened from mechanical irritation.
5. *Injury of greater tuberosity*. A contusion or undisplaced fracture of the greater tuberosity is a frequent cause.

Clinical features. Whatever the primary cause, the clinical syndrome has the same general features, though they vary in degree. With the arm dependent pain is absent or minimal. During abduction of the arm pain begins at about

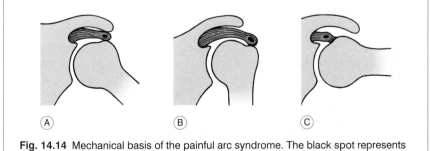

Fig. 14.14 Mechanical basis of the painful arc syndrome. The black spot represents any tender lesion near the supraspinatus insertion. Ⓐ With the arm in mid-abduction the lesion is nipped between the humerus and the acromion. Ⓑ With the arm dependent, the lesion is free from pressure. Ⓒ At full elevation the lesion is again free from pressure.

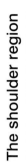

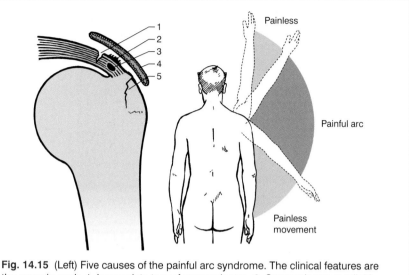

Fig. 14.15 (Left) Five causes of the painful arc syndrome. The clinical features are the same in each. 1. Incomplete tear of supraspinatus. 2. Supraspinatus tendinitis. 3. Calcified deposit in supraspinatus. 4. Subacromial bursitis. 5. Crack fracture of greater tuberosity.

Fig. 14.16 (Right) Painful arc syndrome. The middle arc of abduction is painful whereas the extremes are painless.

45° and persists through the arc of movement up to 160° (Fig. 14.16). Thereafter the pain lessens or disappears. In descent from full elevation pain is again experienced during the middle arc of the range: often the patient will twist or circumduct the arm grotesquely in an effort to get it down with the least pain. The severity of the pain varies from case to case. In cases of calcified deposit in the supraspinatus tendon the pain may be so intense that the patient is scarcely able to move the shoulder, or to sleep, and is driven to seek emergency treatment.

Radiographic features. These vary with the underlying cause. Plain radiographs will reveal a fracture of the greater tuberosity or a calcified deposit (Fig. 14.17). A calcified deposit is distinguished radiologically from an avulsed fragment of bone by the fact that it is homogeneous and does not show the trabeculation characteristic of bone. MR scanning may demonstrate some of the other causes from degeneration and partial tears of the rotator cuff.

Diagnosis. Painful arc syndrome is sometimes confused with arthritis of the acromio-clavicular joint, which also causes pain during a certain phase of the abduction arc. But in acromio-clavicular arthritis the pain begins later in abduction (not below 90°) and increases rather than diminishes as full elevation is reached.

Differentiation between the five primary causes of the syndrome is aided by the history and by radiography. A history of injury suggests a strain of the

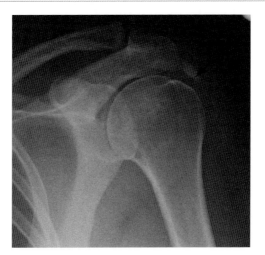

Fig. 14.17 Radiograph of shoulder showing calcification of the soft tissues above the greater tuberosity of the humerus (arrow). The calcified material usually lies within the supraspinatus tendon and is often associated with a painful tendinitis, but can be asymptomatic.

supraspinatus tendon or a lesion of the greater tuberosity, whereas a spontaneous onset suggests tendinitis, calcified deposit or subacromial bursitis. As noted, radiography will confirm or exclude a fracture or a calcified deposit (Fig. 14.17).

Treatment in the acute case. In mild cases treatment is often unnecessary, but when pain is more severe this may be required depending upon the primary cause of the syndrome.

Calcified deposit in supraspinatus tendon. If the pain is intense, as it sometimes is in these cases, relief can usually be gained by direct injection of hydrocortisone into the calcified deposit. If this fails the deposit of hydroxyapatite crystals may be dispersed with an aspiration needle followed by lavage of the subacromial space.

Contusion or crack fracture of greater tuberosity. Reliance should be placed on active use and mobilising exercises.

Strain of supraspinatus, supraspinatus tendinitis, and subacromial bursitis. Most of these cases respond gradually to physiotherapy in the form of ultrasound or interferential therapy, and mobilising exercises.

Treatment in the chronic case. In cases of painful arc syndrome in which severe symptoms persist despite a full trial of efficient conservative treatment, operation may be required. The procedure of acromioplasty excises the acromion process, or preferably its anterior third, together with the coraco-acromial ligament to prevent the possibility of further nipping of inflamed tissue between it and the upper end of the humerus. The operation can be carried out as either an open or closed arthroscopic procedure.

RUPTURE OF LONG TENDON OF BICEPS

The long tendon of the biceps is one of several tendons in the body that are prone to rupture without violent stress or injury. (Others are the supraspinatus tendon and the tendon of extensor pollicis longus.)

Cause. The tendon will not rupture under ordinary stresses unless it is already weak. The predisposing factor is age-degeneration, probably accelerated by oft-repeated friction and angulation at the point where the tendon enters the bicipital groove of the humerus.

Clinical features. The patient is usually a man past middle age. While lifting or pulling with the arm he feels something give way in the region of the front of the shoulder. There is only moderate discomfort, and often the patient neglects to seek early advice. Later he may notice an unusual bulge of the muscle in front of the arm.

On examination soon after the rupture, there is slight tenderness over the bicipital groove of the humerus. When the patient contracts the biceps muscle, as in flexing the elbow or supinating the forearm against resistance, the belly of the long head is seen to bunch up into a short round mass like a ball. There is surprisingly little weakness of elbow flexion or of supination.

Treatment. The disability is usually so slight that operation is not required. When repair is considered necessary, it is sufficient to produce a tenodesis by fixing the distal stump of the tendon to the walls of the bicipital groove. The proximal stump is ignored.

TENOSYNOVITIS OF LONG TENDON OF BICEPS (Biceps tendinitis)

This is an uncommon and rather minor affection characterised by pain and local tenderness in the region of the bicipital groove of the humerus and the long tendon of the biceps. It is generally ascribed to frictional irritation of the tendon within its groove, but it may be associated with degeneration of the tendons that form a cuff at the top of the shoulder.

Clinical features. The complaint is of pain in the front of the shoulder, worse on active use of the arm. Examination reveals local tenderness in the course of the long tendon of the biceps in the bicipital groove of the humerus. The pain can often be exacerbated by moving the shoulder while the tendon is made taut by forced supination of the forearm.

Treatment. Excessive use of the shoulder should be avoided. Physiotherapy by ultrasound, interferential therapy, or short-wave diathermy is worth a trial. Failing this, a local injection of hydrocortisone may be advised.

POLYMYALGIA RHEUMATICA

Polymyalgia rheumatica was described on page 166. It is worth mentioning again here because the soft tissues about the shoulders and the base of the neck are commonly the parts affected. The onset of this disorder of connective tissue is insidious, with aching pain and tenderness in the muscles of the shoulder girdle, neck, and spine, and severe 'stiffness' with substantial restriction of mobility of the shoulders, neck, and spine. There is also constitutional illness, with malaise, mild pyrexia, and night sweats, and elevation of the erythrocyte sedimentation rate. Early treatment by prednisolone in high doses should be advised if there is a suspicion of giant cell arteritis, pending confirmation of the diagnosis by biopsy.

DISORDERS OF THE ACROMIO-CLAVICULAR JOINT

OSTEOARTHRITIS OF THE ACROMIO-CLAVICULAR JOINT

Degenerative arthritis (osteoarthritis) of the acromio-clavicular joint is seen much more often than is osteoarthritis of the gleno-humeral joint. Pathologically, there are degeneration and attrition of articular cartilage, and spurs of bone (osteophytes) are formed at the joint margins.

Clinical features. There is pain, localised accurately to the acromio-clavicular joint and aggravated by strenuous use of the limb – especially in overhead work. *On examination* irregular bony thickening of the joint margins due to osteophytes may be felt. There is no soft-tissue thickening and no increase of local skin temperature. The total range of shoulder movements is not appreciably decreased, but pain in the region of the acromio-clavicular joint is exacerbated at the extremes of movement, especially on elevation of the arm towards the vertical: the arc of movement below 90° is painless, but above 90° pain develops and persists throughout the remainder of the arc to full elevation (compare painful arc syndrome, p. 268).

Imaging. Radiographs show features that are typical of osteoarthritis with narrowing of the cartilage space and marginal osteophytes. MR scans can provide more information on the extent of rotator cuff impingement in the sub-acromial space.

Treatment. Often treatment is not needed, other than modification of everyday activities. In severe cases operation is justified: it should take the form of excision of the lateral end of the clavicle with preservation of the conoid and trapezoid ligaments.

PERSISTENT ACROMIO-CLAVICULAR DISLOCATION OR SUBLUXATION

Persistent upward displacement of the lateral end of the clavicle is a common sequel to traumatic dislocation or subluxation of the acromio-clavicular joint. In most cases the displacement is slight and causes no symptoms, except perhaps for pain or discomfort during overhead work. Exceptionally there is pain, worse during full elevation of the arm. *On examination* the lateral end of the clavicle is unduly prominent, and a distinct step can be felt between it and the surface of the acromion.

Treatment. Usually treatment is unnecessary, but if disabling pain persists operation is advised. A simple and effective method to achieve pain relief is to excise the lateral end of the clavicle. However, in younger patients the resultant instability may be troublesome and it may be preferable to reconstruct the joint by coraco-acromial ligament transfer combined with internal fixation of the coraco-clavicular joint.

DISORDERS OF THE STERNO-CLAVICULAR JOINT

PERSISTENT OR RECURRENT DISLOCATION OF THE STERNO-CLAVICULAR JOINT

Forward dislocation of the medial end of the clavicle may be permanent, or it may recur on certain movements of the arm. Often, but not always, there is a history of precipitating injury. The symptoms are slight: there is a prominence in the region of the joint, with mild local pain. Recurrent displacement of the clavicle in and out of joint during movements of the arm may be an annoying disability. *On examination* the medial end of the clavicle, when displaced, is easily felt as a prominent forward projection. In recurrent dislocation the clavicle can be felt to click out of joint when the shoulders are braced back, and to go back into position when the shoulders are arched forwards.

Imaging. Radiographs reveal the displacement, when present. It is difficult to show the joint clearly on plane films and CT scanning may be necessary to provide fuller information.

Treatment. In many cases treatment is unnecessary, but operation is occasionally justified. The displacement is reduced and the clavicle is held in place by constructing a new retaining ligament from the tendon of the subclavius muscle or an autogenous semitendinosus tendon in a figure-of-eight configuration. Wire fixation must be avoided because of the risk of damage to the underlying major vessels.

EXTRINSIC DISORDERS SIMULATING SHOULDER DISEASE

Pain in the shoulder or arm often has no local cause, but is referred from an extrinsic lesion. Such a possibility must always be considered in differential diagnosis.

DISORDERS OF THE BRACHIAL PLEXUS OR ITS ROOTS

The pain caused by pressure upon the brachial plexus or its roots is commonly attributed erroneously to an affection of the shoulder. Such pain varies in its precise distribution according to the site and nature of the nerve lesion. Usually it radiates from the base of the neck, across the top of the shoulder, and down the front, side, or back of the arm; thence it extends into the forearm, and often into the hand and fingers. Thus in its typical form the pain from a nerve lesion in the neck differs from the pain of a shoulder lesion, which typically does not extend below the elbow. The conditions which can result in brachial plexus symptoms are described in Chapter 12.

Affections that may cause referred symptoms in the distribution of the brachial plexus include prolapsed cervical intervertebral disc, osteoarthritis of the cervical spine, cervical rib, herpes zoster, and tumours involving the spinal cord or the component nerves of the brachial plexus.

DISORDERS OF THE UPPER ARM

Shoulder pain typically radiates distally and is often felt near the insertion of the deltoid muscle. Pain arising locally at this site, for instance from a lesion in the shaft of the humerus, may thus be confused with pain arising at the shoulder itself. Radiographs including the upper half of the humerus will usually help to make the distinction.

DISORDERS WITHIN THE THORAX

Angina pectoris

In a small proportion of cases of angina pectoris the pain is felt predominantly in the shoulder region (usually on the left side). Other features are invariably present to suggest a cardiac origin, and the shoulder shows no clinical abnormality.

Pleurisy

Basal pleurisy is sometimes a cause of shoulder pain which is explained by irritation of phrenic nerve endings, with referred pain in the distribution of the cutaneous branches of the same cervical roots (mainly C4).

Tumour

Pancoast's apical lung carcinoma is a well-known cause of radiating shoulder and upper limb pain, from involvement of the lower trunks of the brachial plexus. Chest radiography is diagnostic.

DISORDERS WITHIN THE ABDOMEN

Cholecystitis

This is a cause of referred pain in the right shoulder, from irritation of the phrenic nerve endings under the diaphragm. The associated abdominal symptoms and signs, and the lack of clinical abnormality in the shoulder, should prevent diagnostic errors.

Subphrenic abscess

This also is an occasional cause of referred shoulder pain. Constitutional symptoms and pyrexia, with normal clinical findings in the shoulder, should indicate this possible cause.

15 | The upper arm and elbow

Apart from injury, disorders of the upper arm and elbow region are generally straightforward and present few special problems. They conform to the general descriptions of bone and joint diseases that were given in Part 2. Thus the humerus is subject to the ordinary infections of bone, and occasionally to bone tumours – especially metastatic tumours. The elbow is liable to every type of arthritis, none is particularly common though rheumatoid arthritis is commoner than osteoarthritis. After the knee, it is the joint most often affected by osteochondritis dissecans and loose body formation. The ulnar nerve lies in a vulnerable position at the back of the medial epicondyle, and the possibility of impairment of nerve function complicating disease or injury of the joint should always be remembered. Replacement arthroplasty of the elbow is undertaken increasingly, but compared with those of hip and knee arthroplasty the results still leave much to be desired, especially from the point of view of the longevity of the new joint.

SPECIAL POINTS IN THE INVESTIGATION OF UPPER ARM AND ELBOW SYMPTOMS

History

The interrogation follows the usual lines suggested in Chapter 1. It is important to ascertain the exact site and distribution of the pain, and its nature. Pain arising locally in the humerus is easily confused with pain arising in the shoulder, which characteristically radiates to a point about half-way down the outer aspect of the upper arm. Elbow pain is localised fairly precisely to the joint, though a diffuse aching pain is often felt also in the forearm. When the ulnar nerve is interfered with behind the elbow the symptoms are mainly in the hand.

In the elbow, a history of previous injury, perhaps long ago in childhood, is often relevant. Injuries in this region are notoriously liable to have late effects in the form of impaired movement, deformity, arthritis, loose body formation, or interference with the ulnar nerve.

Exposure

The whole length of the upper limb must be uncovered. The opposite limb must be similarly exposed for comparison.

Table 15.1 Routine clinical examination in suspected disorders of the upper arm and elbow

1. LOCAL EXAMINATION OF THE ARM AND ELBOW	
Inspection	**Power**
Bone contours and alignment	Flexors
Soft-tissue contours	Extensors
Colour and texture of skin	Supinators
Scars or sinuses	Pronators
Palpation	**Stability**
Skin temperature	Lateral ligament
Bone contours	Medial ligament
Soft-tissue contours	**The median nerve**
Local tenderness	Sensory function
Movements (active and passive)	Motor function (opponens action)
Humero-ulnar joint:	Sweating
Flexion	**The radial nerve**
Extension	Sensory function
Radio-ulnar joint:	Motor function (extension of wrist, thumb, and fingers)
Supination	**The ulnar nerve**
Pronation	Sensory function
? Pain on movement	Motor function
? Crepitation on movement	Sweating

2. EXAMINATION OF POTENTIAL EXTRINSIC SOURCES OF ARM PAIN

This is important if a satisfactory explanation for the symptoms is not found on local examination. The investigation should include:
1. the neck, with the brachial plexus
2. the shoulder

3. GENERAL EXAMINATION

General survey of other parts of the body. The local symptoms may be only one manifestation of a widespread disease

Steps in routine examination

A suggested plan for the routine clinical examination of the upper arm and elbow is summarised in Table 15.1.

Movements at the elbow

The elbow joint has two distinct components: the hinge joint between the humerus above and the ulna and radius below, allowing flexion–extension movement; and the pivot joint between the upper ends of the radius and ulna, allowing rotation of the forearm. It should be remembered that free rotation of the forearm is dependent not only upon an intact superior radio-ulnar joint: it demands also free mobility between the radius and ulna throughout their length, and distally at the inferior radio-ulnar joint. *Flexion–extension*: The normal range is from 0 to 155° (0=anatomical position, with the arm straight). *Supination–pronation*: Rotation movements must be tested with the elbow flexed to a right angle, to eliminate rotation at the shoulder (Fig. 15.1A). The normal range is 90° of supination (palm up) and 90° of pronation (palm down) (Fig. 15.1B). If the range of rotation is restricted possible causes must be sought in the forearm and wrist as well as in the elbow.

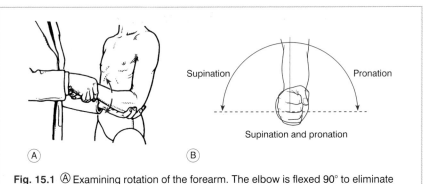

Supination

Pronation

Supination and pronation

(A)

(B)

Fig. 15.1 (A) Examining rotation of the forearm. The elbow is flexed 90° to eliminate rotation at the shoulder. (B) Range of supination and pronation of the forearm.

The ulnar nerve

Because of the vulnerability of the ulnar nerve in its course behind the elbow, tests of ulnar nerve function should be carried out as part of the routine examination of the elbow. Examine for sensibility in the little finger and medial half of the ring finger, and test the ulnar-innervated small muscles of the hand for wasting or weakness: a simple test is to ask the patient to spread the fingers and to bring them together again forcibly, to prevent a card gripped between the middle and ring fingers from being withdrawn. Note whether the skin in the territory of the ulnar nerve sweats equally with the rest of the hand.

The median and radial nerves

The integrity of the median and radial nerves should also be tested. Criteria of integrity of the median nerve are volar sensibility in the lateral three and a half digits, and active power of opposition of the thumb. Integrity of the radial nerve is demonstrated by ability to dorsiflex the wrist and to extend the digits at the metacarpo-phalangeal joints. A distal lesion, affecting the posterior interosseous division of the nerve, may leave wrist extension intact while impairing extension of the digits.

Imaging

Radiographic examination. Radiographs of the humerus must always include antero-posterior and lateral projections, and they should take in both the shoulder joint and the elbow.

Routine radiographs of the elbow comprise an antero-posterior projection with the elbow straight and a lateral projection with the joint semiflexed. In special circumstances additional oblique or tangential projections may be helpful. A radiograph of the forearm bones and of the inferior radio-ulnar joint is also required when rotation of the forearm is impaired.

Other imaging techniques. Radioisotope scanning, CT scanning, and MR imaging may all be helpful in appropriate circumstances.

Extrinsic sources of pain in the upper arm

Pain in the upper arm is commonly referred from a lesion elsewhere—particularly from the shoulder, and from the neck when the brachial plexus or its roots are involved. Shoulder pain usually radiates from the tip of the acromion process to about the middle of the outer aspect of the arm, but it does not extend below the elbow. In contrast, nerve pain from interference with the brachial plexus often extends throughout the length of the arm and forearm into the hand and fingers; and frequently there is accompanying paraesthesiae in the form of tingling, numbness, or 'pins and needles'.

DISORDERS OF THE UPPER ARM

ACUTE OSTEOMYELITIS (General description of acute osteomyelitis, p. 85)

Osteomyelitis is less common in the upper limb than in the lower. Nevertheless the humerus is a well-recognised site of haematogenous infection – especially its upper metaphysis.

Pathology. Except in time of war the humerus is seldom infected directly by organisms introduced from without, for compound fractures are rare. Infection is usually haematogenous, from a focus elsewhere in the body. This type of infection occurs mainly in children, and it usually begins in a metaphysis of the bone – more often the upper metaphysis than the lower. Since

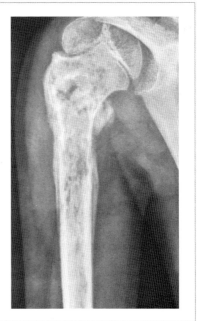

Fig. 15.2 Acute osteomyelitis of upper end of humerus. Radiograph 4 weeks after onset showing marked rarefaction of the bone, with patchy areas of destruction and much subperiosteal new bone formation.

both the upper and the lower metaphyses are partly enclosed within the capsule of the shoulder and of the elbow respectively, a metaphysial infection is liable to spread directly to the adjacent joint, causing pyogenic arthritis (see Fig. 7.2).

Clinical features. There is constitutional illness, with pyrexia. Locally, there is severe pain at the site of infection. *On examination* there is intense and well-localised tenderness over the affected area – usually near one end of the bone. Later, there may be swelling and increased warmth, and a fluctuant abscess may form. The adjacent joint is commonly swollen from an effusion of fluid ('sympathetic' effusion), even if the joint itself is not involved in the infection. In the absence of joint infection, however, movements are restricted only slightly, if at all.

Imaging. *Radiographs* do not show any abnormality at first. After about two weeks there are often localised rarefaction and subperiosteal new bone formation (Fig. 15.2), but these changes may be slight at first. *Radioisotope scanning* shows increased uptake in the affected area.

Investigations and **treatment** are the same as for acute osteomyelitis elsewhere (p. 89).

CHRONIC OSTEOMYELITIS (General description of chronic osteomyelitis, p. 90)

As in other bones, chronic pyogenic osteomyelitis of the humerus is nearly always a sequel to acute osteomyelitis that has been neglected or has responded poorly to treatment. The bone is thickened, often throughout its whole length, and there may be a persistent or intermittent purulent discharge from a sinus, or recurrent flare-ups with local pain and induration. *Radiographs* show irregular thickening with patchy areas of sclerosis and cavitation, and sometimes a sequestrum.

Treatment was described on page 91.

TUMOURS OF BONE

Benign tumours (General description of benign bone tumours, p. 106)

Osteochondroma, osteoid osteoma, and giant-cell tumour can all affect the humerus but none are particularly common at this site.

Giant-cell tumour is uncommon in the humerus, but when it does occur the usual site is at the upper end, where it often extends close up to the articular surface. The tumour occurs chiefly in young adults, and its general characteristics are like those of giant-cell tumour of bone at other sites (p. 109).

Treatment. The high risk of recurrence after simple curettage and bone grafting has to be balanced against the likely disability after radical excision of the whole of the upper end of the humerus. Each case must be considered on its merits, but if the tumour is large there is much to be said for radical local excision of the affected part of the bone and replacement by a custom-made metal prosthesis.

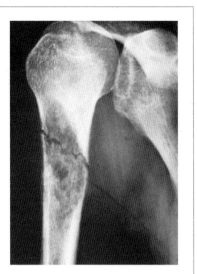

Fig. 15.3 Metastatic tumour in the humerus from primary carcinoma of the lung. This is a common site for metastatic tumours, which often lead eventually to pathological fracture.

Malignant tumours (General description of malignant bone tumours, p. 112)

Primary malignant tumours

Primary malignant tumours of bone are much less common in the upper limb than in the lower, and examples are seen only infrequently. However, osteosarcoma, chondrosarcoma, Ewing's tumour, and multiple myeloma should all be considered as possible causes of painful destructive bone lesions in the humerus.

Metastatic tumours

Metastatic tumours, by comparison, are common, especially in the proximal part of the humerus (Fig. 15.3). Carcinomatous deposits from tumours of the lung, breast, prostate, kidney, and thyroid are common and usually occur near the upper end of the shaft, where there is much vascular marrow. Such metastases are a common cause of pathological fracture and may require internal fixation as well as adjuvant treatment with radiotherapy.

BONE CYST

Both simple bone cysts and aneurysmal bone cysts can occur in the humerus and were described on page 126. The humerus is the commonest site of simple bone cyst, which occurs especially in children or adolescents, and at the upper end of the bone. The cyst replaces the normal bone structure and may lead to pathological fracture as the presenting symptom in over 50% of cases. (Fig. 15.4A). Small cysts may simply be kept under observation, since the majority heal spontaneously in adult life (Fig. 15.4B). A large cyst which might lead to fracture, should first be aspirated and injected with corticosteroid solution or autogenous bone marrow. Most fractures through cysts heal with conservative treatment and internal fixation is rarely required in the humerus.

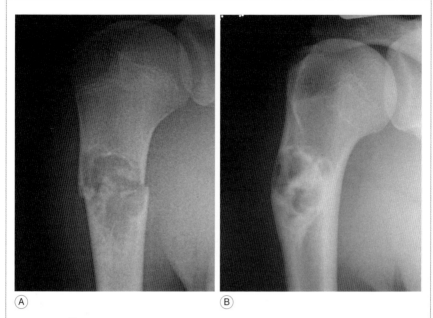

Fig. 15.4 Ⓐ Radiograph showing a pathological fracture through a simple bone cyst in the shaft of the humerus in an adolescent patient. Cortical fragments have fallen into the multilocular cystic cavity. Ⓑ Same patient nine months later showing the fracture has healed spontaneously and the cyst is showing evidence of infilling with dense sclerotic bone.

DISORDERS OF THE ELBOW

CUBITUS VALGUS

The normal elbow, when fully extended, is in a position of slight valgus – usually 10° in men and 15° in women. This is known as the carrying angle. If the angle is increased, so that the forearm is abducted excessively in relation to the upper arm, the deformity is known as cubitus valgus (Fig. 15.5).

Cause. Cubitus valgus is usually a consequence of previous disease or injury in the elbow region. The most frequent causes are:

1. previous fracture of the lower end of the humerus or of the capitulum, with mal-union
2. interference with epiphysial growth on the lateral side, from injury or infection.

Clinical features. Apart from the visible deformity there are no symptoms unless secondary effects develop.

Secondary effects. The most important sequel of cubitus valgus is interference with the function of the ulnar nerve. When valgus deformity is marked, the nerve is angled sharply round the prominent medial part of the joint, and repeated friction may lead to fibrosis of the nerve trunk. Symptoms develop insidiously over a long period: there are tingling and blunting of sensibility

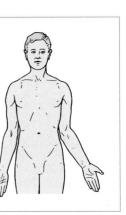

Fig. 15.5 Cubitus valgus (left elbow). The deformity predisposes to friction neuritis of the ulnar nerve.

in the ulnar distribution in the hand, with weakness and wasting of the ulnar-innervated small hand muscles (p. 291).

Treatment. Slight uncomplicated deformity is best left alone. If angulation is severe, correction by osteotomy near the lower end of the humerus is justified. If the function of the ulnar nerve is impaired the nerve should be transposed from its post-humeral groove to a new bed at the front of the elbow.

CUBITUS VARUS

Cubitus varus is the opposite deformity to cubitus valgus. The carrying angle, or normal angle of valgus at the fully extended elbow, is decreased or reversed.

Cause. The causes are similar to those of cubitus valgus:

1. previous fracture with mal-union (especially supracondylar fracture of the humerus)
2. interference with epiphysial growth on the medial side.

Clinical features. There are usually no symptoms other than the visible deformity, which may be embarrassing, especially to a child.

Treatment. Minor degrees of deformity can safely be left uncorrected. If the angulation is severe it may be corrected by osteotomy through the lower end of the humerus.

PYOGENIC ARTHRITIS OF THE ELBOW (General description of pyogenic arthritis, p. 96)

Pyogenic arthritis is usually an acute infection with suppuration, but it may occur in subacute or even in chronic form.

The causation, pathology, clinical features and treatment of the condition are similar to other large joints and are described on page 97.

TUBERCULOUS ARTHRITIS OF THE ELBOW (General description of tuberculous arthritis, p. 98)

Tuberculous arthritis is much less common in the elbow than it is in the large weight-bearing joints such as the hip and knee.

The pathological and clinical features of joint tuberculosis were described on page 98, and further description is not required here. Biopsy may be required to establish the diagnosis.

RHEUMATOID ARTHRITIS OF THE ELBOW (General description of rheumatoid arthritis, p. 134)

One or both elbows are commonly affected in rheumatoid arthritis, usually in conjunction with several other joints, and may result in considerable pain and functional disability.

Pathology. The pathological changes are like those of rheumatoid arthritis elsewhere. Beginning as a chronic inflammatory thickening of the synovial membrane, it tends later to involve the articular cartilage, which may eventually be almost totally destroyed. The subchondral bone may also be eroded by the synovial pannus formation.

Clinical features. As in other joints, the main symptoms are pain, swelling from thickening of the synovial membrane, abnormal warmth of the overlying skin, and impairment of movement, particularly of rotation of the forearm. In the later stages there is commonly a fixed flexion deformity.

Imaging. *Radiographic examination*. At first there are no changes. Later, there is diffuse rarefaction in the area of the joint. In long-established cases the cartilage space is lost and there may be considerable erosion of the bone ends (Fig. 15.6).

CT scanning may be useful in pre-operative planning to determine the amount of bone available for prosthetic support.

Treatment. Primary treatment is along the lines suggested for rheumatoid arthritis in general (p. 137).

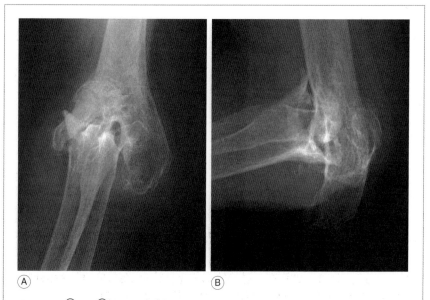

(A)   (B)

Fig. 15.6 Ⓐ and Ⓑ Radiographs of elbow affected by chronic rheumatoid arthritis. There is almost complete destruction of the articular surfaces of radius, ulna and humerus with subluxation of the joints.

Operative treatment. If extensive destruction of the articular cartilage leads to persistent disabling pain with bone destruction and deformity, operation must be considered. If pain is largely at the lateral side of the joint the simple operation of excision of the head of the radius, with a limited synovectomy, often gives good relief. Replacement arthroplasty, by the fitting of a hinged prosthesis with long stems cemented into the humerus and ulna, has now been largely abandoned because of the risk of loosening and fracture. Improved results have been obtained by non-linked replacements of the articular surfaces with metal and plastic liners. The long-term functional results are not as good as with hip and knee replacements, but offer satisfactory pain relief.

OSTEOARTHRITIS OF THE ELBOW (General description of osteoarthritis, p. 140)

Osteoarthritis seldom occurs in an elbow that was previously normal. In nearly every case a predisposing factor has been present for several years. This is usually a damaged articular surface from previous fracture involving the joint, or from osteochondritis dissecans.

Clinical features. There is slowly increasing pain in the elbow, worse on heavy use of the limb. The patient may also notice that movement is impaired. In some cases there are attacks of sudden locking, suggesting the presence of a loose body in the joint. There is often a history of previous injury or disease involving the elbow – for instance, osteochondritis dissecans. *On examination* there is palpable thickening at the joint margins, from osteophytes. Flexion and extension are impaired but rotation is often full. There is coarse crepitation on movement.

Radiographs show narrowing of the cartilage space and pointed osteophytes at the joint margins (Fig. 15.7). Loose bodies (formed from detached osteophytes or from flakes of articular cartilage) may be present.

Treatment. Many patients with early arthritis, causing only intermittent pain and minimal loss of movement, can be managed by re-assurance and modification of activities. Others may require conservative treatment with analgesics and physiotherapy in the form of short-wave diathermy and mobilisation of the joint. Where pain becomes severe on a daily basis, or locking and joint stiffness limit function, surgery is usually indicated. Open or arthroscopic debridement to remove osteophytes and any loose bodies from the joint may be effective, but excision of the radial head may also be required to restore forearm rotation. In only a few cases is prosthetic joint replacement required to replace the humeral and ulnar surfaces using the techniques described for rheumatoid arthritis. It is important that the ulnar nerve is transposed anteriorly at the time of surgery to avoid the risk of later neuropraxia.

NEUROPATHIC ARTHRITIS OF THE ELBOW (General description of neuropathic arthritis, p. 147)

In neuropathic arthritis (Charcot's osteoarthropathy) of the elbow the joint becomes disorganised in consequence of a loss of sensibility to pain. It is a rare form of arthritis.

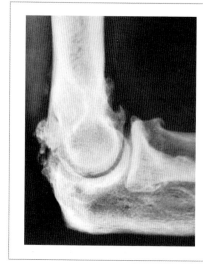

Fig. 15.7 Osteoarthritis of the elbow. Note the narrowed cartilage space and pointed osteophytes at the joint margins. In this case osteoarthritis was secondary to osteochondritis dissecans occurring many years before.

Cause. The usual underlying cause of the disease in the elbow is syringomyelia, but any other affection that leads to loss of sensibility (e.g. diabetic neuropathy) may be responsible.

Pathology, clinical features and treatment are similar to other affected joints. Treatment is conservative with elbow bracing as operation is inappropriate.

HAEMOPHILIC ARTHRITIS OF THE ELBOW (General description of haemophilic arthritis, p. 145)

Haemophilic arthritis affects the elbow more often than any other joint except the knee. As in other joints, the main feature is intra-articular haemorrhage, often recurrent, with consequent irritation and, later, degeneration of the joint.

The clue to the diagnosis is a history of previous bleeding or of a haemophilic tendency in the family. Haemarthrosis without major injury should always arouse suspicion of haemophilia. A prolonged blood clotting time is an important confirmatory finding.

Treatment (for fresh haemarthrosis). If antihaemophilic factor is available it should be given in adequate dosage and the joint should be aspirated. The elbow is supported by crepe bandages and a removable light plaster or plastic splint. Gentle exercises are resumed after 2 weeks. If antihaemophilic factor is not available reliance must be placed on splintage, without aspiration. In this event, particularly after repeated haemarthrosis, permanent damage with fibrosis of the synovial membrane and the formation of intra-articular adhesions must be expected in the long term.

OSTEOCHONDRITIS DISSECANS OF THE ELBOW (General description of osteochondritis dissecans, p. 153)

After the knee, the elbow is the most frequent site of osteochondritis dissecans. The disorder is characterised by necrosis of part of the articular cartilage and of

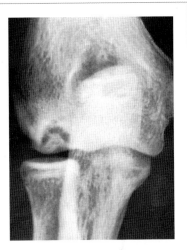

Fig. 15.8 Osteochondritis dissecans. A fragment of the capitulum is separating. This is the typical site of osteochondritis dissecans in the elbow.

the underlying bone, with eventual separation of the fragment to form an intra-articular loose body (Fig. 15.8).

Cause. The precise cause is unknown. Impairment of blood supply to the affected segment of bone and cartilage by thrombosis of an end artery has been suggested. Injury probably plays a part.

Pathology. The part of the elbow affected is nearly always the capitulum of the humerus. The necrotic segment of articular surface varies in size; commonly its surface area is about a centimetre in diameter and its depth less than half a centimetre. A line of demarcation forms between the avascular segment and the surrounding normal bone and cartilage, and after an interval of months the avascular segment separates as a loose body (sometimes two or three), leaving a shallow cavity in the articular surface which is ultimately filled with fibrous tissue. The damage to the joint surface predisposes to the later development of osteoarthritis.

Clinical features. In the early stages, before the fragment has separated, the symptoms are those of mild mechanical irritation of the joint – namely, aching after use and intermittent swelling (from fluid effusion). *On examination* at this stage there is often an effusion of clear fluid into the joint, and there is slight limitation of flexion or extension.

When a loose body has separated, the main features are recurrent sudden painful locking of the elbow and subsequent effusion of fluid.

Imaging. Plain radiographs in the early stages show an area of irregularity on the affected subchondral bone, usually of the capitulum. Later a shallow cavity, whose margins are demarcated clearly from the bone within it, is seen (Fig. 15.8). Eventually the bony fragment separates from the cavity and lies free within the joint, usually in the lateral compartment. MR scanning in the earlier stages of the disease may be valuable in determining the possibility of operative treatment prior to separation of the bony fragment.

Treatment. If the fragment is small, operation is delayed until the fragment of bone and cartilage is ripe for separation or has actually separated. The fragment is then removed. If the fragment is large and is identified prior to separation it may be fixed in place with a fine screw or pin until fixation to the underlying bone occurs.

LOOSE BODIES IN THE ELBOW

Causes. There are four important causes of loose bodies in the elbow:

1. osteochondritis dissecans (1–3 bodies)
2. osteoarthritis (1–3 bodies)
3. fracture with separation of a fragment (1–3 bodies)
4. synovial chondromatosis (50–500 bodies).

PATHOLOGY AND CLINICAL FEATURES

Osteochondritis dissecans was described on page 153 and *osteoarthritis* on page 140.

Loose body after fracture. A fragment may rarely be detached from the capitulum. Sometimes the medial epicondyle is detached and sucked into the joint, retaining its attachments to the flexor muscles. (Strictly this is not a loose body because it retains soft tissue attachments, but it behaves as one.)

Synovial chondromatosis (osteochondromatosis). This is a rare disease of synovial membrane in which numerous synovial villi become pedunculated and transformed into cartilage; eventually they are detached to form a large number of loose bodies, many of which become calcified (Fig. 15.9).

Clinical features. Many so-called loose bodies are 'silent' – that is, they do not cause symptoms. Often in such cases the fragment is not in fact loose, but has soft-tissue attachments that prevent its moving about the joint.

The characteristic symptom of a freely movable loose body is sudden locking of the elbow during movement, with sharp pain. The joint is usually unlocked after an interval, either spontaneously or by the patient's

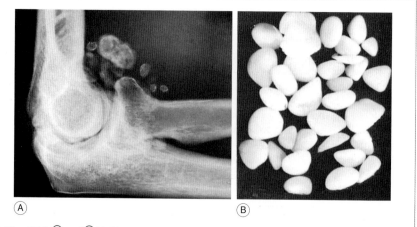

Fig. 15.9 Ⓐ and Ⓑ Multiple loose bodies in the elbow. A case of synovial chondromatosis.

manoeuvres. Several hours later the joint swells because of effusion of fluid within it. The symptoms subside within a few days, but repeated attacks are to be expected.

Examination in the stage of swelling shows the joint to be distended with fluid – a clear, pale, straw-coloured effusion. Between attacks a loose body may sometimes be felt. There is often a history or clinical evidence to suggest the cause of the loose body formation.

Radiographs show the loose body or bodies (Fig. 15.9A) and usually indicate the nature of the primary condition.

Treatment. Symptomless loose bodies may usually be safely left alone; but if a loose body causes locking it should be removed by operation. In cases of synovial chondromatosis, with numerous loose bodies, removal of the bodies should usually be supplemented by excision of as much of the synovial membrane as is easily accessible, to minimise the risk of recurrence.

TENNIS ELBOW (Lateral epicondylitis)

'Tennis elbow' is a common and well-defined clinical entity. It is an extra-articular affection characterised by pain and acute tenderness at the origin of the extensor muscles of the forearm from the lateral epicondyle. A similar but less common condition is 'golfer's elbow' at the origin of the muscles at the medial epicondyle.

Cause. It is believed to be caused by strain of the forearm extensor muscles, particularly the extensor carpi radialis brevis, at the point of their origin from the bone. Although it sometimes occurs after playing tennis or golf, other repetitive activities such as wheelchair use are just as likely to be responsible.

Pathology. It is assumed that there is incomplete rupture of aponeurotic fibres at the muscle origin, which is a region plentifully supplied by nerve endings. Histology shows no evidence of acute inflammation, but an angiofibroblastic tendinosis is suggestive of repetitive micro injury with attempted healing. The elbow and radio-humeral joints are unaffected.

Clinical features. Patients are usually in the 30–50 age group presenting with pain at the lateral aspect of the elbow often radiating down the back of the forearm.

On examination there is tenderness precisely localised to the front of the lateral epicondyle of the humerus (Fig. 15.10). Pain is aggravated by putting the extensor muscles on the stretch – for example, by flexing the wrist and fingers with the forearm pronated. Movements of the elbow are full.

Imaging. *Radiographs* do not show any alteration from the normal except for occasional calcification at the muscle origin in chronic cases. However, MRI scans may demonstrate local oedema and thickening in the extensor muscle origin.

Course. In about 80% of patients the symptoms eventually subside spontaneously after 1–2 years. In cases resistant to modification of activities more active treatment may be required.

Treatment. A large number of treatment methods, both conservative and surgical, have been applied to the condition but none have proved reliable in every case.

Conservative treatment. Where rest and non-steroidal anti-inflammatory drugs have failed to provide relief, injection of the muscle origin with local anaesthetic and hydrocortisone is frequently employed. Repeat injections may be required on one of two occasions, but usually give relief for up to 6 weeks.

The upper arm and elbow

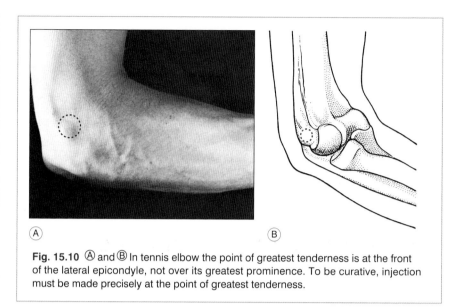

(A)   (B)

Fig. 15.10 Ⓐ and Ⓑ In tennis elbow the point of greatest tenderness is at the front of the lateral epicondyle, not over its greatest prominence. To be curative, injection must be made precisely at the point of greatest tenderness.

However, results from randomised trials with longer follow-up showed no greater improvement than achieved with other conservative measures. Orthotic devices, such as the proximal forearm band splint to reduce tension at the extensor origin are popular with those wishing to continue sporting activities, but their long-term benefit remains uncertain. Other local treatment modalities such as sonic shock wave therapy and eccentric strengthening exercises provide equally uncertain long-term results.

Operative treatment. If severe disabling pain fails to respond to any of these conservative treatments, operation may have to be considered. The operation requires a small incision over the extensor origin which is stripped from its attachment to the lateral epicondyle, thereby detaching the pain-sensitive fibres from the bone while allowing natural healing to occur. With modern technology this procedure can now be carried out through an arthroscope without the need for open release. Long-term results have reported pain relief in over 80% of patients but some local discomfort may persist.

OLECRANON BURSITIS

The bursa behind the olecranon process is liable to traumatic bursitis, septic bursitis, and gout.

Traumatic bursitis. In traumatic bursitis ('student's elbow') the bursa is distended with clear fluid (Fig. 15.11). Treatment at first should be by aspiration, followed by the injection of hydrocortisone into the bursa. If the swelling recurs the bursa should be excised.

Septic bursitis is treated by incision to secure adequate drainage. This should be conbined with an appropriate antibiotic to treat the underlying infecting organism.

Gouty bursitis. In gouty bursitis there is acute or subacute inflammation, and whitish deposits of sodium biurate (tophi) may be visible through the walls of the bursa. If the symptoms are troublesome the bursa may be excised.

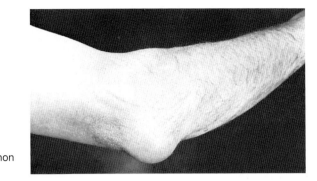

Fig. 15.11 Olecranon bursitis.

FRICTION NEURITIS OF THE ULNAR NERVE

The ulnar nerve is vulnerable where it lies in the groove behind the medial epicondyle of the humerus. Its function may be interfered with either by constriction or by recurrent friction while in tension. Constriction is usually secondary to osteoarthritis, with encroachment of osteophytes upon the ulnar groove. Friction under tension occurs especially when the carrying angle of the elbow is increased (cubitus valgus, p. 282). This latter type is often a late sequel of a supracondylar fracture of the humerus sustained in childhood ('tardy ulnar palsy'). In both cases the nerve undergoes fibrosis, and unless the mechanical fault is relieved without undue delay the changes may eventually become irreversible.

Clinical features. The patient complains of numbness or tingling in the area of sensory distribution of the ulnar nerve, and often of clumsiness in performing fine finger movements, as for instance in such activities as playing musical instruments.

On examination in the fully developed condition the following signs are present: *Sensory*—There is blunting or loss of sensibility along the ulnar border of the hand and in the little finger and medial half of the ring finger. *Motor* – There are wasting and weakness of the ulnar-innervated small hand muscles. *Sweating* – The skin in the ulnar territory is drier than normal because sweating is impaired. In doubtful cases nerve conduction studies may be carried out on the ulnar nerve, to detect any slowing of impulses at the elbow level.

Treatment. Whenever the ulnar nerve is interfered with by a lesion at the elbow operation should be undertaken. The operation will consist in decompression of the nerve by division of the overlying aponeurosis of the flexor carpi ulnaris; or, if deformity is present, by transposing the nerve to a new bed in front of the medial epicondyle of the elbow.

16 The forearm, wrist, and hand

So much in everyday life depends upon the efficient working of the hand, and so great is the practical and economic consequence of its disablement, that the care of the diseased or injured hand has become one of the most vital branches of orthopaedic surgery. It is also one of the most fascinating.

Hand surgery is an art and a science in itself. Indeed it has already become a distinct speciality, demanding a knowledge and experience not only of orthopaedic surgery but also of plastic surgery, microvascular surgery, and neurology.

In the treatment of hand disorders the primary emphasis should always be on restoration of function. Keen judgement is often called for in deciding between the claims of rest and of movement. It should be remembered that the hand tolerates immobilisation badly. Whereas the wrist may be immobilised for many weeks or even months with impunity, to immobilise injured or diseased fingers for a long time is to court disaster in the form of permanent joint stiffness. Although rest may be essential in the early days after a hand injury or in the acute stage of an infection, active finger exercises must be insisted upon as soon as that stage has passed. It is wise to accept it as a general rule that fingers should never be immobilised for longer than two, or at most three, weeks.

SPECIAL POINTS IN THE INVESTIGATION OF FOREARM, WRIST, AND HAND COMPLAINTS

History

It should be remembered that symptoms in the hand are often caused by disorders of the neck (with involvement of the brachial plexus or its roots) and sometimes by disorders at the elbow. Enquiry should always be made into any previous injury or other trouble with the neck or with the upper extremity as a whole.

Exposure

For the local examination the whole forearm should be uncovered to well above the elbow. The sound limb should be exposed likewise for comparison.

Steps in clinical examination

A suggested routine of clinical examination is summarised in Table 16.1.

Table 16.1 Routine clinical examination in suspected disorders of the forearm, wrist, and hand

1. LOCAL EXAMINATION OF THE FOREARM, WRIST, AND HAND

Inspection
Bone contours
Soft-tissue contours
Colour and texture of skin
Scars and sinuses

Metacarpo-phalangeal joints—
Flexion–extension; adduction–
abduction
Interphalangeal joints—Flexion–extension

Palpation
Skin temperature
Bone contours
Soft-tissue contours
Local tenderness

Power
Power of each muscle group in control of:
1. wrist movement;
2. thumb and finger movement; and
3. gripping

Movements (active and passive)
At the wrist:
Radio-carpal joint—Flexion–extension;
adduction–abduction
Inferior radio-ulnar joint—Supination and
pronation
At the hand:
Carpo-metacarpal joint of thumb—Flexion–
extension; adduction–abduction; opposition

Stability
Tests for abnormal mobility

Nerve function
Tests of sensory function, motor function,
and sweating in distribution of median, ulnar,
and radial nerves

Circulation
Arterial pulses, warmth and colour, capillary
return, cutaneous sensibility

2. EXAMINATION OF POSSIBLE EXTRINSIC SOURCES OF FOREARM AND HAND SYMPTOMS

This is important if a satisfactory explanation for the symptoms is not found on local
examination. The investigation should include:
1. the neck and thoracic inlet, with special reference to the brachial plexus
2. the upper arm
3. the elbow

3. GENERAL EXAMINATION

General survey of other parts of the body. The local symptoms may be only one
manifestation of a more widespread disease

Movements at the wrist

Like the elbow, the wrist comprises two distinct components:

1. the radio-carpal joint (including the intercarpal joints), allowing flexion, extension, adduction, and abduction
2. the inferior radio-ulnar joint, allowing supination and pronation.

The movements at each component must be examined independently.

The radio-carpal joint. The normal range of flexion (palmar flexion) is 80° and of extension (dorsiflexion) 90°. The range of adduction, or ulnar deviation, is about 35°, and of abduction, or radial deviation, about 25°. It is impracticable to measure the movements of the intercarpal joints individually, and it is simplest to regard them as integral parts of the radio-carpal joint.

A rapid and reasonably accurate method of comparing the range of flexion–extension movement on the two sides is as follows: To judge the range of extension: The patient places the palms and fingers of the two hands in contact in the vertical plane and lifts the elbows as far as he can while keeping the 'heels' of the hands together (Fig. 16.1). The angle between hand and forearm is easily compared on the two sides. To judge the range of flexion

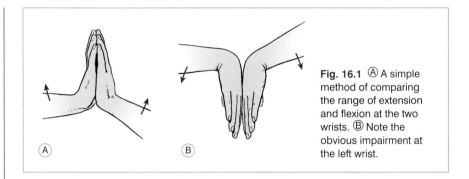

Fig. 16.1 Ⓐ A simple method of comparing the range of extension and flexion at the two wrists. Ⓑ Note the obvious impairment at the left wrist.

the manoeuvre is reversed. The patient places the backs of the hands together, with the fingers directed vertically downwards, and lowers the elbows as far as he can (Fig. 16.1). The angle between hand and forearm is compared on the two sides.

The inferior radio-ulnar joint. The normal range is 90° of supination and 90° of pronation. To determine the range accurately the patient's elbows must be flexed to a right angle in order to eliminate rotation at the shoulder (see Fig. 15.1).

It must be emphasised that impaired rotation does not necessarily denote an abnormality of the wrist: it may equally well be caused by a disorder of the elbow or of the forearm.

Movements of the hand

Movements of the hand occur mainly at three groups of joints:

1. the carpo-metacarpal joint of the thumb
2. the metacarpo-phalangeal joints
3. the interphalangeal joints.

Carpo-metacarpal joint of thumb. This joint allows movement in five directions: flexion, or movement of the thumb metacarpal medially in the plane of the palm; extension, or movement of the thumb metacarpal laterally in the plane of the palm; adduction, or movement of the metacarpal towards the palm in a plane at right angles to it; abduction, or movement of the metacarpal away from the palm in a plane at right angles to it; and opposition, or rotation of the metacarpal to bring the thumb nail into a plane parallel with the palm (Fig. 16.2).

Metacarpo-phalangeal joints of thumb and fingers. These joints allow flexion–extension movement through 90° (the range is variable and often through as little as 30° in the thumb), and a small range of abduction from, and adduction to, the midline of the middle finger.

Interphalangeal joints of thumb and fingers. These are true hinge joints, allowing only flexion and extension. In the fingers, the range of flexion is 90° at the proximal interphalangeal joints, and 45° at the distal interphalangeal joints. In the thumb, the range of movement at the interphalangeal joint is usually about 80°.

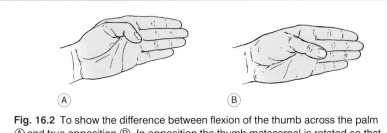

Fig. 16.2 To show the difference between flexion of the thumb across the palm Ⓐ and true opposition Ⓑ. In opposition the thumb metacarpal is rotated so that the thumb nail lies in a plane parallel with the palm.

Power

Test the power of each movement in turn. In the hand this examination demands considerable patience, for each muscle group must be tested individually. Thus in the thumb it is necessary to test the abductors, the adductor, the extensors (longus and brevis), the flexors (longus and brevis), and the opponens. In the fingers test the flexors (profundus and superficialis), the extensor digitorum and extensor indicis, the interossei and the lumbricals. Grip: Test the power of grip, which demands the combined action of the flexors and extensors of the wrist and the flexors of the fingers and thumb.

Nerve function

The state of the median, ulnar, and radial nerves is determined by tests of sensory function, motor function, and sweating. The ulnar nerve normally supplies sensation to the ulnar side of the hand together with the little finger and half the ring finger (Fig. 16.3).

The remainder is largely innervated from the median nerve with some overlap on the dorsum of the hand from the radial nerve (Fig. 16.3). Only a

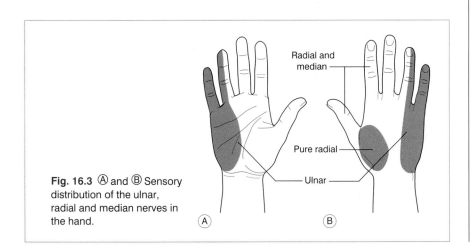

Fig. 16.3 Ⓐ and Ⓑ Sensory distribution of the ulnar, radial and median nerves in the hand.

Radial and median

Pure radial

Ulnar

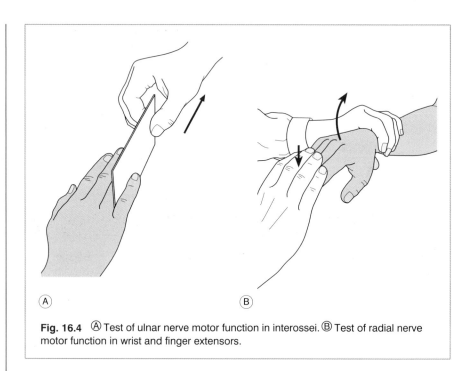

Fig. 16.4 Ⓐ Test of ulnar nerve motor function in interossei. Ⓑ Test of radial nerve motor function in wrist and finger extensors.

small skin area at the base of the thumb is purely supplied by the radial nerve. Intact function of the median nerve is indicated by ability to oppose the thumb to the little finger (see Fig. 16.2). Intact ulnar nerve function is shown by ability to spread the fingers apart and to bring them together again to grip a card between the middle and ring fingers (Fig. 16.4). An index of radial nerve function is the ability to extend the thumb and to extend the fingers at the metacarpo-phalangeal joints.

Circulation

The state of the circulation is assessed from the condition of the arterial pulses, the warmth and colour of the digits, the capillary return at the nail beds, and cutaneous sensibility. It should be remembered that sensibility to touch in the fingers is a most useful index of the adequacy of the circulation. Nerves require a blood supply to enable them to conduct impulses, and if the circulation is interrupted sensibility is quickly lost.

Extrinsic sources of forearm and hand symptoms

It is sometimes difficult to determine whether symptoms and signs in the fore-arm or hand are caused by a local disorder or whether they are referred from a more proximal lesion. This difficulty arises mainly in neurological conditions. For instance, the symptoms of compression of the median nerve in the carpal tunnel may be mimicked closely by a prolapsed cervical disc, and the symptoms of constriction of the ulnar nerve at the elbow may likewise be confused with those from a low cervical disc lesion or a cervical rib. When symptoms in the hand are not satisfactorily explained by the local condition a search must be made for a possible cause in the neck, upper arm, or elbow.

Imaging

Radiographic examination. Routine radiographs should include antero-posterior and lateral projections of the forearm, wrist, and hand. For detailed study of the carpal bones additional oblique projections are required.

If it is suspected that the symptoms may be referred from the neck or proximal part of the limb, radiographs of the appropriate part should be obtained.

DISORDERS OF THE FOREARM

ACUTE OSTEOMYELITIS (General description of acute osteomyelitis, p. 85)

Acute osteomyelitis is rather uncommon in the forearm bones. As in other sites, the infection may be blood-borne (haematogenous) or it may be introduced from without, usually in consequence of a compound fracture. The haematogenous type occurs mainly in children. It affects the radius more often than the ulna, and the lower metaphysis rather than the upper (see Fig. 7.3B).

The clinical features and treatment are like those of acute osteomyelitis elsewhere.

CHRONIC OSTEOMYELITIS (General description of chronic osteomyelitis, p. 90)

As in other bones, chronic osteomyelitis of the radius or ulna follows an acute infection.

Treatment. In most cases treatment should follow the usual lines, reliance being placed on rest and antibacterial drugs for non-suppurative flares of infection, and on thorough drainage operations and sequestrectomy for persistent purulent discharge.

BONE TUMOURS IN THE FOREARM AND HAND

Benign tumours (General description of benign tumours of bone, p. 106)

Any type of benign tumour may occur in the bones of the forearm and hand. Only chondroma and giant-cell tumour require further mention here because of their more common occurrence at these anatomical sites.

Chondroma

Enchondroma, which grows within the bone and expands it, is prone to occur in the metacarpals and phalanges of the hand presenting with deformity or pathological fracture. The tumour may be solitary, but in the condition of multiple enchondromatosis, or Ollier's disease, the tumours may affect many bones in the hand causing ugly swelling and deformity of the fingers (Fig. 16.5).

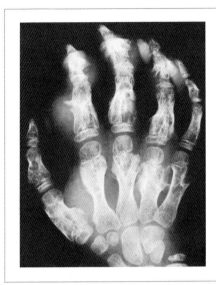

Fig. 16.5 Multiple enchondromata in the metacarpals and phalanges.

Malignant transformation is hardly known in a solitary chondroma of a bone of the hand, but it is a possibility in cases of multiple enchondromatosis, leading to chondrosarcoma.

Treatment. If small, the tumour should be treated expectantly and fractures normally heal with simple splintage. Operation is required only if the tumour is found to be enlarging. Large tumours should be excised and sent for routine histological examination, the bone substance being restored by cancellous bone grafts.

Enchondromas of long bones are less common in the forearm, though these bones may be affected by multiple osteochondroma in the hereditary condition of diaphyseal aclasis (p. 63). These tumours may interfere with the normal growth of the affected bone resulting in shortening and deformity.

Enchondromas occur chiefly in multiple form, in the condition known as dyschondroplasia, Ollier's disease, or multiple chondromatosis. Their special significance in the forearm lies in the fact that the tumours may interfere with the normal growth of the affected bone. If growth is retarded in one bone but proceeds normally in its partner marked curvature of the bones is to be expected, and it may cause ugly deformity, as seen commonly in dyschondroplasia.

Treatment. Severe deformity from uneven growth of the radius and ulna should be corrected by osteotomy, combined when necessary with excision of the distal ulna, or sometimes the head of the radius.

Giant-cell tumour (osteoclastoma)
The lower end of the radius is one of the common sites in the upper limb for the development of a giant-cell tumour, which though classed as benign may show invasive tendencies. The lower end of the ulna is also susceptible. The tumour extends into the former epiphysial region close up to the articular surface (Fig. 16.6).

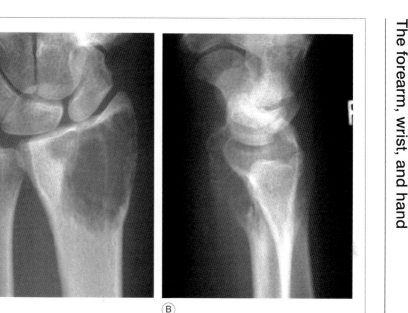

Fig. 16.6 Ⓐ and Ⓑ Radiographs of wrist showing a giant cell tumour in the distal radius. The lucent lesion has ill-defined proximal margins with a narrow zone of transition and lies in a typical subarticular position in the epiphysis.

Treatment. If the tumour is in the lower end of the radius radical excision and replacement by a suitable bone graft is to be recommended. A graft obtained from the upper part of the fibula is suitable because its shape matches that of the original bone. Ideally, the graft should be taken with the supplying artery and veins, which are anastomosed to suitable vessels in the recipient area by a microsurgical technique. If the lower end of the ulna is the part affected the bone should be excised up to a point well proximal to the tumour. The resulting disability is negligible.

Malignant tumours (General description of malignant tumours of bone, p. 112)

The radius and ulna are seldom affected by malignant bone tumours, whether primary or metastatic. When osteosarcoma does occur in the forearm the lower end of the radius is the usual site. Malignant change to chondrosarcoma is more common when there are multiple enchondromas present in the small bones of the hand.

VOLKMANN'S ISCHAEMIC CONTRACTURE[1]

This is a flexion deformity of the wrist and fingers from fixed contracture of the flexor muscles in the forearm.

[1]Richard von Volkmann (1830–1889) German surgeon who was Professor in Halle, Saxony and also served as an army surgeon in the Franco-Prussian War. He described the ischaemic muscle paralysis and contracture in 1881.

Cause. It is caused by ischaemia of the flexor muscles, brought about by injury to, or obstruction of, the brachial artery near the elbow; or by tense oedema of the soft tissues of the forearm constrained within an unyielding fascial compartment.

Pathology. The effects of sudden occlusion of the brachial artery vary. In a few worst cases gangrene of the fingers will follow. Usually, however, the collateral circulation is sufficient to keep the hand alive, but not to nourish adequately the flexor muscles of the forearm or the main peripheral nerve trunks. The ischaemia that follows tense oedema in the anterior fascial compartment of the forearm, a consequence of severe injury in the region, has similar effects. Necrosis of muscle fibres of the forearm flexor group – especially the flexor digitorum profundus and flexor pollicis longus – with subsequent fibrosis and shortening, is the essential feature of Volkmann's contracture. It is often associated with temporary or permanent ischaemic paralysis of the peripheral nerves, especially the median nerve.

Any major fracture in the elbow region or upper forearm may lead to arterial occlusion. That most commonly responsible is a supracondylar fracture of the humerus with displacement, the brachial artery being severed or contused by the sharp lower end of the main shaft fragment (Fig. 16.7). Contusion alone is sufficient to interrupt the flow of blood, because the artery goes into spasm and its lumen may be occluded by thrombosis.

Progressive oedema within the closed anterior fascial compartment of the forearm – for instance after fracture of the forearm bones – is commonly responsible for obstruction of the arterial flow (compartment syndrome).

In some cases the cause of the vascular obstruction is an over-tight plaster or bandage.

Clinical features. The condition is commonest in children. After sustaining a supracondylar fracture of the humerus or some other injury in the elbow region or forearm, the child complains of severe pain in the forearm.

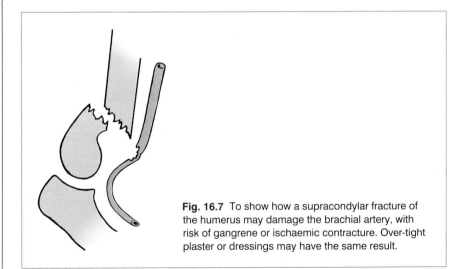

Fig. 16.7 To show how a supracondylar fracture of the humerus may damage the brachial artery, with risk of gangrene or ischaemic contracture. Over-tight plaster or dressings may have the same result.

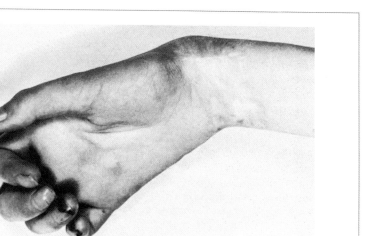

Fig. 16.8 Typical appearance of the hand in established Volkmann's ischaemic contracture.

On examination in the incipient stage, the fingers are white or blue, and cold. The radial pulse is absent. Active finger movements are weak and painful. Passive extension of the fingers is especially painful and restricted. There may or may not be evidence of interruption of nerve conductivity – namely, anaesthesia of the fingers and paralysis of the small muscles of the hand.

In the established condition, which develops gradually within a few weeks of the injury, there is a striking flexion contracture of the wrist and fingers, from shortening of the fibrotic forearm flexor muscles (Fig. 16.8). Sensory and motor paralysis of the hand may persist as complicating factors, but they do not form an essential feature of Volkmann's contracture as such.

Diagnosis. In the incipient stage absence of the radial pulse, with marked unwillingness to extend the fingers because of pain, should always arouse suspicion of Volkmann's contracture. If there are also anaesthesia and paralysis of the hand the diagnosis is practically certain. In the established condition the history and clinical features make the diagnosis clear.

Volkmann's ischaemic contracture bears no real resemblance to Dupuytren's contracture (p. 321), for it affects the wrist as well as all the joints of the fingers, and there is no palpable thickening in the palm. Moreover the contracture is demonstrably brought about by shortening of the flexor muscles, because if the wrist is flexed passively to relax the flexor tendons the range of extension at the finger joints is increased. Conversely, if the tendons are relaxed by flexing the fingers fully the range of wrist extension is increased (Fig. 16.9).

Treatment. In the *incipient stage* the problem is that of dealing with a sudden occlusion of the brachial artery or obstruction to the blood flow within a tightly congested fascial compartment. The case must be handled as an emergency, because the effects of occlusion become irreversible after about six hours. The following action must be taken:

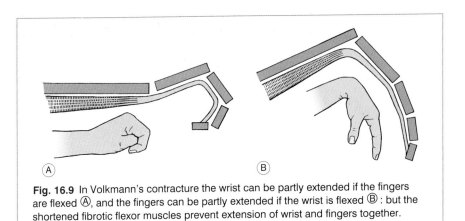

Fig. 16.9 In Volkmann's contracture the wrist can be partly extended if the fingers are flexed Ⓐ, and the fingers can be partly extended if the wrist is flexed Ⓑ : but the shortened fibrotic flexor muscles prevent extension of wrist and fingers together.

First step. All splints, plaster, and bandages that might be obstructing the circulation are removed. In the case of a fracture, gross displacement of the fragments is corrected as far as possible by gentle manipulation and a well-padded plaster splint is applied. Likewise if the elbow is dislocated it must be reduced without delay. Heat cradles or hot bottles are applied over the other three limbs and trunk to promote general vasodilation.

If these measures fail to bring about a return of adequate circulation within half an hour, the next step is taken:

Second step. At operation the anterior fascia of the forearm is exposed and split longitudinally throughout its length to open the fascial compartment, allowing the muscles to bulge through the gap. The brachial artery is then explored. If there is occlusion from kinking or spasm of the artery an attempt is made to relieve it by freeing the vessel and applying papaverine. If this fails, the artery may be distended by the injection of saline between clamps. In the last resort, the artery may have to be opened and damaged intima removed; or the damaged length of artery may be excised and continuity restored by a vein graft. These procedures are best accomplished using magnification techniques, by a surgeon with wide experience of vascular surgery.

In the *established stage* restoration to normal is impossible: reconstructive surgery at best can only improve what function remains. The choice of treatment depends upon the circumstances of each case. In a mild case acceptable function may be restored by intensive exercises guided by a physiotherapist: such cases are however exceptional. In more severe cases the muscle shortening may be counteracted by shortening of the forearm bones, or by detachment and distal displacement of the flexor muscle origin (muscle slide operation).

In selected cases with severe muscle infarction, however, the best results are probably obtained by excision of the dead muscles and subsequent transfer of a healthy muscle (for example, a wrist flexor or a wrist extensor) to the tendons of flexor digitorum profundus and of flexor pollicis longus to restore active flexion of the digits. These muscle transfers may be combined, in appropriate cases, with arthrodesis of the wrist. When the median nerve is irreparably damaged by ischaemia nerve grafting is sometimes successful in restoring limited nerve function.

ARTICULAR DISORDERS OF THE WRIST AND HAND

MADELUNG'S DEFORMITY[1] (Radio-ulnar dyschondrosteosis)

Madelung's deformity (radio-ulnar dyschondrosteosis) is a congenital subluxation or dislocation of the lower end of the ulna, from malformation of the bones. Although it is seemingly a localised disorder there may be minor generalised abnormalities of bone structure, often with short stature.

A similar wrist deformity is more often caused by disease or injury, such as a fracture of the lower end of the radius with proximal displacement of the lower fragment.

The deformity varies in degree from a slight prominence of the lower end of the ulna at the back of the wrist, to complete dislocation of the inferior radio-ulnar joint with marked radial deviation of the hand (Fig. 16.10). The more severe types of deformity may be associated with congenital absence or hypoplasia of the radius.

Treatment. If the disability justifies operation the lower end of the ulna should be excised. In a severe case, with marked radial deviation of the hand, it may be necessary also to fuse the radius (or ulna, if the radius is absent) to the carpus in order to gain satisfactory correction.

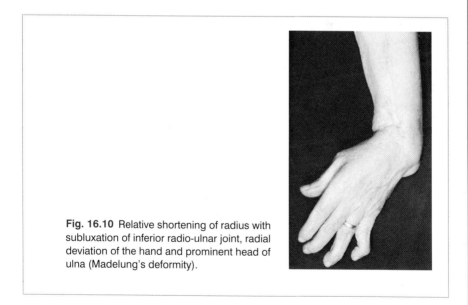

Fig. 16.10 Relative shortening of radius with subluxation of inferior radio-ulnar joint, radial deviation of the hand and prominent head of ulna (Madelung's deformity).

[1]Otto Madelung (1846–1926) German general surgeon who was professor in Strasburg until after the First World War when the city was returned to France and he was forced to retire to Germany. He described the deformity in 1878.

PYOGENIC ARTHRITIS OF THE WRIST AND HAND (General description of pyogenic arthritis, p. 96)

Pyogenic arthritis of the wrist is uncommon. Infection may be haematogenous, or it may be introduced through a penetrating wound. Spread from a focus of osteomyelitis is rare, partly because osteomyelitis itself is uncommon in the forearm bones, and partly because the lower metaphysis of the radius is entirely outside the capsule of the joint. (The lower metaphysis of the ulna is partly intracapsular (see Fig. 7.2).)

In the hand, any of the small joints may be infected by pyogenic organisms. The distal interphalangeal joints of the digits are prone to infection spreading from a suppurative lesion in the adjacent pulp space, or from a penetrating wound. These infections often cause permanent damage to the joint, with impairment of movement or even rigid ankylosis. Radiographs in the late stage of infection may show diffuse rarefaction, loss of cartilage space and some bone destruction.

The clinical features and treatment of pyogenic arthritis are similar to those at other sites.

RHEUMATOID ARTHRITIS OF THE WRIST AND HAND (General description of rheumatoid arthritis, p. 134)

Rheumatoid arthritis commonly affects the wrists and hands and is a major cause of serious loss of function and of ugly deformity. Usually many or all of the joints of the hand are affected, though occasionally the disease may begin in a single joint. Affected joints are swollen from synovial thickening, and movement is restricted. In the later stages articular cartilage and the underlying bone are eroded, and the fingers tend to deviate medially ('ulnar drift'), with dorsal prominence of the metacarpal heads and characteristic visible deformity (Fig. 16.11A). At the wrist joint the disease commonly results in dorsal subluxation and dislocation of the ulnar head accompanied by subluxation of the carpus on the radius and radial deviation of the hand. Radiographs do not show any abnormality at first. Later, there is diffuse rarefaction of the bones. Later still, in progressive disease, destruction of cartilage leads to narrowing of the joint space (Fig. 16.11B), and the subchondral bone may be eroded.

Important though these joint changes are in rheumatoid disease of the hand, equally serious disability may be caused by involvement of the soft tissues. These soft-tissue changes may take several forms, the most important of which are:

1. chronic tenosynovitis
2. rupture of tendons
3. contracture of intrinsic muscles
4. compression of the median nerve.

Chronic tenosynovitis. Masses of greatly thickened vascular synovial tissue envelop the flexor or the extensor tendons over the wrist or in the hand. Proliferation of the tenosynovium combined with nodular formation in the flexor tendon may produce symptoms of trigger finger.

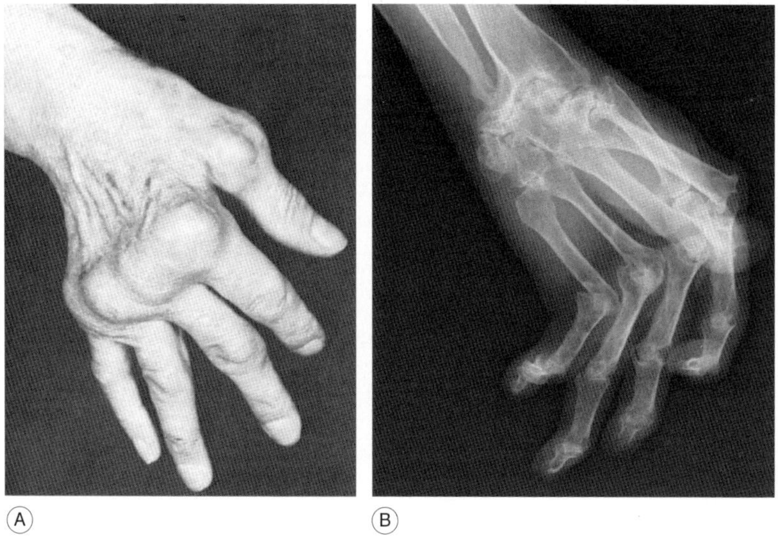

The forearm, wrist, and hand

(A) (B)

Fig. 16.11 Ⓐ Typical appearance of hand in long-established rheumatoid arthritis of wrist, metacarpo-phalangeal and interphalangeal joints. Ⓑ Radiograph of the hand showing advanced erosive arthropathy due to rheumatoid arthritis. There is extensive destruction and subluxation of the radio-carpal, carpal, metacarpo-phalangeal, and interphalangeal joints with typical ulnar deviation of the fingers.

Rupture of tendons. Both the extensor and the flexor tendons are liable to spontaneous rupture, from softening or fraying where they lie within inflamed synovial sheaths. The extensor pollicis longus, extensor digitorum, and extensor digiti minimi are the tendons that most commonly rupture.

Contracture of intrinsic muscles. Fixed contracture of the intrinsic muscles of the hand may follow fibrosis induced by the disease. It leads to inability to flex the interphalangeal joints fully when the metacarpo-phalangeal joint is held extended.

Compression of the median nerve. A secondary effect of the synovial proliferation within the carpal tunnel is that the median nerve may be compressed by the transverse carpal ligament.

Treatment

Management of these complex disabilities of the hand is difficult and often unsatisfactory. The tendency of the disease to progress during months or years of activity means often that the hand becomes seriously crippled. Nevertheless much can be done with modern medical therapy to retard the progress of the disease and to prevent or correct deformity, either by conservative treatment alone or by conservative treatment combined with operation.

Conservative treatment. The general plan of treatment is like that for rheumatoid arthritis as a whole (p. 137). It will usually include the administration of non-steroidal anti-inflammatory drugs, or in more resistant disease second-line drug therapy may be required with gold, penicillamine, or immuno-suppressive agents. Cortisone and related steroids should be avoided if possible because of their undesirable side effects. Physiotherapy is of value: it should take the form of warm water or wax baths, with mobilising exercises and encouragement in active use of the hand. During an acute exacerbation the wrist joint may be immobilised temporarily in a moulded polythene splint or plaster of Paris back slab, but immobilisation is never advised for the joints of the fingers other than with a dynamic active splint.

Operative treatment. In carefully selected patients operation can be a valuable adjunct to conservative treatment, though it can never replace it. It should never be undertaken lightly, but only after careful deliberation and full discussion with the patient as well as the other members of the treatment team. Operations, particularly soft-tissue procedures, are often more rewarding when carried out in the fairly early stages of the disease, before deformity from changes in the joints and soft tissues has become fixed and irreversible. Depending upon the nature of each individual case, operation may take one or more of the following forms.

Synovectomy. Excision of masses of thickened synovial tissue from tendon sheaths or from joints may slow down the destructive progress of the disease, and prevent tendon rupture and joint dislocation.

Arthroplasty. When the metacarpo-phalangeal or interphalangeal joints are badly disorganised arthroplasty by the insertion of a flexible silicone-rubber ('Silastic') prosthesis may sometimes be appropriate (Fig. 16.12). But the patient must be prepared to cooperate in a long programme of rehabilitation afterwards. The improvement gained is often cosmetic rather than functional. The benefit is not always lasting and deformity may recur because of breakage or loosening of the prosthesis.

Arthrodesis. For selected joints that are painful, stiff, deformed, or unstable, arthrodesis in the position of most useful function is sometimes the best solution to the problem. When the wrist joint is badly destroyed, arthrodesis of the wrist in a neutral or slightly palmar flexed position, will provide a stable basis for other reconstructive procedures in the hand. The metacarpo-phalangeal joint of the thumb may require fusion to restore deformity and to provide the stability required for a pinch grip.

Tendon repair or replacement. Ruptured tendons may be repaired by suture or by grafting when practicable, or their lost function may be compensated by a tendon transfer operation (p. 44).

Release of tight intrinsic muscles. Impaired finger movement and grasp from fixed contracture of the intrinsic muscles can be improved by partial division of the aponeurotic insertion of the muscles into the extensor expansion at the back of each finger.

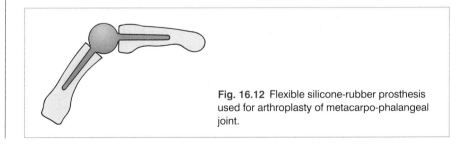

Fig. 16.12 Flexible silicone-rubber prosthesis used for arthroplasty of metacarpo-phalangeal joint.

Carpal tunnel decompression. Division of the transverse carpal ligament and excision of the proliferative synovium will provide adequate decompression for the median nerve when neuropathy is present.

OSTEOARTHRITIS OF THE WRIST (General description of osteoarthritis, p. 140)

Although uncommon compared with osteoarthritis of the hip or knee, osteoarthritis of the wrist is a well-recognised sequel to certain injuries and diseases affecting the joint.

Cause. Although it is essentially a wear-and-tear process osteoarthritis seldom develops in a wrist that was previously normal. The wear and tear is nearly always accelerated by previous injury to, or disease of, the joint surfaces. The commonest predisposing factors are comminuted fracture of the lower end of the radius with involvement of the articular surface, fracture of the scaphoid bone complicated by failure of union or avascular necrosis (osteonecrosis) of the distal fragment, dislocation of the lunate bone, Kienböck's disease of the lunate bone, and long-established ('burnt out') rheumatoid arthritis.

Pathology. The predominant change is degeneration and wearing away of the articular cartilage lining the joint surfaces. The changes eventually involve all the carpal joints as well as the radio-carpal joint.

Clinical features. Months or years after one of the predisposing conditions mentioned, the patient notices gradually increasing pain and stiffness of the wrist, worse on activity. On examination the wrist is slightly thickened from bony irregularity, but the swelling is not marked. The skin temperature is normal. Movements are markedly restricted, and painful if forced at the extremes.

Radiographic features. Radiographs show narrowing of the cartilage space and sharpening or spurring of the bone at the joint margins. The underlying causative condition (for example, an ununited fracture of the scaphoid bone) is usually evident (Fig. 16.13).

Treatment. In mild cases the condition is best left alone, especially if the patient can avoid subjecting the wrist to heavy stress. When active treatment seems necessary, a choice must be made between conservative and operative methods. Conservative treatment can only diminish the symptoms; it can never remove them. Nevertheless it is usually worth a trial. The most useful method is to provide support for the wrist by a detachable splint made from moulded plastic (Fig. 16.14).

Operative treatment sometimes becomes necessary when the disability is severe. The only reliable method is by total arthrodesis of the wrist, with ablation of the radio-carpal and all the intercarpal joints. The inferior radio-ulnar joint and the triangular fibrocartilage are left undisturbed; so rotation of the forearm is preserved.

OSTEOARTHRITIS OF THE JOINTS OF THE HAND

The metacarpo-phalangeal joints and the interphalangeal joints of the hand are frequently the site of osteoarthritis in the elderly. Such manifestations are relatively unimportant and in most cases treatment is not required. Commonly involved are the carpo-metacarpal joint of the thumb (trapezio-metacarpal joint) (Fig. 16.15A) and the distal interphalangeal joints (Fig. 16.15B).

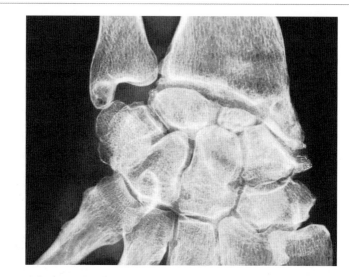

Fig. 16.13 Osteoarthritis of the wrist caused by an ununited fracture of the scaphoid bone. Note the diminished cartilage space, sclerosis, and spurring of bone at the joint margins, mainly at the radial side of the wrist.

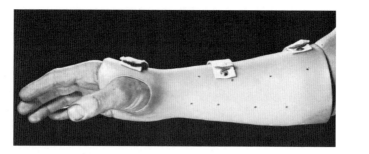

Fig. 16.14 Polythene wrist support. A splint such as this is sometimes used in the conservative treatment of osteoarthritis of the wrist.

Osteoarthritis of the trapezio-metacarpal joint

This is a common affection in women beyond middle age but it may also occur in younger persons, especially when there has been previous injury such as a fracture of the base of the first metacarpal bone involving the joint (Bennett's fracture-subluxation). The arthritis may seriously impair the function of the thumb because of pain.

Clinical features. There is pain, localised to the trapezio-metacarpal joint, on using the thumb. The disability slowly increases over the years until activities such as sewing or knitting – or indeed any active use of the thumb – become virtually impossible.

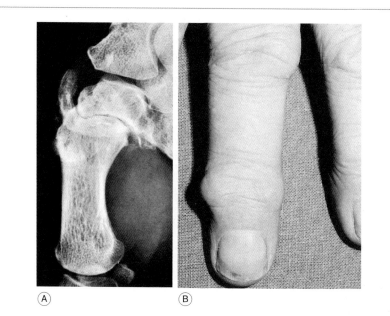

Fig. 16.15 Ⓐ Osteoarthritis of the trapezio-metacarpal joint. Note the marked narrowing of the cartilage space and the large osteophytes. Ⓑ Typical Heberden's nodes, a characteristic feature of degenerative arthritis of the interphalangeal joints.

On examination the trapezio-metacarpal joint is prominent and slightly thickened. Active or passive movements of the thumb metacarpal cause pain. The range of movement at this joint varies widely even in normal individuals; so its measurement is of little practical value, though comparison with the opposite hand may be a guide to the extent to which movement is impaired. In cases of severe arthritis there may be very little remaining movement.

Radiographs show narrowing of the cartilage space and sharpening or spurring of bone at the joint margins (Fig. 16.15A). In many cases the joint is subluxated.

Treatment. In the early stages, with only moderate pain, the condition is best left alone. Conservative treatment is generally disappointing, though sometimes the injection of hydrocortisone into the joint may give worthwhile temporary relief.

Operative treatment. If the symptoms become disabling operation is advisable. The choice lies between arthroplasty and arthrodesis. Arthroplasty is done simply by excising the trapezium, allowing the resulting gap to fill with fibrous tissue. It gives results that are very satisfactory for the usual elderly sufferer from this disorder and should usually be the method of choice. The use of a prosthetic implant is better avoided. If heavy use is to be demanded of the hand in a young person (as in the case of a labourer, for example), arthrodesis of the trapezio-metacarpal joint is sometimes preferred.

Osteoarthritis of interphalangeal joints

This leads to pain and stiffness especially in the distal interphalangeal joints. Characteristically the formation of osteophytes is a prominent feature, with the appearance of ugly swellings known as Heberden's nodes (Fig. 16.15B). Active treatment is not required.

KIENBÖCK'S DISEASE[1] (Osteochondritis of the lunate bone)

Kienböck's disease is an uncommon affection of the lunate bone characterised by temporary softening, fragmentation, and liability to deformation. It tends to predispose to the later development of osteoarthritis of the wrist.

Cause. The precise cause is unknown. A disturbance of blood supply, possibly from thrombosis of a nutrient vessel, is believed to be the essential factor, but how it comes about is not clear. Repeated injury (for example, using the front of the wrist to drive a chisel in carpentry, or operating a pneumatic road drill) has sometimes been noted in the case history, but a causative connection is not fully established.

Pathology. In its behaviour the disease resembles osteochondritis of developing epiphysial centres in children (p. 130), such as Perthes' disease: in effect, it is a form of avascular necrosis (osteonecrosis). The bone becomes granular in texture, small dense fragments being interspersed with softened areas. In this state the bone eventually crumbles, and under the pressure imposed by muscle action and use of the wrist it gradually becomes compressed into a thin saucer-shaped mass. The overlying cartilage dies. After about two years the bone texture is restored to normal, but the bone remains deformed and lacks a smooth cartilaginous covering. The bone behaves like a piece of grit in a bearing and leads gradually to the development of osteoarthritis of the wrist.

Clinical features. There is pain in the wrist, most marked at the centre of the joint over the lunate area. The pain is worse during active use of the wrist. Because of the pain, the strength of grip is impaired.

On examination there is discomfort on pressure over the lunate bone. An important sign is that movements of the wrist are substantially restricted and cause pain if forced.

Radiographs are diagnostic. In the early stages the lunate bone appears slightly more dense than the surrounding bones, and if its depth is compared with that of the lunate bone of the sound wrist it is seen to be reduced, though only slightly at first (Fig. 16.16). Later, the bone has a fragmented appearance, small areas of increased density being scattered through it, and the flattening of the bone becomes obvious. Later still, signs of osteoarthritis of the wrist are evident.

Treatment. Treatment is often rather unsatisfactory. It must depend upon the duration of the symptoms and the degree of damage to the wrist. In the earliest stage, when radiographic changes are only just perceptible, there is probably a place for protecting the wrist in plaster for two or three months in the hope that the condition will resolve through revascularisation of the bone. But once the

[1]Dr Robert Kienböck (1871–1953) Austrian radiologist and Professor in Vienna who began using X-rays in 1897, only 2 years after their discovery by Röntgen.

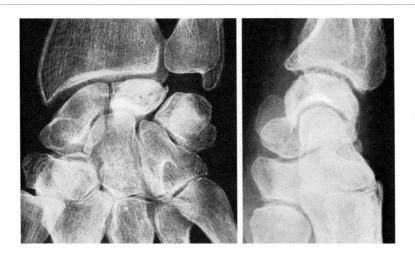

Fig. 16.16 Kienböck's disease of the lunate bone. Note the increased density, fragmentation and beginning compression of the bone.

disease is clearly established surgical treatment is recommended. If the wrist is free from arthritis it is probably best to excise the lunate bone and replace it with a metal prosthesis. This probably gives better results than excision alone, without replacement, but the long-term results are nevertheless uncertain.

In late cases, if severe osteoarthritis is already present, excision of the lunate bone is of no avail. Treatment should then be the same as for osteoarthritis of the wrist (p. 307).

EXTRA-ARTICULAR DISORDERS ABOUT THE WRIST AND HAND

ACUTE INFECTIONS OF THE FASCIAL SPACES OF THE HAND

Acute infections of the hand account for a considerable proportion of the work of a casualty department or emergency room and are of great importance in industrial medicine. Unless they are treated efficiently they can lead to prolonged or even permanent disability, with impairment of working capacity.

Classification

If minor superficial infections are excluded there are six types to be considered:

1. nail-fold infection (paronychia)
2. pulp-space infection (whitlow, felon)
3. other subcutaneous infections
4. thenar space infection
5. mid-palmar space infection
6. tendon sheath infection.

Cause. All types are caused by infection with pyogenic bacteria. The usual causative organism is the *Staphylococcus aureus*, but the *Streptococcus* and occasionally other bacteria may be responsible. Minor injury such as a prick, abrasion, or blister usually provides the route by which infection can enter. Manual work in dirty conditions is clearly a factor that favours infection.

Pathology. The organisms reach the tissue planes by direct implantation from outside, often as the result of a trivial injury such as a prick or abrasion. They set up an acute inflammatory reaction which in many cases goes on to suppuration. Without effective treatment, infection may spread to adjacent tissue planes; occasionally it may give rise to spreading lymphangitis or to septicaemia.

Clinical features. In general, the symptoms of acute hand infections are local pain (often with throbbing), swelling and loss of function. There is often some degree of constitutional disturbance, with pyrexia.

On examination there are obvious swelling, redness of the skin (except in deep infections), and marked local tenderness over the site of the infection. Special features of the individual lesions are described in the following pages.

Principles of treatment. Before suppuration has occurred, the aim of treatment is to abort the infection and avoid the need for operation. The essentials of this expectant treatment are rest for the hand, elevation of the limb, and antibiotic drugs. In a minor case it may be sufficient to support the hand in a sling, but in a severe case rest is best assured by a light plaster back-splint, and elevation may be maintained by suspending the limb in a roller towel attached above the side of the bed. The question of antibiotics is difficult because the sensitivity of the organism is not at first known. Flucloxacillin is usually given, often in conjunction with ampicillin. Regrettably, patients are not often seen early enough to permit success from this expectant treatment.

When suppuration has already occurred, as indicated by severe throbbing pain, intense local tenderness, pyrexia, loss of function, and loss of sleep, the abscess should be drained surgically without further delay. Surgery must be done with adequate facilities, under regional nerve block or general anaesthesia and with tourniquet control. An adequate incision must be used to allow adequate abscess drainage but must not endanger important underlying structures. After adequate drainage has been secured the wound may be packed lightly open with vaselined gauze for two days. Thereafter, dry dressings are used and active finger exercises are encouraged.

Within the limits imposed by these principles there is often more than one way of performing the actual drainage operation. However, it should be stressed that a knowledge of the anatomy of the fascial spaces[1] of the hand is indispensable for the correct treatment of hand infections.

---

[1]The term 'space' as used in this connection is a misnomer. It refers to the interval or plane between adjacent tissues, and in the normal hand it is only a potential space.

SPECIAL FEATURES OF INDIVIDUAL LESIONS

Nail-fold infection (paronychia)

This is one of the commonest but least serious types of hand infection. The subcuticular plane beneath the nail fold is potentially continuous, at the base and sides of the nail, with the subungual space deep to the nail. Infection beginning in the nail fold may therefore easily spread under the nail (Fig. 16.17), and the resulting abscess cannot be drained effectively unless part of the nail is removed.

Clinical features. There are pain, redness, and swelling at one or both sides of the nail fold and at the base of the nail. There is local tenderness over the reddened area. If suppuration has extended deep to the nail there is marked tenderness on pressure upon the nail.

Complications: These are:

1. extension to the pulp space
2. chronic paronychia, following inadequate treatment of the acute infection.

Treatment. In this type of infection conservative measures are often successful if begun within a few hours of the onset. When local suppuration has occurred the subcuticular abscess is drained by raising the cuticle from the nail or by raising it as a short flap after incising it vertically at one or both corners (Fig. 16.18A). If pus has extended under the nail the proximal third of the nail must also be removed.

Pulp-space infection (whitlow)

This is almost as common as nail-fold infection. The interval between the front of the distal phalanx and the skin is traversed by tough fibrous partitions, which subdivide the space into numerous fat-filled cells (like the cells of a honeycomb) disposed at right angles to the skin surface (Fig. 16.17). Infection occurring in this tough tissue is virtually within a closed compartment: tissue pressure rises rapidly and accounts for early throbbing pain.

Clinical features. The pulp is swollen, tense and tender. Severe throbbing pain, with exquisite localised tenderness, suggests that suppuration is present.

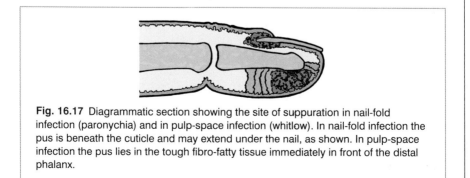

Fig. 16.17 Diagrammatic section showing the site of suppuration in nail-fold infection (paronychia) and in pulp-space infection (whitlow). In nail-fold infection the pus is beneath the cuticle and may extend under the nail, as shown. In pulp-space infection the pus lies in the tough fibro-fatty tissue immediately in front of the distal phalanx.

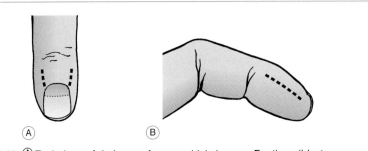

Fig. 16.18 Ⓐ Technique of drainage of paronychial abscess. For the mildest infections it is sufficient to raise the cuticle alone without incising it; but better drainage is secured by a vertical incision through the cuticle, on one or both sides. When pus has extended beneath the nail it is necessary also to remove the proximal third of the nail (shaded area). Ⓑ Incision for drainage of pulp abscess. The incision is deepened across the pulp, in front of the phalanx, and the abscess cavity is cleared out under direct vision.

Complications: These are:

1. osteomyelitis of the terminal phalanx, often leading to necrosis and sequestration of its distal half
2. pyogenic arthritis of the distal interphalangeal joint
3. very rarely, spread of infection to the flexor tendon sheath (suppurative tenosynovitis).

Treatment. Conservative measures are seldom successful except in the earliest stages. Surgical drainage is effected well by a lateral incision just in front of the plane of the terminal phalanx (Fig. 16.18B); it is deepened transversely across the pulp of the finger but should not extend proximally beyond a point half a centimetre distal to the terminal skin crease lest the flexor tendon sheath be inadvertently opened. An alternative method is to incise directly into the pulp over the centre of the abscess, a technique that is to be preferred if the abscess is already threatening to point at the surface.

Subcutaneous infections (other than pulp-space infections)

These infections are common. Infection may occur in the subcutaneous plane at any point in the hand. Common sites are the middle or proximal segment of a finger, and the web spaces between the digits. Less common sites are the palm of the hand and the dorsum of the hand. These superficial spaces are clearly demarcated from the deep palmar spaces next to be described, and must not be confused with them.

Clinical features. The infection may arise in any part of the hand or fingers. There is localised swelling with redness and tenderness. In many cases the infection has spread through the skin from a subcuticular infection or blister.

Complications are:

1. sloughing of skin over the lesion
2. spread to the deep space or to the flexor tendon sheaths.

Treatment. Surgical drainage is by a short incision appropriately placed to reach the abscess without harming important structures or leaving an awkward scar. In the case of a web-space infection the incision should not divide the skin fold of the web: a short transverse incision in the palm just proximal to the skin fold is adequate (see Fig. 16.20B).

Thenar space infection

This is a well-defined entity but it is very uncommon. It may arise by extension from a subcutaneous lesion or a tendon sheath infection. The thenar space lies deeply under the lateral (radial) half of the hollow of the palm. It is the interval between the adductor pollicis muscle behind and the flexor tendon of the index finger and the first and second lumbrical muscles in front. Medially it is separated from the mid-palmar space by a fibrous septum that extends deeply from the fascia on the deep surface of the flexor tendons to the fascia covering the interossei and adductor pollicis muscle (Figs 16.19 and 16.20A). The space is prolonged forwards into the delicate sheath that surrounds the first lumbrical muscle. It sometimes communicates also with the second lumbrical canal. The lumbrical canals thus provide a potential communication between the subcutaneous web spaces and the thenar space: in practice, however, it is rare for infection to spread along this route.

Clinical features. The radial half of the palm is ballooned out and the swelling extends to the dorsal aspect of the web between thumb and index finger. *Treatment*: Drainage is by an incision at the dorsal aspect of the first web space (Fig. 16.20B).

Mid-palmar space infection

This is also uncommon. It resembles the thenar space infection, but the swelling is confined to the ulnar half of the palm. It usually arises by extension from a subcutaneous lesion or a tendon sheath infection. The mid-palmar space

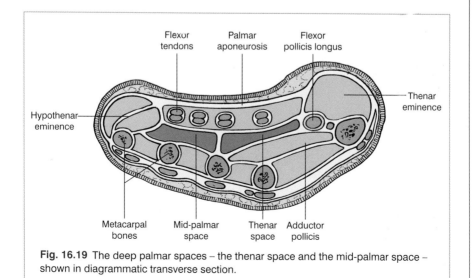

Fig. 16.19 The deep palmar spaces – the thenar space and the mid-palmar space – shown in diagrammatic transverse section.

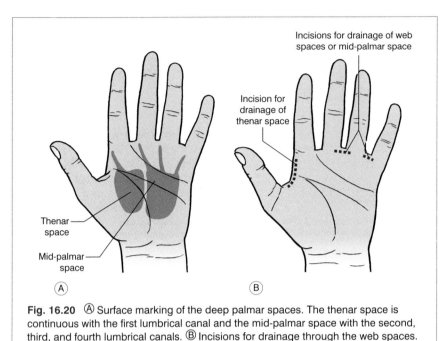

Fig. 16.20 Ⓐ Surface marking of the deep palmar spaces. The thenar space is continuous with the first lumbrical canal and the mid-palmar space with the second, third, and fourth lumbrical canals. Ⓑ Incisions for drainage through the web spaces.

lies under the medial (ulnar) half of the hollow of the palm. It is the interval between the interossei and metacarpal bones behind and the flexor tendons (in their sheaths) of the middle, ring, and little fingers in front (Fig. 16.19). Laterally, it is separated from the thenar space by the fibrous septum already described. The space is prolonged forwards into the sheaths of the second, third, and fourth lumbrical muscles (Fig. 16.20A). Again, despite the potential communication between a web space and the mid-palmar space along the lumbrical canals, web-space infection very seldom spreads deeply to involve the palm.

Clinical features. The ulnar half of the palm is ballooned out. Movements of the fingers are restricted and painful.

Treatment. Drainage can be established through the web space between the middle and ring fingers or through that between the ring and little fingers (Fig. 16.20B).

Tendon sheath infection

This is rare, but important because prompt treatment is essential if the function of the finger is to be preserved. Distinction must be made between the tough fibrous sheaths, which exist only in the digits, and the flimsy synovial sheaths, which line the fibrous sheaths and, in the case of the thumb and little finger, extend proximally into the palm. In acute infections of the tendon sheaths (acute infective tenosynovitis) the pus is within the synovial sheath and it is confined only by the limits of the sheath. The flexor sheaths of the index, middle, and ring fingers end proximally at the level of the transverse palmar skin crease (Fig. 16.21A). The sheaths of the thumb and little finger extend

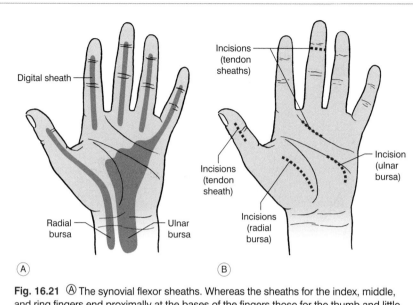

Fig. 16.21 Ⓐ The synovial flexor sheaths. Whereas the sheaths for the index, middle, and ring fingers end proximally at the bases of the fingers those for the thumb and little finger extend upwards to become continuous with the radial bursa and the ulnar bursa respectively. Ⓑ Incisions for drainage and irrigation of tendon sheaths and bursae.

proximally through the palm to end two or three centimetres above the level of the wrist. The proximal part of the sheath for the thumb is known as the radial bursa. The sheath for the little finger opens out proximally into the ulnar bursa, which encloses the grouped tendons of flexor digitorum superficialis and flexor digitorum profundus (Fig. 16.21A).

Clinical features. The finger is swollen throughout its length, and acutely tender over the flexor tendon sheath. It is held semiflexed and the patient is unwilling to extend it because of pain.

Complications: These are:

1. necrosis of the tendons and adhesions between tendon and sheath, causing permanent stiffness of the finger in semi-flexion
2. spread of infection to involve the radial bursa (from the flexor sheath of the thumb), or the ulnar bursa (from the sheath of the little finger).

Treatment. Systemic antibiotic therapy is begun immediately. The sheath is opened at its proximal end in the palm and at its distal end (Fig. 16.21B), and irrigated with antibiotic solution through a fine tube passed along the sheath; the tube is withdrawn and the wounds are packed lightly open.

If the radial bursa or the ulnar bursa is infected it must be drained and irrigated through an additional incision in the palm (Fig. 16.21B).

CHRONIC INFECTIVE TENOSYNOVITIS (Including compound palmar ganglion)

Chronic inflammation of tendon sheaths in the lower forearm and hand may occur in response to low-grade infection, usually tuberculous. It is entirely distinct from acute tenosynovitis and is not preceded by it. It is now seen only rarely in Western countries except in some patients with chronic rheumatoid arthritis.

Pathology. The flexor tendon sheaths in the lower forearm and hand are those most commonly affected. The affected sheaths are greatly thickened and show the changes of chronic inflammation. There may be histological evidence of tuberculosis in the thickened tissue. The sheaths often contain an excess of fluid and there may be collections of small fibrinous bodies. The tendons themselves are affected only slightly.

Clinical features. There is a gradual onset of swelling, with mild aching pain, in the region of the affected tendon sheaths – usually the flexor sheaths of the lower forearm and hand. The function of the fingers and thumb is impaired with moderate restriction of flexion and extension of the digits. The swelling is confined to the line of the tendon sheaths in the front of the forearm and the proximal part of the palm (Fig. 16.22). In many cases fluctuation can be elicited between the forearm swelling and the swelling in the palm. This physical sign led to the use of the term compound palmar ganglion, though this is a misnomer as the common ganglia around the wrist joint arise from the synovial cavity of the joint and not the tendon sheath.

If an active tuberculous lesion is found elsewhere in the body it is reasonable to infer that the tenosynovitis is also tuberculous.

Treatment. In mild cases in which the function of the fingers and thumb is not impaired conservative treatment is advised. In tuberculous cases a course of the appropriate antibacterial drugs is given (see p. 102).

In severe cases operation is recommended. It consists in excising thoroughly all the thickened and oedematous synovial membrane. After operation finger movements are encouraged and practised daily under the supervision of a physiotherapist. A useful range of finger movement is usually restored, but permanent inability to flex the fingers fully into the palm may have to be accepted.

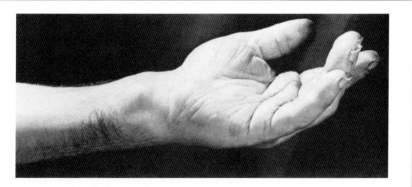

Fig. 16.22 Compound palmar ganglion. The swellings in the palm and at the front of the wrist are continuous deep to the flexor retinaculum, and fluctuation can be elicited between them.

SOFT-TISSUE TUMOURS IN THE HAND (General description of soft-tissue tumours, p. 157)

Soft-tissue tumours are uncommon in the hand but special mention must be made of an unusual tumour that is the second most common cause of swelling in the hand after simple ganglion cyst. This is the giant-cell tumour of tendon sheath (localised nodular tenosynovitis).

Giant-cell tumours of tendon sheath

This is a benign tumour that is related to the more diffuse pigmented villonodular synovitis in terms of its histological appearances. It presents in patients aged 30–50 years as a painless localised slow-growing mass on the volar aspect of the finger. It arises from the sheath of a tendon and, as it enlarges, it burrows between the tissue planes to eventually form a bulky mass which almost surrounds the finger like a collar. Histologically it is composed of cells of many forms, including round cells, giant cells of foreign-body type, xanthoma cells containing cholesterol, and fibroblasts. Treatment is by complete marginal excision of the mass, which may be difficult because of its proximity to the tendon and underlying bone.

GANGLION (Simple ganglion)

A ganglion is the commonest cystic swelling at the back of the wrist.

Pathology. Conflicting views have been put forward on the origin of ganglia. Some believe that they represent a degenerative process. Others claim that they are benign tumours of tendon sheath or joint capsule. The cyst wall is of fibrous tissue and there is no true endothelial lining. It is connected at some point with a joint capsule or tendon sheath, but there is no communication between the joint cavity or tendon sheath and the interior of the cyst. The cyst is usually unilocular. The contained fluid is clear and viscous.

Clinical features. Ganglia are commonest at the back of the wrist, where they are often seen in adults of any age (Fig. 16.23). They also occur, less commonly, at the front of the wrist, or in the palm or fingers. Ordinarily there are no

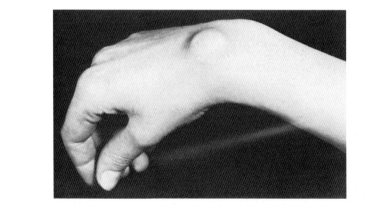

Fig. 16.23 A simple ganglion at the back of the wrist. This is the commonest site.

symptoms other than the swelling itself and, sometimes, discomfort or slight pain. On examination the swelling may be soft and obviously cystic, but more often it is tense. It is often mistaken for a bony prominence – but careful tests will show that it is fluctuant.

Complications. A ganglion arising deeply in the wrist or palm may interfere mechanically with the ulnar or the median nerve or their branches. There will be motor and usually sensory impairment in the distribution of the particular branch affected.

Treatment. A ganglion is harmless and in the absence of pain or complications it may safely be left alone. Sometimes the ganglion can be dispersed subcutaneously by firm local pressure. This rather dramatic treatment is harmless and temporarily effective, but the ganglion may slowly reappear. An alternative method of providing temporary relief is to aspirate the cyst with a wide-bore needle. Lasting cure can be ensured only by complete excision of the ganglion – not always an easy task because the thin-walled sac often tracks deeply between the tendons, where it may be torn and a fragment left behind, leading to recurrence. In children there is a tendency to spontaneous resolution; so the question of excision may be deferred.

A ganglion that is interfering with a peripheral nerve demands operative excision without delay.

CARPAL TUNNEL SYNDROME (Compression of median nerve in carpal tunnel)

Constriction of the median nerve as it passes beneath the flexor retinaculum is the commonest compression neuropathy in the arm, resulting in discomfort in the hand, especially in middle-aged or elderly women.

Cause. In the majority of cases no primary cause can be discovered, but any space-occupying lesion within the carpal tunnel may be responsible. Recognised causes are chronic inflammatory thickening of the tendon sheaths (as in rheumatoid arthritis), osteoarthritis of the wrist, deformity or malunion after fracture of the lower end of the radius, and myxoedema.

Pathology. The median nerve lies beneath the flexor retinaculum in company with the flexor tendons of the hand. If the available space within this strong-walled tunnel is reduced the nerve is compressed against the flexor retinaculum. When the retinaculum is divided in such a case the nerve may be found constricted and flattened where it lay behind it. The ulnar nerve does not pass behind the flexor retinaculum; so it is not liable to compression in this way.

Clinical features. The condition is commonest in women in or beyond middle life. The symptoms are sensory and motor. There is tingling, numbness, or discomfort usually in the radial three and a half digits (that is, in the normal distribution of the median nerve), and there is a feeling of clumsiness in carrying out fine movements such as those concerned in sewing. Distressing tingling is often prominent during the night and the patient may have to work the fingers or shake the hand to gain relief, making this an almost diagnostic symptom.

On examination the findings vary with the degree and duration of the compression. At first there are no objective clinical findings. Later there may be blunting of sensibility in the median nerve distribution. In a severe case there may eventually be evident wasting and weakness of the median-innervated small muscles of the hand, particularly abductor pollicis brevis. The Durkan test may be positive when direct compression of the median nerve at the carpal tunnel for 30 seconds reproduces numbness and tingling in one or more of the radial digits.

Investigations. Electrophysiological nerve conduction testing may show decreased conduction velocity in the affected part of the median nerve. This is a reliable confirmatory test if the clinical diagnosis is in doubt.

Diagnosis. Care must be taken to exclude other causes of neurological disturbance in the hand, especially those arising in the neck from interference with the brachial plexus, and lesions of the median nerve elsewhere in its course.

Treatment. A trial may be made of conservative treatment by supporting the wrist at night for three weeks with a simple splint in a neutral position. When the symptoms arise in pregnancy, relief that lasts until after delivery (when the symptoms usually subside spontaneously) may be gained by the injection of hydrocortisone alongside the nerve at wrist level. This may be tried also in other cases and may cure the symptoms in 50% of patients. If it is unsuccessful full relief is assured by dividing the flexor retinaculum to decompress the nerve. This is a simple operation that may be done either through an open incision or (with slightly greater risk to the motor branch of the median nerve) by an endoscopic technique.

DUPUYTREN'S[1] CONTRACTURE (Contracture of the palmar aponeurosis; Dupuytren's disease)

This is an easily recognised condition characterised in the established phase by flexion contracture of one or more of the fingers from thickening and shortening of the palmar aponeurosis.

Cause. This is unknown. There is a hereditary predisposition. In a predisposed person injury possibly plays a part but its exact significance is uncertain. There is an increased incidence of the disorder among epileptics, but this is possibly related to the use of anticonvulsant drugs rather than to an underlying genetic association between the two diseases.

Pathology. The palmar aponeurosis (palmar fascia) is normally a thin but tough membrane whose fibres radiate from the termination of the palmaris longus tendon at the front of the wrist to gain insertion into the proximal and middle phalanges of the fingers. It lies immediately beneath the skin. In Dupuytren's contracture the aponeurosis, or part of it, becomes greatly thickened (often to half a centimetre or more), and it slowly contracts, drawing the fingers into flexion at the metacarpo-phalangeal and proximal interphalangeal joints. The medial (ulnar) half of the aponeurosis is affected most, and serious flexion deformity is usually confined to the ring and little fingers, with only moderate deformity of the middle finger (Figs 16.24 and 16.25). The joints themselves are unaffected at first, but in long-established cases secondary capsular contractures occur. The flexor tendons in the palm are in no way affected.

The plantar aponeurosis in the foot is occasionally affected, but in the foot the lesion usually takes the form of a firm nodule under the instep rather than of a contracture involving the toes (Fig. 16.26). Other parts that may be affected include the penis. Thus although the hands are primarily affected, the condition is sometimes much more widespread (Dupuytren's disease).

Clinical features. The affection is much more common in men than in women. Often both hands are affected. The earliest sign is a small thickened nodule in the

[1]Baron Guillame Dupuytren (1777–1835) A French surgeon who rose from humble beginnings to become Surgeon-in-chief at the Hotel Dieu in Paris. He described many pathological conditions including the contracture in 1833.

The forearm, wrist, and hand

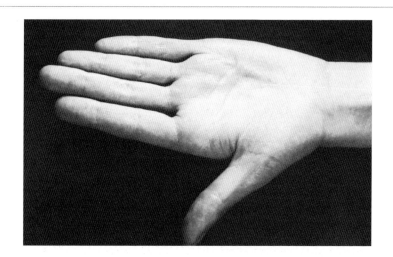

Fig. 16.24 Early Dupuytren's contracture. There is a nodule of thickened aponeurosis in the palm, opposite the base of the ring finger, with slight puckering of the skin; but so far there is no flexion contracture of the fingers.

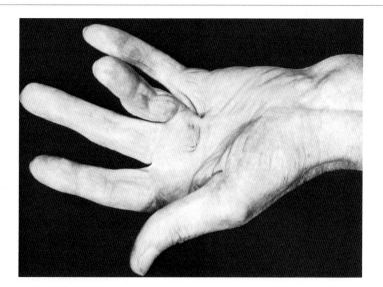

Fig. 16.25 A typical example of Dupuytren's contracture of the palmar aponeurosis in which the ring finger has been drawn down into flexion. Note the tight band of thickened aponeurosis immediately under the skin. The band has sometimes been mistaken for a contracted flexor tendon.

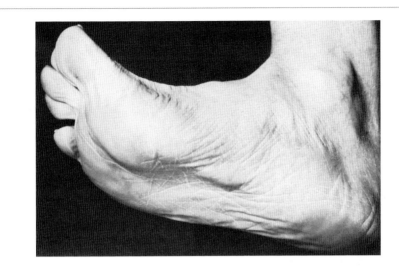

Fig. 16.26 Typical nodule in the sole of the foot in Dupuytren's disease.

mid-palm opposite the base of the ring finger (Fig. 16.24). The area of thickening gradually spreads from this point, giving rise eventually to firm cord-like bands that extend into the ring finger or little finger, or both, and prevent full extension of the metacarpo-phalangeal and proximal interphalangeal joints (Fig. 16.25). The skin is closely adherent to the fascial bands, and is often puckered. The flexion deformity becomes progressively worse in the course of months or years.

In some cases these changes in the palm are accompanied by thickening over the dorsum of the interphalangeal joints (knuckle pads). The feet may also show nodules in the sole (Fig. 16.26). Occasionally the penis is distorted by thickened bands.

Diagnosis. The thickened bands of palmar aponeurosis must not be mistaken for contracted flexor tendons. It is easily confirmed that the bands are distinct from tendons because they do not move when the fingers are flexed and extended.

Treatment. The only effective treatment is by operation, though a number of proteolytic drugs administered by injection are under trial. However, operation is not necessary in every case: a contracture that is not progressing rapidly is often better left alone, especially in an elderly patient. Surgery is usually required if the flexion contractures exceed 30° at the metacarpo-phalangeal, or 15° at the interphalangeal joints. Operation entails excision of the thickened part of the palmar aponeurosis by painstaking dissection to avoid damage to digital nerves. Simple division of the taut contracted bands is less satisfactory because the contracture tends to recur. In selected cases multiple releases of metacarpo-phalangeal contractures through small separate incisions may give permanent improvement in over 50% of patients. In advanced cases the contractures may involve the overlying palmar skin and there may be a need to use skin grafting following radical excision. An alternative is to apply a splint to maintain the correction and allow the skin to heal by secondary intention.

RUPTURE OR SEVERANCE OF TENDONS IN THE HAND

Most tendon divisions in the hand are caused by cuts with sharp objects such as glass or knives. Certain tendons are prone to rupture: thus the extensor tendon of a finger is easily torn from its insertion into the distal phalanx by sudden forced flexion of the finger; and the extensor pollicis longus tendon is liable to rupture spontaneously after fractures of the lower end of the radius in consequence of its becoming frayed where it crosses the roughened bone. In rheumatoid arthritis, also, spontaneous rupture – especially of an extensor tendon – is common.

Clinical features and diagnosis. Loss of function of a tendon is obvious clinically. When the findings are correlated with the history the diagnosis is usually clear.

Treatment. This varies according to the tendon affected and the site of severance or rupture (see below and Fig. 16.27). Sometimes treatment is unnecessary or undesirable, but more often operative reconstruction is to be advised: the tendon is either sutured directly or replaced by a free tendon graft or by a tendon transfer, according to circumstances (see pages 46 and 44 for the principles of these methods).

SPECIAL FEATURES OF INDIVIDUAL LESIONS

Injuries of flexor tendons

Division within a fibrous flexor sheath of a finger. Severance at this site presents the most difficult problem of all tendon injuries. The prognosis is

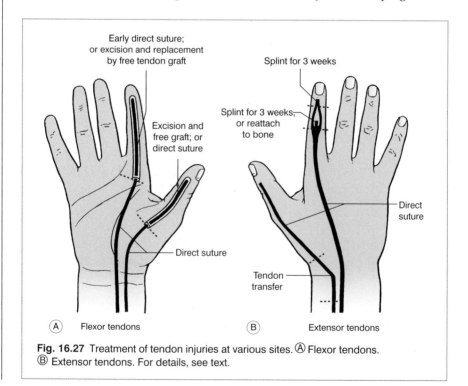

Fig. 16.27 Treatment of tendon injuries at various sites. Ⓐ Flexor tendons. Ⓑ Extensor tendons. For details, see text.

uncertain after operative repair or reconstruction because of the proclivity of the tendon to adhere to the sheath.

Treatment. If a flexor superficialis tendon alone is divided and the flexor profundus is intact treatment may not be required, for there is virtually no disability.

If a flexor profundus tendon alone is divided, the flexor superficialis being intact, the loss of active flexion at the distal interphalangeal joint can often be accepted. Attempted repair of the tendon is usually better avoided because of its uncertain results. Arthrodesis of the distal interphalangeal joint in slight flexion reduces the disability to a negligible level.

If both tendons are divided, operative repair or later reconstruction is advised. When the injury is recent (within one week) and the wound clean, and when good conditions and skilled staff are available, primary repair is the method of choice.

Technique. Direct suture of the severed ends demands high technical skill and long experience. Both the superficialis tendon and the profundus tendon should be repaired with loupe magnification, an atraumatic technique, and using semi-absorbable fine 4-0 suture material.

For delayed repair because of late presentation, or where there is extensive damage or loss of tendon tissue, it may be necessary to use a free tendon graft. The standard method is to remove the flexor superficialis tendon entirely (to make more room in the sheath) and to replace the whole of the digital part of the flexor profundus tendon by a free tendon graft (from the palmaris longus or from a toe extensor) sutured proximally to the profundus tendon in the palm or at wrist level, and inserted distally into a drill hole in the distal phalanx (Fig. 16.28). This method eliminates the need for a tendon junction within the sheath, which carries the risk of adhesions that may cause disabling stiffness.

Division of flexor pollicis longus in the thumb. The problem is less difficult than that presented by division of both flexor tendons in a finger. Repair may

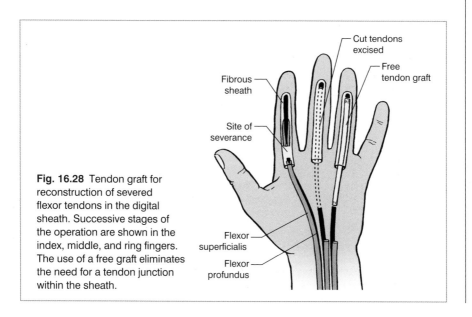

Fig. 16.28 Tendon graft for reconstruction of severed flexor tendons in the digital sheath. Successive stages of the operation are shown in the index, middle, and ring fingers. The use of a free graft eliminates the need for a tendon junction within the sheath.

Cut tendons excised

Free tendon graft

Fibrous sheath

Site of severance

Flexor superficialis

Flexor profundus

be made by direct suture, by advancement of the tendon, or by replacement of the digital part of the tendon by a free graft as described for the fingers.

Division of flexor tendons in the palm or wrist. Direct suture is advised. It may be done primarily if the wound is clean. The prognosis is good if a single tendon is affected but it is uncertain in cases of multiple tendon divisions at the front of the wrist, especially if the nerves are also injured.

Injuries of extensor tendons

Severance of extensor tendons at the back of the hand. This injury has a good prognosis. There is a tendency to spontaneous union with recovery of normal function. *Treatment*: Primary suture should be undertaken if the injury is recent. If there has been delay, freshening and direct suture of the divided ends is advised. Repair of a spontaneously ruptured extensor tendon in rheumatoid arthritis has a less satisfactory prognosis because the tendon is of impaired quality. Nevertheless, operative repair should usually be attempted.

Rupture of extensor pollicis longus tendon may complicate fracture of the lower end of the radius. The tendon gives way after becoming frayed by repeated movement over the roughened lower end of the radius. Spontaneous rupture may also occur in drummers. The extensive fraying makes direct suture unsatisfactory. *Treatment*: A clean rupture should be sutured end-to-end. If the tendon is frayed, as is usually the case, a tendon transfer operation is to be preferred. The tendon of extensor indicis is divided at the level of the neck of the second metacarpal bone, re-routed towards the thumb, and sutured to the freshened distal stump of the extensor pollicis longus tendon (Fig. 16.29).

Rupture of middle slip of extensor expansion. This is caused by sudden forced flexion of the proximal interphalangeal joint, the middle slip of the

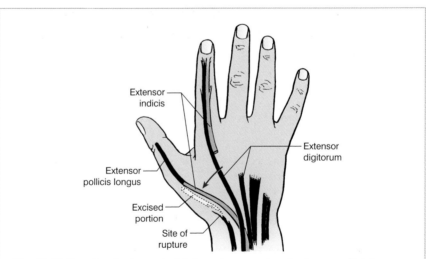

Fig. 16.29 Transfer of extensor indicis to replace a ruptured extensor pollicis longus. The tendon of extensor indicis is divided opposite the neck of the second metacarpal, re-routed towards the thumb, and sutured to the freshened distal stump of the extensor pollicis longus. This transfer is to be preferred to direct suture when the ends of the ruptured tendon are frayed.

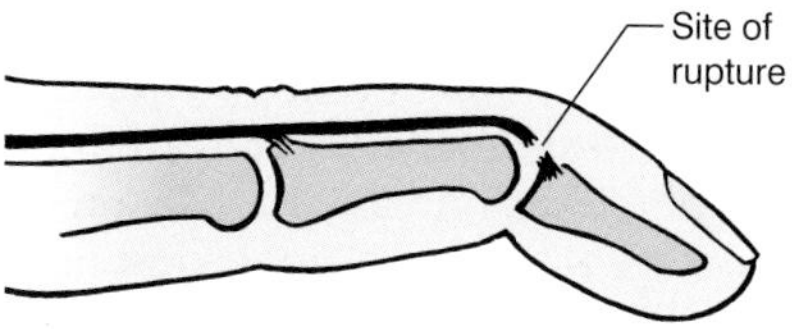

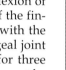

Fig. 16.30 Mallet finger (baseball finger). The extensor tendon is avulsed from its insertion. The terminal joint cannot be extended fully.

Site of rupture

extensor expansion being torn from its attachment to the middle phalanx. The patient is unable to extend the proximal interphalangeal joint fully. The distal joint becomes hyperextended. *Treatment*: The choice lies between immobilisation on a splint in the straight position for three weeks, or operative repair. In a fresh case simple splintage probably gives the better results, though restoration of full function is seldom achieved.

Avulsion of extensor tendon from distal phalanx of a finger. This is known as 'mallet' finger or 'baseball' finger. It is caused by sudden forced flexion of the distal interphalangeal joint – for instance, by a blow on the tip of the finger from a ball. In a few cases a small fragment of bone is avulsed with the tendon. The patient is unable fully to extend the distal interphalangeal joint (Fig. 16.30). *Treatment*: Immediate treatment is to splint the finger for three weeks with the distal interphalangeal joint fully extended. Splintage must be continuous and uninterrupted if a good result is to be achieved. The avulsed tendon always unites back to the bone, but often with lengthening, in which case some deformity persists. However, the disability is usually insignificant and acceptable.

ACUTE FRICTIONAL TENOSYNOVITIS (Peritendinitis crepitans; paratendinitis crepitans; repetitive stress syndrome)

This is an easily recognised clinical condition common in young adults whose occupations demand repetitive movements of the wrist and hand.

Cause. It is attributed to friction between the tendons and the surrounding paratenon, from over-use of the hand. It is entirely distinct from infective tenosynovitis.

Pathology. The tendons most often affected are those of the deep muscles at the back of the forearm, especially the extensors of the thumb and the radial extensors of the wrist. There is a mild inflammatory reaction about the tendon and its coverings, with local swelling and oedema.

Clinical features. After unusually active use of the wrist or hand over a period of days or weeks pain is felt at the back of the wrist and lower forearm, and swelling is noticed. The pain is aggravated by use of the hand.

On examination there is localised swelling in the line of the affected tendons – usually the extensors of the thumb or wrist. If the examiner's hand is placed over the swelling while the patient flexes and extends the wrist and digits a characteristic fine crepitation is felt: it is caused by the fibrin-covered tendon gliding within the inflamed paratenon. This typical crepitation is diagnostic of frictional tenosynovitis.

Treatment. Initially, a trial should be made of local injection of hydrocortisone. If this is unsuccessful, the wrist and forearm should be immobilised in plaster of Paris for three weeks, the fingers being left free. This affords sufficient rest to allow the inflammation to resolve. Excessive use of the fingers and thumb should be avoided for two months.

Comment. The condition described above is a distinct clinical entity with incontrovertible evidence of organic pathology. In recent years the label 'repetitive stress syndrome' has been applied, too often, to a range of rather vague and purely subjective symptoms affecting the hand, or sometimes the whole arm, in persons occupied for long periods in repetitive tasks such as keyboard operation and computer work. In most such cases it is difficult to separate a genuine physical disability (if indeed it exists at all) from the psychological or 'functional' overlay that is often a prominent feature of such conditions.

DE QUERVAIN'S[1] STENOSING TENOVAGINITIS (Tenovaginitis of the abductor pollicis longus and extensor pollicis brevis)

This is a common and well-recognised condition characterised by pain over the styloid process of the radius and palpable thickening in the course of the abductor pollicis longus and extensor pollicis brevis tendons.

Cause. The precise cause is unknown. Excessive friction from overuse may be a factor, because the condition seems prone to follow repetitive actions such as wringing clothes, or in more recent times excessive typing or manipulations.

Pathology. The fibrous sheaths of the abductor pollicis longus and extensor pollicis brevis tendons are thickened where they cross the tip of the radial styloid process. The tendons themselves appear normal as does the synovial lining of the sheath. The condition is possibly analogous to that other common form of tenovaginitis, 'trigger' finger (see below).

Clinical features. The condition is five times commoner in women than men, predominantly in middle age. The main symptom is pain on using the hand, especially when movement tenses the abductor pollicis longus and extensor pollicis brevis tendons (as in lifting a saucepan or a teapot). On examination there is local tenderness at the point where the tendons cross the radial styloid process (Fig. 16.31). The thickened fibrous sheaths are usually palpable as a firm nodule. Passive adduction of the wrist or thumb causes the patient to wince with pain.

Treatment. Conservative treatment with rest by splintage, or the injection of hydrocortisone and local anaesthetic into the tendon sheath, produces recovery in over 80 per cent of patients. Where pain and disability continue an operation to divide the thickened sheaths of the affected tendons provides a certain cure.

[1]Fritz de Quervain (1868–1940) Swiss general surgeon who was Professor of Surgery in Berne. Described the chronic tenovaginitis which bears his name in 1895.

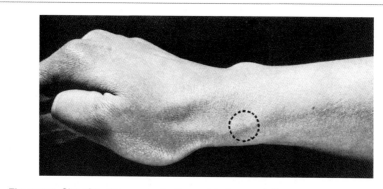

Fig. 16.31 Site of tenderness in de Quervain's tenovaginitis.

'TRIGGER' FINGER; SNAPPING FINGER
(Digital tenovaginitis stenosans)

In this rather common condition thickening and constriction of the mouth of a fibrous digital sheath interfere with the free gliding of the contained flexor tendons.

Cause. This is unknown.

Pathology. The proximal part of the fibrous flexor sheath at the base of a finger or thumb is thickened and the mouth of the sheath is constricted. The contained tendons become 'waisted' opposite the constriction, and swollen proximal to it. The swollen segment enters the mouth of the sheath only with difficulty when an attempt is made to straighten the finger from the flexed position (Fig. 16.32).

Clinical features. The condition occurs:

1. in the fingers of the middle-aged (especially women)
2. in the thumb in infants or young children.

The adult type. There is complaint of tenderness at the base of the affected finger and of locking of the finger in full flexion (Fig. 16.33). The locking can be overcome either by a strong effort or by extending the finger passively with the other hand, when the flexion is released with a distinct snap. *On examination*

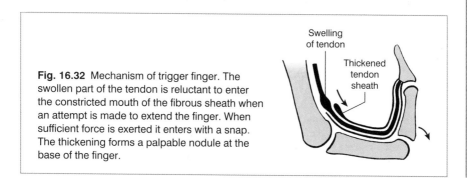

Fig. 16.32 Mechanism of trigger finger. The swollen part of the tendon is reluctant to enter the constricted mouth of the fibrous sheath when an attempt is made to extend the finger. When sufficient force is exerted it enters with a snap. The thickening forms a palpable nodule at the base of the finger.

Swelling of tendon

Thickened tendon sheath

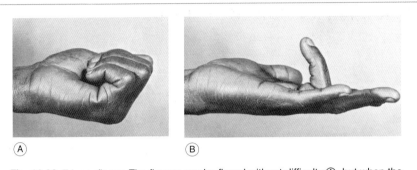

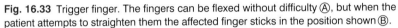

Fig. 16.33 Trigger finger. The fingers can be flexed without difficulty Ⓐ, but when the patient attempts to straighten them the affected finger sticks in the position shown Ⓑ.

there is a palpable nodule, usually slightly tender, at the base of the affected finger or thumb – that is, over the mouth of the fibrous flexor sheath. The snapping cannot be reproduced well on passive movements; it can be demonstrated only when the patient extends the finger fully with its own muscles or assists extension with the other hand.

The infantile type (contracted thumb of infants). The infant is unable to straighten the thumb, which is locked in flexion. On examination it may be possible to extend the thumb passively with a snap, but in many cases the flexed position of the joint cannot be corrected even by moderate force. A palpable nodule is present at the base of the thumb in the position of the mouth of the fibrous flexor sheath – that is, at the level of the head of the metacarpal bone. It should be noted that because the deformity is often resistant to correction this condition in infants is often mistaken for a dislocated thumb or for a congenital deformity.

Treatment. Conservative treatment by injection of local steroid at the site of the palpable nodule may sometimes achieve full relief. When this fails both the adult and the infantile type can be cured by the simple operation of incising the mouth of the fibrous flexor sheath longitudinally.

EXTRINSIC DISORDERS SIMULATING DISEASE OF THE FOREARM OR HAND

DISORDERS OF THE NECK

Certain disorders of the neck interfere with the brachial plexus or its roots, and thereby produce their predominant symptoms – or even their only symptoms – in the lower arm or hand. By far the commonest of such disorders are osteoarthritis of the cervical spine (cervical spondylosis) and prolapse of a cervical intervertebral disc. Less common as causes of peripheral symptoms are cervical rib, tumours of the spinal column or of the spinal cord, and soft-tissue tumours involving nerves.

TUMOUR AT THE THORACIC INLET

A mass at the thoracic inlet is an occasional cause of peripheral symptoms in the upper limb. The commonest cause is an apical tumour of the lung (Pancoast's tumour) involving the nerves of the brachial plexus.

DISORDERS OF THE UPPER ARM

Rarely, a disorder of the upper arm may produce its chief effects in the lower arm or hand, usually through the medium of the major nerve trunks. A well-known example is crutch palsy, in which there is weakness or paralysis of the extensor muscles of the wrist, fingers, and thumb from repeated pressure of an axillary crutch upon the radial nerve in the axilla. These complications are avoided if elbow crutches can be used instead of axillary crutches.

DISORDERS OF THE ELBOW

Affections of the elbow may be associated with vague referred pain in the forearm. Almost always, however, the local symptoms in the elbow overshadow the referred symptoms; so mistakes in diagnosis are unlikely.

17 | The hip region

Disorders of the hip are common both in children and in adults. Prominent among childhood affections are developmental (congenital) dislocation of the hip and Perthes' disease (osteochondritis) of the head of the femur. The hip is subject to all types of arthritis, but in adults osteoarthritis is overwhelmingly the most prominent affection.

Practically and economically, injuries and diseases of the hip are important because they so often cause prolonged suffering and serious disablement – even total incapacity. Academically, the region is of interest for several reasons: the mechanics of the joint are complex; it is one of the most difficult joints to examine with accuracy; and – of special significance to students – cases of hip disease are often presented as tests of clinical acumen in the examinations in surgery. Time spent on learning how to examine the hip correctly will usually be well rewarded.

SPECIAL POINTS IN THE INVESTIGATION OF HIP COMPLAINTS

History

The characteristics of hip pain. Pain in the region of the hip is notoriously misleading, for often it is referred from the spine or pelvis and has no connection with the hip joint itself. Therefore one must always be cautious in attributing such pain to a hip lesion without first investigating the possibility of an extrinsic cause.

Pain arising in the hip is felt mainly in the groin and in the front or inner side of the thigh. Pain is often referred also to the knee; indeed pain in the knee is sometimes the predominant feature. In contrast, the 'hip' pain that is referred from the spine is felt mainly in the gluteal region, whence it often radiates down the back or outer side of the thigh.

True hip pain is made worse by walking, whereas gluteal pain referred from the spine is aggravated by activities such as stooping and lifting, and it is often eased by walking.

Age incidence of hip disorders. Many of the important disorders of the hip occur in childhood, and often at a particular period of childhood. So true is this with some disorders that the age of the patient at the onset of symptoms affords some indication of the likely nature of the trouble, as shown in Table 17.1. (For ease of memorising, round figures have been given in the table but some latitude must be allowed.)

Table 17.1 Usual age incidence of common hip disorders at time of diagnosis

Age at time of diagnosis (years)	Disease
0–2	Developmental (congenital) dislocation
2–5	Tuberculous arthritis; transient synovitis
5–10	Perthes' disease; transient synovitis
10–20	Slipped upper femoral epiphysis
20–50	Osteoarthritis (secondary to previous injury or disease)
50–100	Osteoarthritis (primary)

Exposure

For the proper examination of the hip the patient should be stripped except for a pelvic slip or underpants and, in women, a bra. The first part of the examination is conducted with the patient lying supine; afterwards the patient is examined standing and walking.

Steps in clinical examination

A suggested routine for clinical examination of the hip is summarised in Table 17.2.

Setting the pelvis square

This is an important preliminary step. Determine from the position of the anterior superior iliac spines whether or not the pelvis is lying square with the limbs (Fig. 17.1). If it is not, an attempt is made to set it square. If this is impossible it means that there is incorrectable adduction or abduction at one or other hip (or, rarely, a severe and rigid curvature of the spine): in that event the fact that the pelvis is tilted should be noted and borne in mind during the subsequent steps of the examination.

Measuring the length of the limbs

Methods of measuring the lower limbs are often confusing to the uninitiated, but it is important that they should be properly understood. Accuracy in measurement is of more than academic significance; it is of practical importance when corrective operations or adjustments to the shoes are contemplated. Limb length can be measured clinically within an error of one centimetre. If greater accuracy is needed, radiographic measurement (scanography) is recommended.

It is necessary to measure, first, the real or *true length* of each limb. Secondly, it is necessary to determine whether there is any *'apparent'* or *false discrepancy* in the length of the limbs from fixed pelvic tilt (Fig. 17.2). Whereas it is always necessary to measure the true length, it is necessary to measure 'apparent' discrepancy only when there is an incorrectable tilt of the pelvis.

Measurement of true length. Ideally it would be desirable to measure from the normal axis of hip movement – that is, the centre of the femoral head – but since there is no surface landmark at that point it is impracticable to do so clinically. The measurement is therefore taken from the nearest convenient landmark – namely, the anterior superior spine of the ilium. Distally, measurement is usually made to the medial malleolus.

Table 17.2 Routine clinical examination in suspected disorders of the hip

1. LOCAL EXAMINATION OF THE HIP REGION

(Patient supine)

Position of pelvis

Determine the lie of the pelvis and set it square with the limbs if possible

Inspection

Bone contours and alignment

Soft-tissue contours

Colour and texture of skin

Scars or sinuses

Palpation

Skin temperature

Bone contours

Soft-tissue contours

Local tenderness

Measurement of limb length

Real or true length:

Measure from anterior superior iliac spine to medial malleolus

(angle between pelvis and limbs to be equal on each side)

If discrepancy found, determine site of shortening (or lengthening):

(a) Above trochanter (Bryant's triangle; Nelaton's line; Schoemaker's line)

(b) Below trochanter (measure each bone)

'Apparent' or false discrepancy:

Measure from xiphisternum to medial malleolus. (Limbs to be parallel and in line with trunk)

Examination for fixed deformity

Including Thomas's manoeuvre for detection and measurement of fixed flexion deformity

Movements (active and passive)

Flexion

Abduction; abduction in flexion

Adduction

Medial (internal) rotation

Lateral (external) rotation

Power (tested against resistance of examiner)

Estimate strength of each muscle group: flexors, extensors, abductors, adductors, rotators

Examination for abnormal mobility

Test for longitudinal (telescopic) movement

Click test (in new-born)

(patient standing)

Examination for postural stability

Trendelenburg's test

Gait

2. EXAMINATION OF POTENTIAL EXTRINSIC SOURCES OF HIP SYMPTOMS

This is important if a satisfactory explanation for the symptoms is not found on local examination. The investigation should include:

1. the spine and sacro-iliac joints
2. the abdomen and pelvis
3. the knee
4. the major blood vessels (arterial circulation)

3. GENERAL EXAMINATION

General survey of the other parts of the body. The local symptoms may be only one manifestation of a widespread or generalised disease

It should be noted that the anterior superior spine is well lateral to the axis of hip movement. This is of no consequence if the angle between limb and pelvis is the same on each side. But it will render the measurements fallacious if the angle between limb and pelvis is not the same on each side. This will be understood best by reference to Fig. 17.3A. It will be seen that abduction of a limb brings the medial malleolus nearer to the corresponding anterior superior spine, whereas adduction of the limb carries the medial malleolus away from the anterior superior spine. Thus if measurements are made while the patient lies with one hip adducted and the other abducted (a common posture in cases of hip disease) inaccurate readings will be obtained: the length will be exaggerated on the adducted side and underestimated on the abducted side.

Fig. 17.1 First step in the clinical examination of the hip: determining the lie of the pelvis.

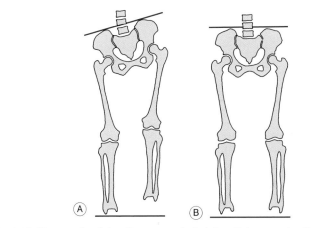

A   B

Fig. 17.2 'Apparent' or false discrepancy in limb length is caused entirely by incorrectable lateral tilting of the pelvis, which effectively abducts one hip and adducts the other hip Ⓐ. If the pelvis is square with the limbs there can be no 'apparent' discrepancy in limb length Ⓑ.

The rule is, therefore, that to obtain an accurate comparison of their true length by surface measurement the two limbs must be placed in comparable positions relative to the pelvis. Thus if one limb is adducted and cannot be brought out to the neutral position, the other limb must be adducted through a corresponding angle by crossing it over the first limb before the measurements are taken (Fig. 17.3B). Similarly, if one hip is in fixed abduction the other must be abducted through the same angle before the measurements of true length are made.

Fixing the tape measure at the anterior superior spine. A flat metal end (as found on the ordinary tailor's measure) is essential. The metal end is placed immediately *distal* to the anterior superior spine and is pushed up against it. The thumb is then pressed firmly backwards against the bone and the tape end together (Fig. 17.4). This gives rigid fixation of the tape measure against the bone and minimises any error in measurement.

Taking the reading at the medial malleolus. The tip of the index finger is placed immediately distal to the medial malleolus and pushed up against it. The thumb nail is brought down against the tip of the index finger so that the tape measure is pinched between them (Fig. 17.5). The point of measurement is indicated by the thumb nail.

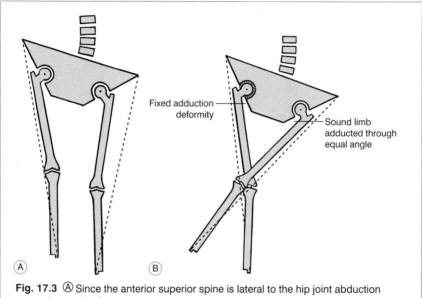

Fig. 17.3 Ⓐ Since the anterior superior spine is lateral to the hip joint abduction approximates the foot to it and adduction carries the foot away from it. For this reason measurements of true length, taken from the anterior superior spine, are inaccurate if the angle of abduction or adduction is not equal on the two sides. Ⓑ Correct way of measuring the true length when there is a fixed adduction deformity of one hip. The other hip must be adducted through an equal angle. (Position of tape measure shown by interrupted lines.)

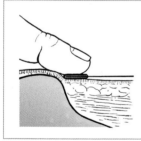

Fig. 17.4 Fixing the tape measure at the anterior superior spine.

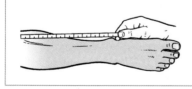

Fig. 17.5 Taking the measurement at the medial malleolus.

Determining the site of true shortening. If measurements reveal real shortening of a limb it is necessary to determine whether the shortening is above the trochanteric level (suggesting an affection in or near the hip), or below the trochanteric level (suggesting a disorder of the limb bones).

Shortening above the greater trochanter. Tests for shortening above the trochanteric level are: the measurement of Bryant's triangle, Nelaton's line, or Schoemaker's line.

In modern practice these tests are seldom used, since the information they provide can be supplied from simpler clinical observations or more accurately from radiographic measurements. They all depend on comparing the relative distance between the tip of the greater trochanters and the iliac crests. This can be quickly achieved with the patient supine, by using both hands with the thumbs placed on the greater trochanters and the tips of the index fingers on the anterior superior iliac spines. Any discrepancy between the two sides should then become apparent.

Shortening distal to the trochanter. True shortening is sometimes caused by an abnormality below the trochanteric level, such as a congenital defect of development, impaired epiphysial growth, or a previous fracture with overlapping of the fragments. To investigate this possibility individual measurements should be made of the femur (tip of greater trochanter to line of knee joint) and of the tibia (line of knee joint to medial malleolus) on each side and by flexing the knees to 90° and observing whether the shortening lies above the knee or below it (Gallenzi test).

Measurement of 'apparent' discrepancy in limb length. 'Apparent' or false discrepancy in limb length is due entirely to incorrectable sideways tilting of the pelvis (Fig. 17.2A). The usual cause is a fixed adduction deformity at one hip, giving an appearance of shortening on that side, or a fixed abduction deformity, giving an appearance of lengthening. Exceptionally, fixed pelvic obliquity is caused by severe lumbar scoliosis.

To measure apparent discrepancy the limbs must be placed parallel to one another and in line with the trunk. Measurement is made from any fixed point in the midline of the trunk (for example, the xiphisternum) to each medial malleolus (Fig. 17.6).

If there is a discrepancy of true length it must be allowed for when 'apparent' discrepancy is determined. As already noted above, there is no need to measure for apparent discrepancy if the pelvis lies square with the limbs, as determined from the position of the two iliac crests.

Examination for fixed deformity

Contracture of the joint capsule or of muscles may cause fixed deformity at the hip, preventing its being placed in a neutral position. Fixed flexion, fixed adduction, and fixed lateral rotation are common in some forms of arthritis.

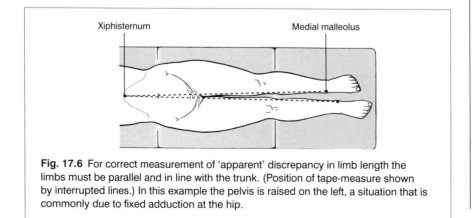

Fig. 17.6 For correct measurement of 'apparent' discrepancy in limb length the limbs must be parallel and in line with the trunk. (Position of tape-measure shown by interrupted lines.) In this example the pelvis is raised on the left, a situation that is commonly due to fixed adduction at the hip.

Xiphisternum   Medial malleolus

Fixed adduction deformity. This is detected by judging the relationship between pelvis and limbs. It will already have been noted at an earlier stage of the examination. If fixed adduction is present the transverse axis of the pelvis (as indicated by a line joining the two anterior superior spines) cannot be set at right angles to the affected limb, but lies at an acute angle with it.

Fixed abduction deformity. The angle between the transverse axis of the pelvis and the limb is greater than 90°.

Fixed flexion deformity. This is determined by a manoeuvre known as Thomas's test.

Principle of Thomas's test. If there is a fixed flexion deformity at the hip the patient compensates for it, when lying on the back, by arching the spine and pelvis into exaggerated lordosis, as shown in Fig. 17.7A. This allows the affected limb to lie flat on the couch. To measure the angle of fixed flexion deformity it is necessary to correct the lumbo-pelvic lordosis. This is done by flexing the pelvis (and with it the lumbar spine) by means of the fully flexed sound limb (Fig. 17.7B).

Technique of the manoeuvre. One hand is placed behind the lumbar spine (between it and the couch) to assess the degree of lumbar lordosis. If there is no lordosis when the affected limb lies flat on the couch there can be no fixed flexion deformity and there is no need to proceed with the test. If there is excessive lordosis, as indicated by arching of the back (Fig. 17.7A), it is corrected in the following way: The *sound* hip is flexed to the limit of its range. The limb is then pushed further into flexion, thereby rotating the pelvis on a horizontal transverse axis until the arching of the spine is obliterated. During this manoeuvre the thigh of the disordered limb, if in fixed flexion, is automatically raised from the couch as the lumbar lordosis is reduced (Fig. 17.7B). The angle through which the thigh is raised from the couch is the angle of fixed flexion deformity.

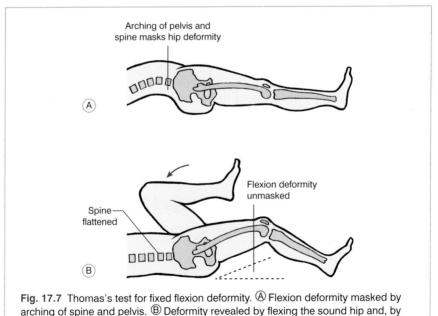

Fig. 17.7 Thomas's test for fixed flexion deformity. Ⓐ Flexion deformity masked by arching of spine and pelvis. Ⓑ Deformity revealed by flexing the sound hip and, by continuing the flexion force, correcting the arching of spine and pelvis.

Fixed rotation deformity. The most reliable index of the rotational position of the thigh is the patella, which normally points forwards when the hip is in the neutral position. If there is fixed lateral rotation or fixed medial rotation the limb cannot be rotated to the neutral position, with the patella directed forwards. The angle by which it falls short of the neutral when rotated as far as possible is the angle of fixed rotation deformity.

Movements

The accurate determination of hip movements demands much care, because restriction of hip movement is easily masked by movement of the pelvis. It is therefore essential to place one hand upon the pelvis to detect any movement there, while the other guides and supports the limb.

Flexion. The range of hip flexion is best demonstrated by flexing the hip and knee together; not by lifting the leg with the knee straight. Movement of the pelvis is best detected by grasping the crest of the ilium (Fig. 17.8). Only in this way is it possible to distinguish between true hip movement and the false flexion imparted by rotation of the pelvis. The normal range of true hip flexion is about 130°, but it varies according to the build of the patient.

Abduction. The limb to be tested is supported by one hand while the other hand bridges the pelvis from anterior superior spine to anterior superior spine (Fig. 17.9). In this way true abduction at the hip can be differentiated from the false abduction that is imparted by tilting of the pelvis. The normal range of true abduction at the hip is 30° to 35° (more in children).

Abduction in flexion. This is often the first movement to suffer restriction in arthritis of the hip. The patient flexes his hips and knees by drawing the heels towards the buttocks. He then allows the knees to fall away from one another towards the couch (see Fig. 17.11B). The normal range is about 70° (90° in young children).

Adduction. The limb to be examined is crossed over the other limb. Again care must be taken to differentiate between true adduction and the false movement imparted by tilting of the pelvis. The normal range of adduction is about 25–30°.

Lateral rotation and medial rotation. Judge the range by an imaginary pointer thrust axially into the patella, not by the position of the foot. The normal range both of medial and of lateral rotation is about 40°.

Extension. Contrary to what has often been written, the range of extension at the hip is nil. Extension of the hip joint beyond the neutral position is prevented by the strong anterior capsule and reinforcing Y-shaped ligament. Seeming backward movement of the thigh is in fact contributed entirely by rotation of the pelvis and extension of the spine, not by extension at the hip joint proper.

Examination for abnormal mobility

In cases of marked instability of the hip longitudinal movement or 'telescoping' can sometimes be demonstrated – especially in children with developmental (congenital) dislocation of the hip. To carry out the test the limb is grasped firmly in one hand and alternately pushed and pulled in its long axis, the trunk being steadied by the examiner's other hand upon the iliac crest.

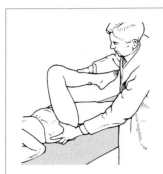

Fig. 17.8 Testing hip flexion. The right hand supports the limb while the left hand grips the ilium to detect incipient rotation of the pelvis. Hip and knee are flexed together.

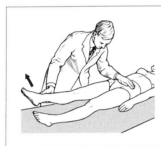

Fig. 17.9 Testing abduction of the hip. The right hand supports the limb while the left, bridging the two anterior superior spines, is ready to detect tilting of the pelvis. Adduction is tested in the same way.

In infants it is important to examine for dislocation by the click tests of Ortolani and Barlow. These are described on page 344.

Examination for postural stability: the Trendelenburg test

The Trendelenburg manoeuvre is a test of the stability of the hip, and particularly of the ability of the hip abductors (gluteus medius and gluteus minimus) to stabilise the pelvis upon the femur when the subject is standing upon the one leg.

Principle of the test. Normally, when one leg is raised from the ground the pelvis tilts upwards on that side, through the action of the hip abductors of the standing limb (Fig. 17.10A). (This automatic mechanism allows the lifted leg to clear the ground in walking.) If the abductors are inefficient they are unable to sustain the pelvis against the body weight and it tilts downwards instead of rising up on the side of the lifted leg (Fig. 17.10B).

Technique. Stand behind the patient. Instruct him first to stand upon the sound limb and to raise the other from the ground. Having thus got the idea of what he is required to do, he should now stand on the affected leg and lift the sound leg from the ground. By inspection, or by palpation with a hand upon the iliac crest, observe whether the pelvis rises or falls on the lifted side. Remember that the limb upon which the patient stands is the one under test. If the pelvis rises on the opposite side (normal) the test is negative (Fig. 17.10A). If it falls, the test is positive (Fig. 17.10B); in other words the abductor muscles are incapable of stabilising the pelvis upon the femur.

Causes of positive Trendelenburg test. There are three fundamental causes:

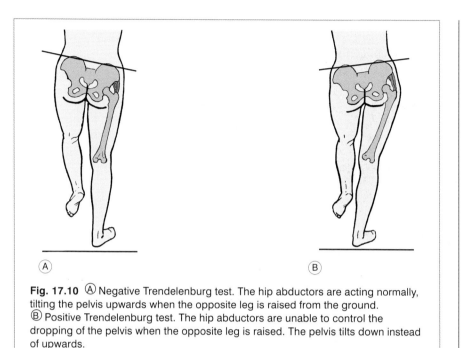

Fig. 17.10 Ⓐ Negative Trendelenburg test. The hip abductors are acting normally, tilting the pelvis upwards when the opposite leg is raised from the ground. Ⓑ Positive Trendelenburg test. The hip abductors are unable to control the dropping of the pelvis when the opposite leg is raised. The pelvis tilts down instead of upwards.

1. paralysis of the abductor muscles (example – poliomyelitis)
2. marked approximation of the insertion of the abductor muscles to their origin by upward displacement of the greater trochanter, so that the muscles are slack (examples – severe coxa vara; developmental dislocation of the hip)
3. absence of a stable fulcrum about which the abductor muscles can act (example – ununited fracture of the femoral neck).

Sometimes two of these factors may operate together: for instance, in a case of upward dislocation of the hip there may be an unstable fulcrum as well as approximation of the origin of the abductor muscles to their insertion.

Gait

Watch how the patient stands and observe his gait on walking. Note that a patient with an unstable or painful hip prefers to use a stick in the *opposite* hand, and tends to shorten the period of weight-bearing on the affected limb ('antalgic gait'). Characteristic gait patterns that are recognised include:

1. antalgic gait (weight-bearing minimised to reduce pain)
2. short-leg gait
3. Trendelenburg gait (patient leans towards the opposite side to lift the sound leg clear of the ground).

The patient's ability to negotiate stairs must also be tested. A disability of the hip often precludes the normal rhythm of ascent and descent: on ascending, the foot of the sound leg is advanced first, and that of the affected side is then brought up to it. On descent, the affected leg is put down first and the sound leg is brought down to it.

Extrinsic causes of pain in the hip region

If examination of the hip itself fails to reveal abnormalities sufficient to account for the patient's symptoms, possible causes outside the hip must be investigated. Attention should be directed particularly to the spine and sacro-iliac joints (including a neurological survey of the lower limbs), to the abdomen and pelvis (including rectal or bimanual examination if necessary), and to the vascular system (state of the peripheral pulses).

Imaging

Radiographic examination. *Plain radiographs* should include an antero-posterior projection showing the whole pelvis with both hips, and lateral films of each hip separately. It is recommended that the lateral films be obtained by slightly abducting the affected hip and directing the X-ray beam horizontally beneath the opposite flexed thigh. In special cases there is a place for *arthrography* (that is, radiography after the injection of radio-opaque fluid into the joint). When there is a possibility that the symptoms may be referred from the back radiographs of the spine and sacro-iliac joints must be obtained.

Radioisotope bone scanning. This is of value especially in the diagnosis of inflammatory lesions in or about the hip. It may also be helpful in the early detection of metastatic neoplastic deposits in the pelvis or upper end of the femur.

Computerised tomography (CT scanning) provides clear cross-sectional images of the pelvis or thigh and is useful in special circumstances. For instance, it can show accurately the orientation (degree of anteversion) of the acetabulum or of the neck of the femur. Or it may be used to outline bony or soft-tissue tumours in or about the pelvis or hip (see Fig. 2.3, p. 15).

Magnetic resonance imaging (MRI) is of particular value in showing the extent of soft-tissue changes – for instance in the case of an invasive tumour. It may also allow early detection of bone necrosis in the femoral head.

Ultrasound is now used increasingly in babies and young infants for the detection of developmental dysplasia before ossification of the femoral head allows radiological assessment.

Arthroscopy. Arthroscopic inspection of the interior of the hip is a useful supplementary method of investigation in adults, and it is now used increasingly in diagnosis and treatment.

DEVELOPMENTAL DYSPLASIA OF THE HIP

The term *developmental dysplasia* of the hip includes congenital dislocation of the hip, nearly always diagnosed either within a few days of birth or within the first two years of life; and dysplasia of the hip in adults, characterised by shallow configuration of the acetabulum, defective congruity between the femoral head and the socket, and a predisposition to osteoarthritis in middle or later life. Despite a trend towards re-naming congenital dislocation of the hip as developmental dysplasia of the hip, the title 'congenital dislocation' of the hip is so well established that it seems unnecessary to discard it. That title is therefore retained here for dislocation diagnosed in infancy.

CONGENITAL DISLOCATION OF THE HIP

This is a spontaneous dislocation of the hip occurring either before or during birth or shortly afterwards. In Western races it is one of the commonest of the congenital skeletal deformities affecting 1 in 1000 neonates: it is also of special importance because neglect or inefficient treatment incurs the penalty to the patient of lifelong crippling.

Cause. Much remains to be learnt, but it now seems to be clear that a number of factors are concerned in the causation – some genetic and some environmental. One such abnormality acting alone may not always be sufficient in itself to bring about dislocation, and it may well be that a combination of factors is often at work.

1. *Genetically determined joint laxity.* Generalised ligamentous laxity is found in a proportion of the patients, and may also be present in a parent or relatives. It leads to lack of stability at the hip, so that dislocation may easily occur in certain positions of the joint.
2. *Hormonal joint laxity.* It is possible that in females a ligament-relaxing hormone ('relaxin') may be secreted by the fetal uterus in response to oestrone and progesterone reaching the foetal circulation. This may cause instability in the same way as does genetically determined joint laxity. It is possible, also, that laxity of the hip ligaments from this cause might help to explain the greater incidence of dislocation in girls (the relaxing agent is not produced in boys). This factor requires further investigation.
3. *Genetically determined dysplasia of the hip.* There is little doubt that defective development of the acetabulum, and probably also of the femoral head, can be inherited as a distinct entity. The defect appears always to be bilateral, and is probably as common in boys as in girls. It predisposes to dislocation, which indeed may often occur before birth. If dislocation does not occur, the defect may show itself in adult life in the form of unduly shallow acetabula, with a tendency to subluxation and later osteoarthritis (acetabular dysplasia: see p. 352).
4. *Breech malposition.* The incidence of hip dislocation is slightly greater when the infant is delivered by the breech than with normal delivery. It is possible that the act of extending the hips during delivery may precipitate dislocation when there is already a predisposition to it from ligamentous laxity or acetabular dysplasia.
5. *Post-natal positioning.* The higher incidence of DDH in Inuit Eskimos who strapped their babies to a board with their hips adducted, compared to African tribes who carry their children on their backs with their hips abducted, indicates that the position that the hip is held in post-natally can have a major effect on acetabular development.

The relative importance of these various factors is not fully understood. Present evidence suggests, however, that there may be two distinct types of congenital dislocation of the hip. The first type is caused predominantly by ligamentous laxity – whether genetically determined or hormonal – in which dislocation occurs as it were accidentally when some precipitating movement such as extension of the hips during delivery is the adjuvant cause, the dislocation in this type often being unilateral and readily correctable. The second type is due predominantly to genetically determined dysplasia of the acetabulum, which is always bilateral and often much more difficult to treat.

Pathology. *The femoral head*: In a case of persistent dislocation the bony nucleus appears late and its development is retarded. The femoral head is dislocated upwards and laterally from the acetabulum. *The femoral neck*: In most cases the neck is anteverted (directed forwards) beyond the normal angle for infants of 25°. *The acetabulum*: The ossific centre for the roof of the acetabulum, like that for the femoral head, is late in developing. The bone slopes upwards at a steep angle instead of forming a nearly horizontal roof for the acetabulum. The cartilaginous part of the roof is often well formed at first, but if the dislocation is allowed to persist development does not proceed normally, and the socket assumes a shallow contour with steeply sloping roof. *The fibro-cartilaginous labrum*: The peripheral labrum which normally increases the depth of the developing acetabular socket is often folded into the cavity of the acetabulum to become a 'limbus' and may impede complete reduction of the dislocation *The capsule*: This is gradually elongated as the femoral head is displaced upwards.

Clinical features. Girls are affected six times as often as boys. In one-third of all cases both hips are affected. Unless it is specially looked for in infancy – as it always should be – abnormality may not be noticed until the child begins to walk. Walking is often delayed, and there is a limp or a waddling gait.

On examination at that time, the main features in unilateral cases are asymmetry (notably of the buttock folds), shortening of the affected limb (Fig. 17.11A), and restricted abduction in flexion. In bilateral cases the striking features are widening of the perineum and marked lumbar lordosis. The range of joint movements is full except for abduction in flexion, which is characteristically slightly restricted (Fig. 17.11B). In most cases the affected limb is abnormally mobile in its long axis (telescopic movement).

Imaging. *Plain radiographs* show three important features (Fig. 17.12):

1. The ossific centre for the head of the femur is late in appearing and its development is retarded
2. the bony acetabular roof has a pronounced upward slope
3. the femoral head (as judged from the position of the ossific centre) is displaced upwards and laterally from its normal position in the centre of the acetabulum.

These changes are not always shown conclusively before the age of 4 months.

Arthrography (radiography after injection of opaque fluid into the joint) is useful in showing the outline of the cartilaginous elements of the joint.

Ultrasound scanning allows the position of the femoral head and acetabular socket to be determined in the new-born, when radiographic examination tends to be inconclusive.

Diagnosis. *In the new-born.* Nearly always – though there are a few exceptions – dislocation or instability of the hip may be detected in the first few days of life by the diagnostic screening tests of Barlow or Ortolani (Fig. 17.13). In both tests the surgeon faces the child's perineum and grasps the upper part of each thigh between fingers behind and thumb in front, the child's knees being fully flexed and the hips flexed to a right angle (Fig. 17.14).

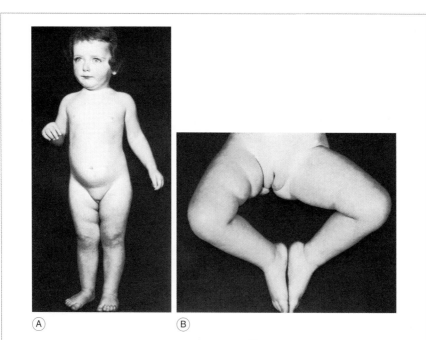

(A)   (B)

Fig. 17.11 Congenital dislocation of the right hip. (A) The right lower limb was slightly shorter than the left, as suggested here by the typical extra skin folds in the thigh. (B) shows the reduced range of abduction of the affected hip – another typical and important diagnostic feature.

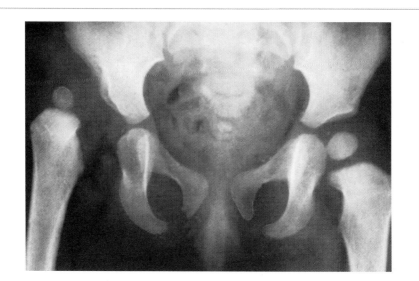

Fig. 17.12 Congenital dislocation of the right hip in a child of 2. The three points to note are the retarded development of the capital epiphysis, the steeply sloping acetabular roof, and the lateral and upward displacement of the upper end of the femur.

While each thigh in turn is steadily abducted towards the couch the middle finger applies forward pressure behind the greater trochanter (Ortolani), and alternately the thumb, placed anteriorly, applies backward pressure while the thighs are adducted (Barlow). One of two abnormal states may be detected:

1. a dislocated femoral head snaps back into the acetabulum with a palpable and audible jerk or jolt (Ortolani)
2. backward pressure with the thumb dislocates a joint that is unstable (Barlow).

The manoeuvre must be combined with assessment of the range of abduction in flexion at each hip (Fig. 17.11B). If abduction is restricted it may indicate persistent or irreducible dislocation, and in such a case the absence of the characteristic jerk or jolt may mislead the observer into believing that all is well. In such a case, if unilateral, shortening may be observed when the knees are placed together, with the hips flexed.

In newborn infants radiography may be inconclusive because the high proportion of radiolucent cartilage in the femoral head and acetabulum makes interpretation difficult. It becomes diagnostic after the age of about 4 months. As the necessary skill in the technique is more widely acquired, ultrasound scanning has become increasingly important in diagnosis in early infancy.

In older children. Delay in beginning to walk or abnormality of gait in early childhood should always arouse suspicion. The most important clinical sign in children 1 or 2 years old is a restricted range of abduction when the hip is flexed (Fig. 17.11B). If for any reason suspicion arises that all is not well with the hips, radiographic examination must be insisted upon. In these older children radiography is always conclusive.

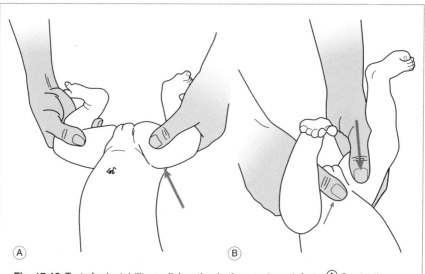

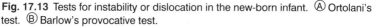

Fig. 17.13 Tests for instability or dislocation in the new-born infant. Ⓐ Ortolani's test. Ⓑ Barlow's provocative test.

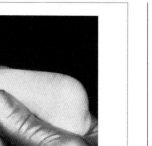

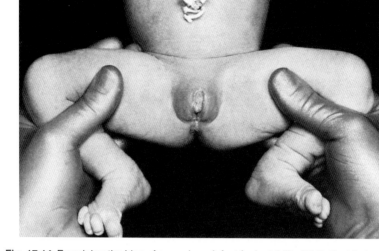

Fig. 17.14 Examining the hips of a new-born infant for instability. While the hip is abducted through the full range forward pressure is applied by the middle finger behind the greater trochanter. For details, see text.

Course and prognosis. The earlier the dislocation is reduced the better the prognosis. Even under the best conditions only about half or two-thirds of the patients treated after the first year of life can be expected to remain permanently free from trouble. Gradual redislocation or subluxation is all too frequent, and pain from secondary degenerative changes often develops in middle adult life.

It is therefore important that, through careful examination of every newborn infant, congenital dislocation be detected within the first week of life, when simple treatment can nearly always assure normal development of the hip.

Treatment

This varies according to the age of the patient when advice is sought. Four groups will be discussed:

1. neonatal cases (instability or dislocation)
2. age 6 months–6 years
3. age 7–10 years
4. adolescents and adults.

Neonatal cases (within 6 months of birth). These are the cases in which instability or dislocation is found on neonatal screening, either by the Ortolani–Barlow test or by ultrasound examination. In most of these cases the hip becomes stable spontaneously within 3 weeks. Accordingly, there is much to be said for delaying a decision on definitive treatment until the time of reassessment three weeks after birth, when it will be found that a large proportion of the infants do not need treatment. In the interval between the first examination and the reassessment at 3 weeks the limbs are left free, though it seems sensible to advise the use of bulky double nappies to encourage abduction of the hips.

If at 3 weeks the hip is found to be stable, treatment is unnecessary, and the parents may be tentatively reassured. Nevertheless it is important that the child should be reviewed at the age of 5 or 6 months, when radiography gives conclusive findings, and again at 1 year of age.

If on the other hand the hip is still unstable at 3 weeks, splinting in the reduced position in moderate (not extreme) abduction for 3 months is recommended. Splintage may be by plaster of Paris or more frequently using the Pavlic harness (Fig. 17.15), which is more flexible than the previously used Denis-Browne or Van Rosen splints. The dynamic Pavlic splint has an adjustable harness that can maintain the hips in flexion while limiting adduction. Splintage should be continued for a minimum of 6 weeks or for as long as instability persists, though this carries an increasing risk of the development of avascular necrosis of the femoral head.

Age 6 months–6 years. This still forms a substantial group, but with more regular diagnosis in early infancy the proportion of patients treated as late as this should progressively decrease. There are three essential principles of treatment:

1. to secure concentric reduction
2. to provide conditions favourable to continued stability and normal development
3. to observe the hips regularly in order to detect any failure of normal development of the acetabulum and to apply appropriate treatment when necessary.

Reduction of dislocation. It is desirable whenever possible to obtain reduction by non-operative means, operation being used only when conservative methods fail. In practice, it is found that closed reduction is often possible in

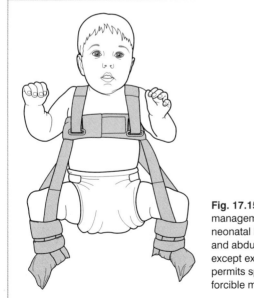

Fig. 17.15 Pavlik harness used for the management of the unstable hip in the neonatal baby. It holds both hips in flexion and abduction allowing all movements except extension and is worn full-time. It permits spontaneous reduction without forcible manipulation.

babies up to 18 months of age, but that thereafter the proportion that require operation progressively increases, so that operative reduction becomes almost routine after the age of 3 years.

Closed reduction. The standard practice is to apply weight traction to the limbs with the child either on a frame or in gallows (Bryant's) suspension, and while traction is maintained, gradually to abduct the hips, a little more each day, until 80° of abduction is reached after 3–4 weeks. Cross traction by slings round the upper thighs may then be applied. In many cases reduction is obtained by this method alone. If, however, the hip is not reduced at 4 weeks an attempt is made to complete the reduction by gentle manipulation under anaesthesia. It is essential that reduction be complete, so that the femoral head fits the socket concentrically. If necessary, arthrography, CT scanning, or magnetic resonance imaging may be employed to establish whether reduction is complete or whether interposed soft tissue is blocking it.

If full reduction is secured, the limbs are immobilised for an initial period in plaster of Paris, usually in a position of moderate medial rotation and moderate abduction (Fig. 17.16): extreme positions must not be used. This has superseded the 'frog' position of right-angled flexion and abduction, formerly widely used, which has been found to prejudice the blood supply of the capital epiphysis of the femur, with risk of necrotic changes resembling those of Perthes' disease.

Operative reduction. If reduction is not obtained by traction and abduction, with or without manipulation, or when a soft-tissue obstruction to reduction has been demonstrated by arthrography, operation should be undertaken without delay. At operation, it will usually be found that full engagement of the femoral head in the acetabulum is prevented by inturning of the acetabular labrum (limbus), or occasionally by a voluminous ligament of the femoral head or a tight psoas tendon. Any such obstruction is removed or released to allow the femoral head to be fully engaged. While the femoral head is exposed to view, note should be made of the angle of anteversion of the femoral neck. This

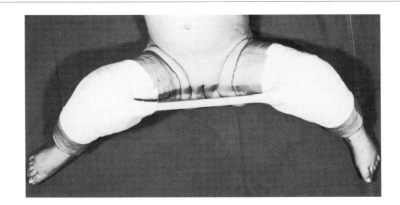

Fig. 17.16 A method of holding the hips in moderate abduction and medial rotation. Extreme positions of abduction or rotation are nowadays avoided because of the risk of damaging the blood supply to the capital epiphysis of the femur.

will often be found to be increased beyond the normal angle of 25°. At the completion of the operation the limbs are immobilised in plaster in the same way as after closed reduction.

Maintenance of stability. A major hazard to continued stability in a child whose hip dislocation has been concentrically reduced comes from excessive anteversion of the femoral neck, which is a common if not a constant feature in children beyond 18 months of age. Excessive anteversion has its main adverse effect when the child assumes the erect posture for walking: with the hip extended excessive anteversion brings the femoral head anteriorly, and radiographs may show it to lie eccentrically in the acetabulum. If uncorrected, this initial subluxation may progress eventually to redislocation.

The diagnosis of excessive anteversion is simple if operative reduction has been undertaken, for with the hip exposed the angle of anteversion can be measured under direct vision. When reduction has been by closed methods, however, diagnosis presents some difficulty – indeed to some extent it may be a matter of guesswork. Methods of radiographic measurement are available but they are not always easy to apply successfully in a small child and have been largely superseded. A more empirical method is often used: antero-posterior radiographs are taken with the hip first in the neutral position and then medially rotated. A more central position of the capital epiphysis in the acetabulum when the hip is medially rotated suggests that excessive anteversion is prejudicing stability. Definitive information on the angle of anteversion can best be gained from computerised tomography (CT scanning) or magnetic resonance imaging.

There are two methods of correcting excessive anteversion:

1. non-operative
2. operative (rotation osteotomy).

Non-operative management of anteversion. Long-continued harnessing of the hips in flexion and moderate abduction, a limited amount of walking being allowed, has been found to favour spontaneous correction of anteversion. Correction may, however, take a year or more.

Rotation osteotomy. Excessive anteversion is easily corrected by rotating the femur through an osteotomy at its upper end. The femur is divided a little below the trochanteric level to allow the shaft fragment to be rotated laterally in relation to the upper end of the femur. The fragments are then fixed with a plate and screws. After operation immobilisation in plaster is maintained until union occurs – usually a matter of about 6 weeks. Thereafter all splintage is discarded.

Counteracting defective development of the acetabulum. In a proportion of cases – greater when treatment has been started late than when it has been begun in the first year of life – the acetabulum fails to develop normally from the stimulus of the femoral head within it, and remains unduly shallow. The femoral head is not well contained within it, being partly uncovered by the acetabular roof. If this deficiency is not corrected the femoral head may become slowly displaced upwards, so that the joint is subluxated, the head no longer articulating congruously with the socket. The treatment of such acetabular deficiency is operative, and it should be carried out as soon as it is observed that this adverse situation has arisen. Mention will be made of four of the several operations that are available for improving the acetabulum:

1. osteotomy of the innominate bone (Salter's pelvic osteotomy)
2. pericapsular osteotomy of the ilium (Pemberton's pelvic osteotomy)
3. shelf acetabuloplasty (Wainwright's shelf operation)
4. Chiari's displacement osteotomy of the ilium.

Osteotomy of the innominate bone (Salter). The iliac bone is divided completely just above the acetabulum, the cut emerging at the greater sciatic notch. The whole of the lower half of the bone, bearing the intact acetabulum, is then sprung outwards and forwards, hinging at the symphysis pubis (Fig. 17.17A). The effect is that the femoral head is more fully covered by the roof of the acetabulum, and stability of the hip is correspondingly increased. This operation is most suitable for young children in whom the acetabular socket and femoral head are congruent.

Pericapsular osteotomy of ilium (Pemberton). This operation has a similar aim of providing increased cover for the femoral head by the roof of the acetabulum. A curved osteotomy is made part-way across the thickness of the pelvic wall from the outer aspect of the ilium a few millimetres proximal to the attachment of the capsule to the upper margin of the acetabulum. The osteotomy extends to the triradiate cartilage, which forms a flexible hinge about which the roof of the acetabulum is deflected downwards over the femoral head. The triangular osteotomy gap is held open by bone obtained

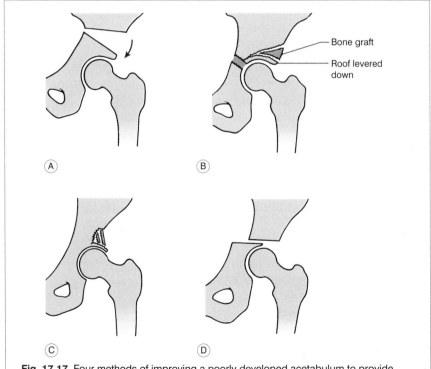

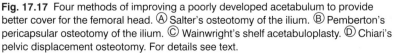

Fig. 17.17 Four methods of improving a poorly developed acetabulum to provide better cover for the femoral head. Ⓐ Salter's osteotomy of the ilium. Ⓑ Pemberton's pericapsular osteotomy of the ilium. Ⓒ Wainwright's shelf acetabuloplasty. Ⓓ Chiari's pelvic displacement osteotomy. For details see text.

locally from the ilium (Fig. 17.17B). This operation is most suitable for young children in whom the acetabular socket is relatively shallow compared to the shape of the femoral head.

Cortical turn-down acetabuloplasty (Wainwright). This so-called shelf operation also has the aim of increasing the surface area of the acetabular roof. A sizeable area of the outer table of the ilium is turned down as a flap into contact with the upper and outer aspect of the capsule of the hip joint (Fig. 17.17C). The flap, thus reflected, is held in place by strut grafts. This operation is suitable mainly for adolescents and young adults.

Chiari's pelvic displacement osteotomy. The iliac bone is divided almost transversely immediately above the acetabulum, and the lower fragment (bearing the acetabulum) is displaced medially (Fig. 17.17D). The cut surface of the upper fragment thus forms an extension of the acetabular roof, with capsule and newly formed fibrous tissue intervening. The operation is suitable mainly for adolescents and young adults.

Age 7–10 years. In these older children with untreated dislocations, the first point to be decided is whether or not treatment should be undertaken at all. In some of these children with well-developed false acetabula symmetrically placed on both sides, functional disability is slight, and appearance and gait may be acceptable. Accordingly it may often be wise to advise against attempted reduction of the dislocation. In contrast, there are others with high-lying femoral heads and poorly developed false sockets who can benefit greatly from operative reduction up to the age of 10 years or sometimes even later. This applies particularly when the dislocation is unilateral. Treatment in such cases entails open reduction of the dislocation, to accomplish which the femur may have to be shortened in the subtrochanteric region. Any excessive anteversion of the femoral neck is corrected at the same time by rotation at the site of bone resection. Either at the same time, or preferably later, one of the operations mentioned above for deepening the acetabulum (the Wainwright shelf operation or the Chiari operation) may be carried out. An obvious advantage of reducing the dislocation in these older children is that conditions are made suitable for replacement arthroplasty should the need for it arise in later life, whereas this presents substantial difficulties if a high dislocation remains unreduced.

Age 11 years onwards. After the age of 10 years, and often in younger children, treatment of freshly diagnosed congenital dislocation of the hip is not advised unless secondary degenerative changes lead to severe pain. If increasing pain justifies operative treatment, the choice of method depends largely upon whether the dislocation affects one or both hips. If only one hip is affected total replacement arthroplasty may sometimes be practicable once adult life is reached; but if not, consideration should be given to the advisability of arthrodesis, which can offer a satisfactory solution. If both hips are affected (Fig. 17.18), if it is practicable, replacement arthroplasty is usually to be preferred.

DYSPLASIA OF THE HIP IN ADULTS

The gene that is responsible for many cases of congenital dislocation of the hip may also cause dysplasia, or failure of normal development of the joint, that may not become apparent in childhood.

Hip dysplasia in adults may become symptomatic at any time from early adult life up till middle age, or later. The common presenting symptom is

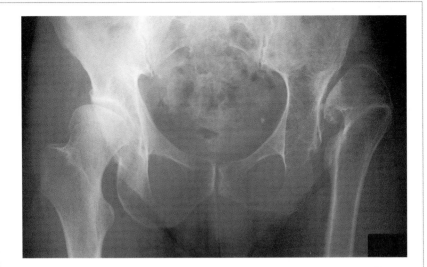

Fig. 17.18 Bilateral untreated developmental hip dysplasia in an adult. The left hip is completely dislocated, with failure of normal acetabular development, and the right hip shows dysplastic changes.

pain, usually in one hip, but often occurring later, or in lesser degree, in the opposite hip as well. Examination shows good mobility of the hip, but often with complaint of pain at the extremes of the range, especially of flexion and abduction. On radiological examination the affected acetabulum is seen to be shallow, often with a steeply sloping roof (Fig. 17.19). The femoral head does not fit concentrically in the acetabulum: it may be shown to be displaced slightly upwards and outwards, so that Shenton's line – the normally smooth arch formed by the medial/inferior border of the femoral neck prolonged into the inferior border of the pubic ramus – is broken.

Dysplasia of the hip is important not only because it may cause pain and instability in its own right, but because it predisposes to the later development of degenerative arthritis, usually in middle life, with slowly increasing pain and difficulty in walking.

Treatment. Operative treatment is often appropriate, but it should be deferred until the disability becomes severe enough to demand it. The choice of operation is usually between osteotomy of the upper end of the femur to displace the femoral head and neck into more varus (Fig. 17.20), and pelvic osteotomy above the acetabulum to increase the coverage of the femoral head and improve stability of the hip (Fig. 17.17D). In patients with established arthritic changes total replacement arthroplasty of the hip may have to be recommended, even in patients who are relatively young.

TRANSIENT SYNOVITIS OF THE HIP (Traumatic synovitis; transient arthritis; observation hip; irritable hip)

The so-called transient arthritis or synovitis of childhood is a short-lived affection of the hip of uncertain pathology, characterised clinically by pain, limp, and limitation of hip movements.

The hip region

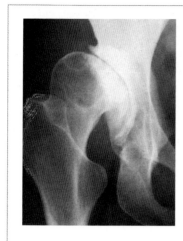

Fig. 17.19 Congenital dysplasia of the hip in a woman aged 42. Note that the acetabulum is very shallow. The femoral head is ill-formed and higher than normal. The cartilage space is greatly narrowed, indicating degenerative arthritis.

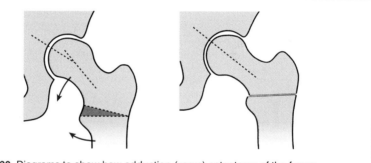

Fig. 17.20 Diagrams to show how adduction (varus) osteotomy of the femur improves the containment of the femoral head in the acetabulum. *Left* – Site of bone wedge to be removed. *Right* – Gap closed after removal of wedge, so that femoral neck is turned down into varus. The osteotomy has the effect that the upper part (head and neck) of the femur is abducted in the socket, while the femoral shaft remains in the neutral position.

Cause. This is unknown. Injury is possibly a factor but the evidence in support of it is slender.

Pathology. This is unknown. Possibly there is a mild inflammation of the synovial membrane, initiated by minor injury; or perhaps a viral infection.

Clinical features. The condition is virtually confined to children under 10, especially boys. The child complains of pain in the groin and thigh and he is noticed to limp, sparing the affected leg. *On examination* the only physical sign is limitation of hip movements. *Radiographs* do not show any alteration from the normal.

Diagnosis. Transient arthritis of the hip is important only because it resembles clinically the earliest stages of pyogenic arthritis, tuberculous arthritis or of Perthes' disease, before the characteristic radiographic features of those conditions have become apparent. Transient arthritis should be diagnosed only after the hip has recovered – never while the symptoms and signs are present. While the symptoms and signs last, the case should be regarded as one of suspected infective arthritis or Perthes' disease and the child investigated fully to exclude these diagnoses. Ultrasound scanning may be indicated to identify any joint effusion which would require aspiration. Full recovery within a few weeks excludes more serious disease and justifies a retrospective diagnosis of transient synovitis.

Course. Full recovery, with return of a normal range of hip movements, invariably occurs within three to 6 weeks.

Treatment. Rest in bed until the pain has settled and movements have been restored is the only treatment required.

PYOGENIC ARTHRITIS OF THE HIP (General description of pyogenic arthritis, p. 96)

Pyogenic arthritis of the hip is uncommon. It occurs mostly in children, in whom it is often secondary to osteomyelitis of the upper end of the femur. Its features resemble those of pyogenic arthritis elsewhere; but in infants there are particular characteristics that require special description.

Pathology. Organisms (usually staphylococci or streptococci) may reach the joint directly through the blood stream, or the infection may spread from an adjacent focus of osteomyelitis of the femur. Rarely, a penetrating wound is responsible. In new-born babies the infection may enter through the umbilicus. There is an acute inflammatory reaction in the joint tissues, with an effusion of turbid fluid or pus. In favourable cases healing with restoration to normal can occur, but often the joint is permanently destroyed or damaged, and in older children and adults bony ankylosis may occur.

In infants bony ankylosis does not occur because the femoral head and the acetabulum are composed almost entirely of cartilage rather than of bone, but there may be total destruction of the developing femoral head, with secondary dislocation of the hip (pathological dislocation) (Tom Smith's disease[1]). The femur may remain short, from destruction of the upper femoral growth cartilage. Additional shortening will occur if the dislocation is allowed to persist and the femur to slide upwards on the ilium; so the discrepancy in length may be substantial by the time adolescence is reached.

Clinical features. The clinical features differ so much in infants and in older patients that separate descriptions are required.

Pyogenic arthritis of infants. The onset is within the first year of life. Often there has been a known septic lesion somewhere on the body (for example, umbilical sepsis), but it may have caused little anxiety. Then the child becomes unwell and pyrexial.

---

[1] Sir Thomas Smith (1833–1909) Surgeon at St.Thomas's and Great Ormond Street Children's Hospitals in London described acute arthritis of infants in 1874.

On examination it is not always apparent at first that the hip is the seat of the trouble. But careful examination will show thickening in the hip area, and movements of the joint are restricted, and disturb the child. Sometimes an abscess points at the skin surface in the buttock or thigh.

Imaging. In the early stages there is no alteration in the plain radiographs, but *ultrasound scanning* may show the hip joint to be distended with fluid (Fig. 7.13, p. 99). If the infection progresses to the stage of destroying the capital epiphysis of the femur, the ossific nucleus fails to appear as it should before the age of one year. In such a case subsequent radiographs may show gradual dislocation of the hip. This 'pathological' dislocation is distinguished from congenital dislocation by the facts that the acetabular roof is of normal shape and that the capital epiphysis is permanently absent (Fig. 17.21). *Radioisotope scanning* reveals increased uptake in the region of the hip.

Pyogenic arthritis in older children and adults. The onset is acute or subacute, with pain in the hip made worse by attempted weight-bearing, reluctance to walk, and severe limp. There is constitutional illness with pyrexia. *On examination* there may be some fullness about the hip region from swelling of the joint. All movements of the hip are markedly restricted, and painful if forced.

Imaging. There may be no change on plain radiographs in the early stages, but ultrasound will demonstrate the presence of an effusion (Fig. 7.13, p. 99). There may be evidence of osteomyelitis in the upper metaphysis of the femur. Later, if the infection persists, there is rarefaction of bone about the hip, and the cartilage space is narrowed, indicating destruction of articular cartilage. Finally, there may be bony ankylosis of the joint (Fig. 17.22).

Radioisotope bone scanning shows increased uptake in the region of the hip.

Investigations in both the infantile and childhood forms of suspected septic arthritis are similar. There is a polymorphonuclear leucocytosis and the erythrocyte sedimentation rate and C-reactive protein level are raised. Blood cultures are taken and if ultrasound shows a joint effusion, aspiration of the

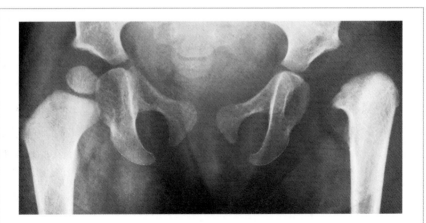

Fig. 17.21 Old pyogenic arthritis of left hip in an infant (Tom Smith's disease). The epiphysis of the head of the femur has been destroyed and the hip is dislocated. Note the almost normal appearance of the acetabular roof, which helps to distinguish this from a congenital dislocation. The normal hip is shown for comparison.

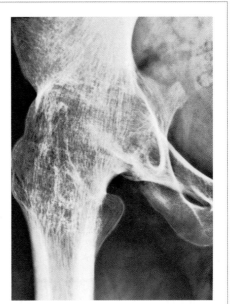

Fig. 17.22 Bony ankylosis of the hip caused by pyogenic arthritis. The infection spread to the hip from a focus of osteomyelitis in the upper metaphysis of the femur. This is a common outcome of pyogenic arthritis in older children and adults.

joint is urgent yielding pus or turbid fluid from which the causative organism and its antibiotic sensitivities may be identified.

Treatment. Treatment is by appropriate antibiotic therapy, initially intravenously with a broad-spectrum cephalosporin, which can be changed later depending upon the nature of the infecting organism. Arthrotomy to permit open drainage and saline irrigation of the joint is preferred to daily aspiration in preventing the formation of adhesions and residual infection. Rest for the joint and relief of muscle spasm are best ensured initially by weight traction through adhesive skin strapping applied to the leg. When the infection has been overcome active movements are encouraged.

Pathological dislocation complicating pyogenic arthritis of infants, with total destruction of the upper femoral epiphysis. Definitive treatment of this rare but crippling condition must await adolescence. In childhood the aim of treatment is to prevent progressive upward displacement of the femur and thereby to minimise shortening. Provided the infection has settled, operation should be undertaken to deepen the acetabulum, to place the upper end of the femur within it and, if necessary, to lever down a 'shelf' of ilium over it, on the lines of the Pemberton osteotomy illustrated in Figure 17.17B. In adolescence, when the bones are nearing full development, arthrodesis may be recommended if the hip is painful. If the hip has fused spontaneously (Fig. 17.22) the situation is best accepted, provided that fusion has occurred in a good functional position.

TUBERCULOUS ARTHRITIS OF THE HIP (General description of tuberculous arthritis, p. 98)

The hip is one of the joints most frequently affected by tuberculosis. In Western countries, however, its incidence has declined so sharply that it is now seldom seen, and it is mainly confined to poorer countries or to immigrants from such countries.

Clinical features. The patient is usually a child – often 2 to 5 years old – or a young adult, often with a history of contact with a person with active pulmonary tuberculosis. The symptoms are pain and limp. The general health is usually impaired. *On examination* a thickening is often palpable in the region of the hip. All movements of the hip are limited, often markedly, and attempts to force movement provoke pain and muscle spasm. The gluteal and thigh muscles are wasted. A 'cold' abscess is sometimes palpable in the upper thigh or buttock. A tuberculous lesion may be apparent elsewhere in the body.

Imaging. *Radiographic features*. At first the changes are slight, but later there are fuzziness of the joint margins and narrowing of the cartilage space, indicating erosion of the articular cartilage (Fig. 17.23).

MRI scanning can show signs of oedema in bone and soft tissues and will demonstrate the effusion and cold abscess. *Radioisotope bone scanning* shows increased uptake in the region of the hip.

Diagnosis. This is mainly from transient synovitis, Perthes' disease (osteochondritis), low-grade pyogenic arthritis, and rheumatoid arthritis. Important features supporting a diagnosis of tuberculosis are: the presence of a tuberculous lesion elsewhere; a positive Mantoux reaction in children; a 'cold' abscess; a high erythrocyte sedimentation rate; and the typical histological appearance on biopsy of the synovial membrane.

Course and prognosis. In a reasonable proportion of cases, especially in children, the infection is aborted by treatment and a sound joint is preserved, provided there has been no destruction of cartilage or bone when treatment is begun.

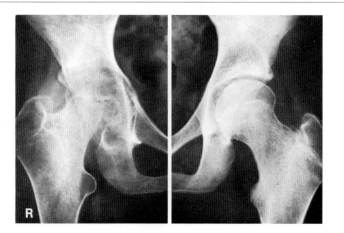

Fig. 17.23 Tuberculous arthritis of right hip in a more advanced stage. The cartilage has been destroyed and the articular surfaces of the acetabulum and femoral head have lost their sharp definition. The joint is permanently destroyed. The normal hip is shown for comparison.

Treatment. Essentially, treatment is the same as that for other tuberculous joints. The mainstay of treatment is a prolonged course of antibacterial agents, as described on page 102.

Local treatment is initially by rest for the hip, either in traction or in plaster. The subsequent treatment depends upon the progress made. If radiographs show no destruction of cartilage or bone, and if there is no evidence of deterioration full activity is gradually resumed.

On the other hand, if at the end of 3 or 6 months' treatment radiographs show marked destruction of cartilage or bone (Fig. 17.23), there is no possibility of preserving the joint intact. The choice then lies between total replacement arthroplasty and arthrodesis. Arthroplasty should only be undertaken when the disease is quiescent, and will require the reintroduction of antibacterial drugs to cover the period of operation. In children such operations should be deferred until adolescence.

RHEUMATOID ARTHRITIS OF THE HIP (General description of rheumatoid arthritis, p. 134)

The hip joints often escape in cases of rheumatoid arthritis; but when they are affected the consequent disability is severe. The main features of the disease are like those of rheumatoid arthritis in general, as described on page 134.

Clinical features. The changes may affect one or both hips, in common with several other joints. The main symptoms are pain and limitation of movement, aggravated by activity.

On examination swelling is not obvious because the joint is so deeply situated; for the same reason the temperature of the overlying skin is not increased as it is in rheumatoid affection of the more superficial joints. The range of all hip movements is impaired and movement is painful if forced. Fixed flexion deformity or adduction deformity may develop. The gluteal and thigh muscles are wasted.

Imaging. *Radiographic features*. In the earliest stages there are no radiographic changes. Later, there is diffuse bone rarefaction in the area of the joint. Later still, destruction of articular cartilage leads to narrowing of the cartilage space between femur and acetabulum, often with inward protrusion of the softened medial wall of the acetabulum (Fig. 17.24).

Investigations. The erythrocyte sedimentation rate is increased during the active stage. The latex fixation test and the Rose–Waaler test may be positive.

Course. The disease becomes inactive after months or years, but the hip is seldom restored to normal. In long-established cases degenerative changes are superimposed upon the original inflammatory condition, giving rise to secondary osteoarthritis (Fig. 17.24A).

Treatment. Medical treatment is the same as that for rheumatoid arthritis in general (p. 137). Local treatment for the hip joints depends upon the activity and severity of the inflammatory reaction. When the reaction is moderate or mild, exercises under physiotherapy supervision and active use within the limits of pain are encouraged. Intra-articular injections of hydrocortisone have sometimes given relief, but they cannot safely be repeated.

Operative treatment is justified when pain is severe and walking is limited to a few yards. Replacement arthroplasty (see Fig. 17.27A, p. 363) is the method of choice and can be expected to give as good results as in patients with osteoarthritis, though involvement of other joints in the lower limb may continue to impair mobility.

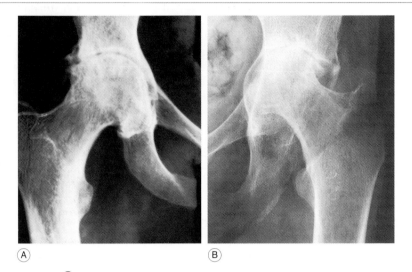

(A)   (B)

Fig. 17.24 Ⓐ Long-established rheumatoid arthritis of the hip, with destruction of the cartilage space. The marginal osteophytes indicate that osteoarthritis is becoming superimposed upon the old rheumatoid disease. Ⓑ The left hip of another patient, showing marked protrusion of the femoral head into the softened acetabulum (protrusio acetabuli).

OSTEOARTHRITIS OF THE HIP (General description of osteoarthritis, p. 140)

Osteoarthritis of the hip is a common cause of severe disablement, especially in the elderly. It is not uncommon even in younger patients, when it is usually secondary to previous injury or disease. Indeed operations for the relief of osteoarthritis of the hip now make up a substantial part of the work of an orthopaedic department.

Cause. It is sometimes regarded as a wear-and-tear process; but in fact it reflects an inability of articular cartilage fully to repair itself. Any injury or disease that damages the joint surfaces initiates or accelerates the process of degeneration. Common examples of such predisposing causes are fracture of the acetabulum, Perthes' osteochondritis, slipped upper femoral epiphysis, and ischaemic necrosis (osteonecrosis) of part of the femoral head from any cause. In another group degeneration of the joint is secondary to a developmental imperfection (dysplasia) or congenital subluxation. In many cases there is no evidence of an underlying cause, and for want of any other explanation such cases are regarded as primary or idiopathic.

Pathology. The articular cartilage is worn away, especially where weight is transmitted. The underlying bone becomes hard and eburnated with subarticular cyst formation. Hypertrophy of bone at the joint margins leads to the formation of osteophytes.

Clinical features. The patient is usually elderly; but when osteoarthritis is secondary to previous hip disease or to injury it often arises in middle life or even earlier. There is pain in the groin and front of the thigh; often also in the knee. The pain is made worse by walking and eased by rest. Later, there may

The hip region

be complaint of stiffness, which manifests itself in everyday life by inability to reach the foot to tie the shoe laces or cut the toe nails. The symptoms tend to increase progressively month by month and year by year until they eventually cause severe painful limp and incapacity for normal activities.

On examination all hip movements are impaired. Limitation of abduction, adduction, and rotation is marked, but a good range of flexion is often preserved. Forced movements are painful. Fixed deformity (flexion, adduction, or lateral rotation, or a combination of these) is common (see Fig. 17.26).

Radiographic features. The changes are characteristic. There is diminution of the cartilage space, with a tendency to sclerosis of the subchondral bone and cyst formation (Figs 17.25 and 17.26). Hypertrophic spurring of bone (osteophyte formation) is usually seen at the joint margins.

Treatment. The treatment required depends upon the severity of the disability. Mild osteoarthritis is best left untreated. In cases of moderate severity conservative treatment may suffice, but in severe cases operation is often advisable.

Conservative treatment. Clearly no form of conservative treatment can possibly influence the distorted anatomy of the joint. At best such treatment is only palliative; it may alleviate but cannot abolish the pain. Four methods will be mentioned:

1. *'Relative' rest*. By this is meant a modification of the patient's mode of life by change of occupation or adjustment of duties so that the work thrown upon the hip is reduced. The use of a stick (cane) or walking aid and the correction of shortening by a shoe raise also come into this category, and they often afford considerable relief.
2. *Drugs*. Mild analgesic medication is often helpful, especially when the pain disturbs sleep, though non-steroidal inflammatory drugs are not as effective as in rheumatoid arthritis.
3. *Physiotherapy*. Local deep heat by short-wave diathermy, with exercises to strengthen the muscles and to preserve mobility, often provides temporary relief.

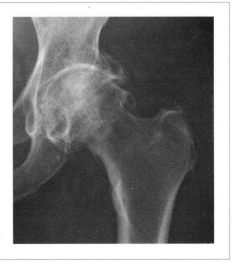

Fig. 17.25 Radiograph of idiopathic osteoarthritis of the hip. There is narrowing of the joint space, a subchondral cyst is seen in the medial femoral head, and large osteophytes are evident at the lateral margin of the acetabulum and on the lateral side of the femoral head.

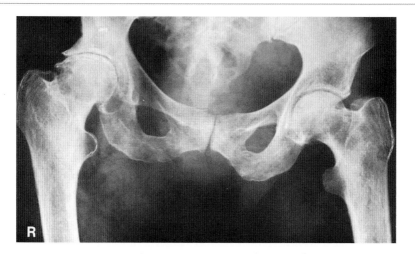

Fig. 17.26 Advanced osteoarthritis of right hip. Note the adduction deformity – a common feature that causes apparent shortening of the limb from tilting of the pelvis. As in Figure 17.25, the characteristic features are narrowing of the joint space, subchondral bone sclerosis, and marginal osteophytes.

4. *Injections into the joint.* The injection into the joint of hydrocortisone, with or without a local anaesthetic solution, has been tried, and in a few cases temporary relief has been claimed. However, repeated injections may accelerate joint destruction and are not to be recommended.

Operative treatment. Operation may be required if pain is severe – especially if it hinders sleep and interferes seriously with the patient's capacity for walking or work. Three types of operation must be considered:

1. arthroplasty (Fig. 17.27)
2. upper femoral osteotomy (Fig. 17.28A)
3. arthrodesis

though the last two are now seldom used.

Arthroplasty. The method most commonly used in primary management is total replacement arthroplasty (Figs 17.27A and 17.29A). Excision arthroplasty (Fig. 17.28B) is now only used as a salvage operation after other methods of treatment have failed, particularly when replacement arthroplasty has failed on account of infection.

In *total replacement arthroplasty* both the femoral and acetabular articular surfaces are replaced by artificial materials. The introduction of this technique in the 1960s resulted from two important innovations: the development of new metal and polymer biomaterials which could provide low friction articulations while remaining inert in the body, and the use of an acrylic filling compound, or polymethylmethacrylate cement, to fix the implants to the bone. One of the earliest, and still most successful designs was that of Charnley, which replaced the femoral head with a much smaller stainless steel head on a stem fixed into the femoral shaft with acrylic cement. This articulated with a thick hemispherical socket or cup of high-density polyethylene, which was also fixed to the bone of the

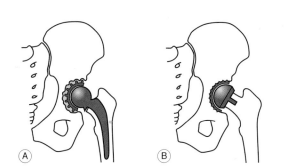

Fig. 17.27 Ⓐ Total replacement arthroplasty. The femoral head is of metal, the socket of plastic. Ⓑ Resurfacing (double cup) arthroplasty. Matching metal shells are used to resurface the femoral head and acetabular socket with cemented or cementless fixation.

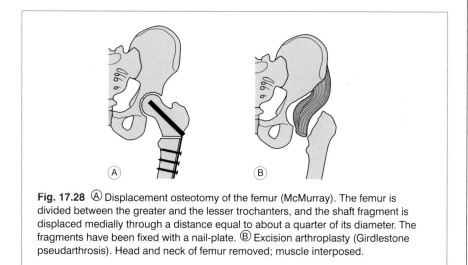

Fig. 17.28 Ⓐ Displacement osteotomy of the femur (McMurray). The femur is divided between the greater and the lesser trochanters, and the shaft fragment is displaced medially through a distance equal to about a quarter of its diameter. The fragments have been fixed with a nail-plate. Ⓑ Excision arthroplasty (Girdlestone pseudarthrosis). Head and neck of femur removed; muscle interposed.

deepened acetabulum with acrylic cement (Fig. 17.29A). This, and similar prostheses, provided restoration of pain-free hip movement and function, which could be expected to continue for more than 10–15 years in over 90% of patients. Replacement arthroplasty is now accepted as one of the most successful operations in terms of restoring the quality of life in patients for most years. However, like all surgical procedures it has risks and complications. In the early years of its use the most feared of these was postoperative infection, either early or late. The rate of this complication has now been reduced to around 1% by the use of routine prophylactic antibiotics combined with sterile operating environments utilising clean air laminar flow ventilation. A more challenging long-term problem is the progressive aseptic

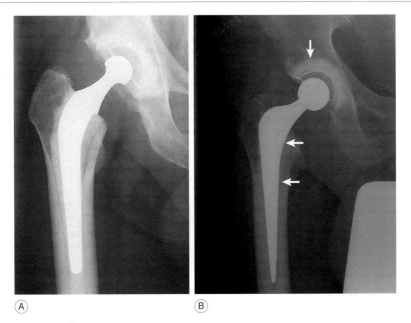

(A)　　　　　　　　　　　(B)

Fig. 17.29 Ⓐ Total replacement arthroplasty of hip. The hemispherical socket, of polyethylene, is not seen, but its mouth is indicated by the wire marker. Ⓑ AP radiograph of hip in patient 10 years after total hip replacement. There is a dark lucent line (arrowed) between the cemented cup and the bone of the acetabulum. The femoral shaft also shows endosteal bone resorption around the proximal and mid portion of the stem. This is indicative of loosening of both prostheses.

loosening of the prosthetic components which may occur (Fig. 17.29B) in some patients and results in a cumulative failure rate of 1% each year. This is associated with bone destruction around the implants which was thought to result from a granulomatous tissue reaction to the wear particles liberated from the weight-bearing surfaces.

In the intervening years, there have been many attempts to improve on this basic design to provide longer implant survival, particularly when the technique is used in younger patients. These have included attempts at 'cementless' mechanical fixation of implants using prostheses with porous metal surfaces to encourage bone ingrowth, and the development of new biomaterials such as ceramics or better polyethylenes with improved wear characteristics.

Another concept that has been reintroduced is the resurfacing or 'double cup' arthroplasty (Figs 17.27B and 17.30). This uses matching shells to resurface the femoral head and reline the reamed acetabular socket. Earlier attempts with this technique in the 1970s, using conventional metal and polyethylene components, had resulted in early failure because of rapid wear of the thin acetabular component. This problem has now been overcome by the use of improved metal-on-metal shells. The operation is only indicated in younger more active patients under the age of 60 where preservation of bone stock is required for

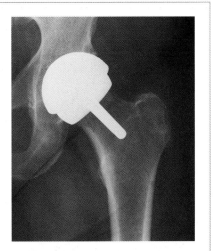

Fig. 17.30 Metal-on-metal 'double cup' hip resurfacing prosthesis.

potential later revision. Short-term results are now as good as with conventional replacement arthroplasty, but the operation, which is more technically demanding, should only be used for selected patients by those skilled in its use until results from longer follow-up become available.

Upper femoral osteotomy (McMurray displacement osteotomy). This operation was a standard method of treatment before total replacement arthroplasty was developed, but it is now little used. It may still be useful in patients under 55 with moderately early osteoarthritis where pain is a major problem but there is still an adequate range of functional movement, including 90° of flexion. The femur is divided between the greater trochanter and the lesser trochanter, and the lower (shaft) fragment is displaced medially through about a quarter of its diameter (Fig. 17.28A). Internal fixation of the fragments by nail-plate and screws is usually employed. Relief of pain is often satisfactory in over 70% of patients and preoperative joint movement is retained. The question of why an upper femoral osteotomy should relieve the pain of an osteoarthritic hip has not been answered satisfactorily. It is possible that in some way the remodelling of bone trabeculae necessitated by the displacement stimulates repair processes in the damaged articular cartilage; or it may alter the vascularity of the femoral head. Certainly in a favourable case the cartilage thickens appreciably in the first two or three years after operation, as shown radiologically. The other advantage of the operation is that it can still be converted to a hip replacement arthroplasty later, should the result prove disappointing in the long term.

Arthrodesis. The joint is fused in a position of 15–20° of flexion but without any abduction, adduction, or rotation. There is complete relief of pain, and good function is possible so long as the other hip, the knees and the spine are normal. It is only applicable in younger patients under 40 with distorted hip anatomy and is inappropriate for patients in countries where squatting is the normal habit.

In *excision arthroplasty* (Girdlestone pseudarthrosis) a false joint is created by excising the head and neck of the femur and the upper half of the wall of the acetabulum, and suturing a mass of soft tissue (such as the gluteus medius muscle) in the gap thus created, to act as a cushion between the bones (Fig. 17.28B). This is essentially a salvage operation, originally designed for chronic infections, and should only be used when alternatives have failed or are inappropriate.

It usually provides pain relief, but at the expense of substantial shortening and instability, necessitating the permanent use of a stick for walking and a considerable shoe raise.

PERTHES'[1] DISEASE (Legg–Perthes' disease; coxa plana; pseudocoxalgia; osteochondritis of the femoral capital epiphysis)

Perthes' disease is osteochondritis of the epiphysis of the femoral head. The general features of osteochondritis were described in Chapter 8 (p. 130). Like most examples of osteochondritis, Perthes' disease is an affection of childhood. The femoral head is temporarily softened and may become deformed. The main importance of the condition is that it may lead to the development of osteoarthritis of the hip in later life.

Cause. A temporary, and possibly repeated, local disturbance of blood supply is believed to be the major factor, but the precise cause of the vascular disturbance is unknown.

Pathology. The bony nucleus of the epiphysis of the femoral head undergoes necrosis either in whole or in part, presumably from ischaemia. This sets up a sequence of changes which occupies two to three years. The first stage is that of ingrowth of new blood vessels and removal of dead bone by osteoclasts. In the second stage, which is not distinct but overlaps the first stage so that both processes are going on together, new bone is laid down on the dead trabeculae, gradually reconstituting the bony nucleus. The third stage is that of remodelling: this may continue for several years. This sequence of necrosis and replacement of bone is patchy rather than uniform, so that the nucleus has an appearance of fragmentation as seen in the radiographs. During this period structural rigidity is lost, and deformation of the epiphysis may occur from pressure across the joint.

In the early phases of the cycle of changes growth of the bony element of the epiphysis is temporarily arrested, but the cartilage surrounding the bony nucleus, which forms a considerable proportion of the femoral head, continues to grow and so is disproportionately thick (Fig. 17.31), though sometimes revascularisation and healing will restore a relatively normal femoral head Fig. 17.32). Nevertheless it may sometimes follow the bone in suffering deformation, so that the femoral head as a whole may become much flattened (Fig. 17.33). At the same time there is often some enlargement of the femoral head. As the acetabulum grows, it tends to follow the contours of the femoral head, so that it may end up abnormally large and shallow (Fig. 17.34).

[1]George Clemens Perthes (1869–1927), German surgeon and early pioneer of radiotherapy and the pneumatic tourniquet, identified the radiological appearance of the disease in 1898.

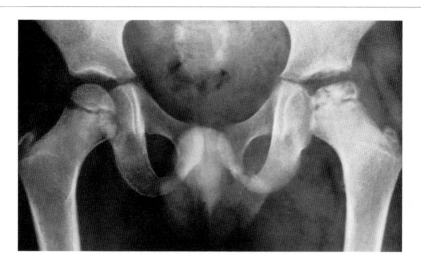

Fig. 17.31 Perthes' disease of the left hip. Note the shrunken appearance of the bony nucleus of the femoral epiphysis, the corresponding increase in depth of the cartilage space, the patchy changes of density, and the suggestion of fragmentation.

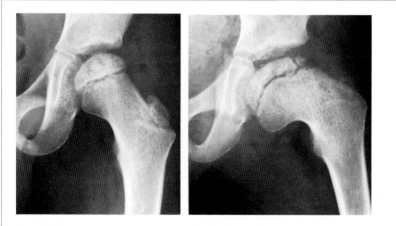

Fig. 17.32 Same patient as in Figure 17.31 two years after the onset of symptoms. The shape of the head is virtually normal, and the femoral neck is of normal length. There is little risk of osteoarthritis.

Fig. 17.33 In this patient, despite prolonged relief from weight-bearing, the femoral head is markedly flattened and the femoral neck is short. The deformity of the femoral head predisposes to osteoarthritis in later life.

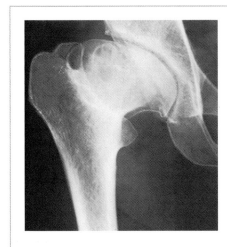

Fig. 17.34 Old untreated Perthes' disease. The femoral head is markedly flattened and the femoral neck is short. There is already some narrowing of the cartilage space, suggesting early osteoarthritis.

In consequence of interrupted growth at the epiphysial plate the femoral neck – and the limb as a whole – may be shorter than on the normal side, though the discrepancy is not great.

Clinical features. The disease occurs mainly in children of 5 to 10 years. It usually affects only one hip. The child complains of pain in the groin or thigh, and is noticed to limp. There is no disturbance of general health. *On examination* the only striking sign is moderate limitation of all hip movements, with pain and spasm if movement is forced.

Imaging. *Radiographic features.* The earliest radiographic changes are usually, though not always, present by the time advice is sought. There is a slight decrease in the depth of the ossific nucleus of the femoral head, whereas the clear cartilage space is often increased in depth: in other words the bony nucleus seems to have shrunk within its surrounding bed of cartilage (Fig. 17.31). The nucleus becomes denser than that of the normal side, though the density is patchy rather than uniform, so that there is an appearance of fragmentation. In severe cases the nucleus becomes progressively more flattened. Eventually the texture of the bone returns to normal (Fig. 17.32), but if flattening has occurred the femoral head is permanently deformed (Figs 17.33 and 17.34). *Radioisotope scanning* shows failure of uptake of the isotope in the region corresponding to the bony nucleus of the femoral head, but the changes are better demonstrated even at a very early stage by *MRI scanning*.

Diagnosis. Perthes' disease is distinguished from tuberculous arthritis, which it may resemble clinically, mainly by the radiographs. A normal erythrocyte sedimentation rate and blood count, and good general health, are other distinguishing features.

Prognosis. The disease has no direct adverse effect upon the general health. The main risk is to the future function of the affected hip joint, because if the femoral head suffers permanent deformation there is a risk of secondary osteoarthritis in later life, often in the fifth or sixth decade (Fig. 17.34).

The outcome depends largely upon whether the whole of the epiphysis is affected or whether part of it escapes, as it often does. In the latter case the prognosis is favourable (Fig. 17.32), whereas if the whole epiphysis is affected marked flattening of the femoral head may occur despite the most careful treatment (Fig. 17.33). The state of the cartilaginous part of the head, as determined from arthrography or from comparison of MRI scanning of both hips, is also important in prognosis. If head height is well preserved, the outlook is favourable, whereas if there has been early collapse of cartilage permanent deformation of the head is to be expected. In general, the outlook is more favourable in younger children than in older children.

Treatment. It has to be admitted that the treatment of Perthes' disease is often disappointing: no universally satisfactory method has yet been evolved. Indeed it has sometimes been questioned whether treatment has any effect on the final state of the hip.

The former method of preventing weight-bearing pressure upon the softened femoral head by prolonged recumbency (often for 2 years or more) has long been abandoned because the results were not commensurate with the severe disruption of home life that this treatment entailed. Other methods of trying to prevent pressure upon the head while still allowing the child to be up and about, such as slings or ischial-bearing calipers, have also fallen into disfavour because they are seldom effective and because they may embarrass the child psychologically.

The present trend is to grade the cases according to the likely outcome, so far as the shape of the femoral head is concerned, as judged from the radiographic features in the early stages and to regulate the treatment accordingly. In the 'favourable' category are placed those with only half the head affected (as seen in the lateral radiographs) and with no sign of lateral extrusion of part of the femoral head from under the roof of the acetabulum. In the 'unfavourable' grade are placed those with the whole head affected or with some lateral extrusion of the head beyond the roof of the acetabulum. In general, patients with a favourable prognosis do not require treatment other than by rest for a few weeks to allow the pain to subside – though it is essential that they attend periodically for radiological review. In contrast, those with an unfavourable prognosis, with the femoral head in danger of becoming badly deformed, are advised to have surgical treatment to prevent this.

Present thought is that treatment, when needed, should be by 'containment' of the femoral head within the acetabulum. This means that the femoral head must be centred within the acetabulum so that the two are co-axial, and thus the whole circumference of the femoral head is embraced by the socket. The socket then acts as a mould, to keep the head hemispherical while it is in the softened state.

In practice, ensuring maximal containment of the femoral head demands that the femoral head and neck (or the whole limb) must be abducted in relation to the acetabulum, to make them co-axial. This has sometimes been achieved by splinting the limbs in 20° or 30° of abduction, but the child is thus greatly handicapped in walking. Most surgeons therefore prefer to realign the femoral head and neck by dividing the femur below the greater trochanter and deflecting the neck downwards to coincide with the central axis of the acetabulum (see Fig. 17.20). Alternatively, the acetabulum itself may be redirected after osteotomy of the innominate bone (see Fig. 17.17D, p. 351).

OSTEONECROSIS (Non-traumatic avascular necrosis) OF THE FEMORAL HEAD

Necrosis of the bone of the femoral head may be a complication of trauma, particularly fracture of the femoral neck, but may also occur without a history of injury. This non-traumatic or idiopathic osteonecrosis is thought to be the result of an ischaemic episode affecting the bone and marrow tissue, and may cause progressive collapse of the femoral head in young adults.

Cause. The aetiology of this uncommon condition is still unclear, though several factors have been proposed as the mechanism of ischaemia, including intra-osseous hypertension, fat embolism, and intravascular coagulation. There is often a history of steroid therapy or alcohol addiction, and the condition may also develop in patients receiving immuno-suppression therapy following organ transplantation. It may also be associated with inherited haemoglobinopathies, such as sickle cell disease; and it may occur as a complication of Gaucher's disease (p. 72).

Pathology. The bone necrosis does not involve the entire femoral head, but commonly occupies a wedge-shaped segment beneath the superior weight-bearing surface. This may result in a subchondral fracture with subsequent collapse of the articular surface and a progression to secondary osteoarthritis. Surrounding the segment of bone necrosis there is a dense margin showing histological changes of an inflammatory response, with vascular granulation tissue suggesting a repair mechanism.

Clinical features. The patient, usually young or middle-aged, will present with increasing pain, which is frequently bilateral, in the hip or thigh during standing or walking. There is often a history of steroid therapy, excessive alcohol intake, or one of the other medical risk factors. Initially the range of hip movement is maintained, though painful at its extremes. Later, when bony collapse has occurred, there may be marked restriction of hip movement, with secondary contractures and limb shortening.

Investigation. In the early stage of the disease plain radiography may be normal (Fig. 17.35A), though magnetic resonance imaging (MRI) may show a low-intensity focus in the affected femoral head (Fig. 17.35B). Bone scintigraphy using a technetium-labelled isotope may reveal an area of increased or decreased uptake in the femoral head at the site of developing necrosis, but is less sensitive than an MRI scan.

A full haematological and biochemical screen should be undertaken to identify any associated disease.

Radiographic features. One of the earliest radiographic signs of developing osteonecrosis may be narrowing of the joint space, with flattening of the weight-bearing surface of the head and an underlying area of sclerosis in the bone. Progression to subchondral fracture results in a crescent sign of lucency beneath the superior articular surface with a dense segment in the underlying femoral head (Fig. 17.36). In the advanced stages of the disease there may be secondary arthritic changes, with progressive collapse of the femoral head.

Treatment. Treatment is usually surgical and is determined by the stage and extent of the disease. If diagnosed early, prior to femoral head collapse, an attempt can be made to encourage revascularisation by drilling the affected segment through a trans-trochanteric approach, with the possible addition of bone grafting to provide both an osteogenic stimulus and mechanical support. In more advanced disease, where some bony collapse has occurred, an osteotomy of the femoral neck may allow better containment of the femoral head and restoration of an intact articular weight-bearing surface. Once secondary

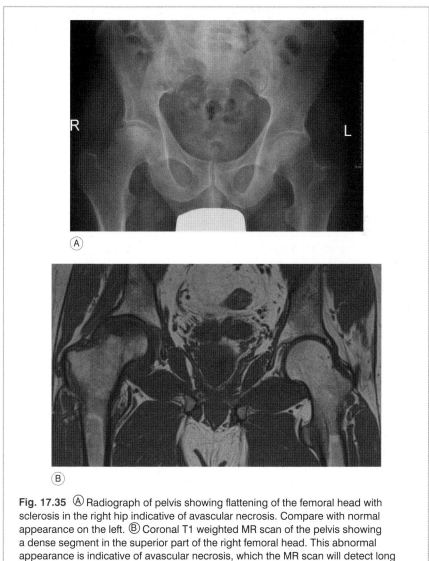

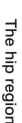

Fig. 17.35 Ⓐ Radiograph of pelvis showing flattening of the femoral head with sclerosis in the right hip indicative of avascular necrosis. Compare with normal appearance on the left. Ⓑ Coronal T1 weighted MR scan of the pelvis showing a dense segment in the superior part of the right femoral head. This abnormal appearance is indicative of avascular necrosis, which the MR scan will detect long before there are changes seen on plain radiographs.

osteoarthritis is established, removal of the femoral head and total replacement arthroplasty of the hip is the only surgical option.

SLIPPED UPPER FEMORAL EPIPHYSIS (Adolescent coxa vara; epiphysial coxa vara)

This is an affection of late childhood in which the upper femoral epiphysis is displaced from its normal position upon the femoral neck. The displacement occurs at the growth plate (epiphysial line), and it is common for it to occur on both sides (though seldom simultaneously).

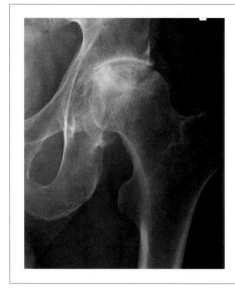

Fig. 17.36 Radiograph of hip showing late avascular necrosis of the femoral head with evidence of collapse of the articular surface and an underlying crescent of sclerotic bone.

Cause. This is unknown. The condition is often associated with overweight from endocrine dysfunction or from other causes, but in other cases the patient is of normal build.

Pathology. The junction between the capital epiphysis and the neck of the femur loosens. With the downward pressure of weight-bearing and the upward pull of muscles on the femur the epiphysis is displaced from its normal position. Displacement is always backwards and downwards, so that the epiphysis comes to lie at the back of the femoral neck (Fig. 17.37).

The displacement usually occurs gradually, but occasionally a sudden displacement is caused by injury, such as a fall. Left undisturbed, the epiphysis fuses to the femoral neck in the abnormal position. The consequent deformity of the articular surface then predisposes to the later development of secondary osteoarthritis.

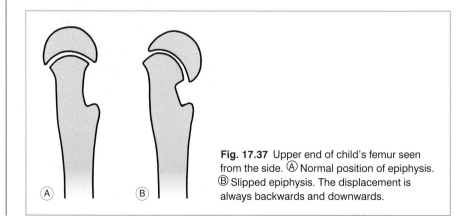

Fig. 17.37 Upper end of child's femur seen from the side. Ⓐ Normal position of epiphysis. Ⓑ Slipped epiphysis. The displacement is always backwards and downwards.

The hip region

Clinical features. The patient is between 10 and 20 years of age. In about half the cases there is evidence of an endocrine disturbance leading to marked overweight. In a little less than half the cases both hips are affected, though seldom simultaneously. Typically, there is a gradual onset of pain in the hip, with limp. Sometimes the pain is felt mainly in the knee, which may confuse the diagnosis. Rarely, these symptoms develop acutely after an injury, such as a fall.

On examination the physical signs are characteristic, for there is selective limitation of certain hip movements, the other movements being full or even increased. The movements that are restricted are flexion, abduction, and medial rotation. Lateral rotation and adduction are often increased, and the limb tends to lie in lateral rotation. Forcing movement in the restricted range exacerbates the pain.

Radiographic examination. Even a slight displacement of the epiphysis is recognisable, provided good *lateral* radiographs are obtained. It must be stressed that a slight displacement is easily overlooked if antero-posterior films alone are examined (Fig. 17.38). Lateral radiographs are essential. In the lateral film the epiphysis is seen to be tilted over towards the back of the femoral neck (Fig. 17.39),[1] the posterior 'horn' being lower than the anterior, whereas in the normal hip they are level.

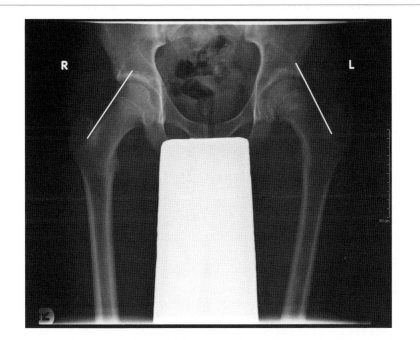

Fig. 17.38 AP radiograph of the pelvis in a child with an early slipped femoral epiphysis of the left hip. The epiphysis has slipped medially and backwards. This subtle abnormality is identified by drawing a line along the superior margin of the femoral neck. On the normal right side a small portion of the epiphysis is seen to extend above the line. On the abnormal left side, when the line is drawn there is no part of the epiphysis lying above it.

[1]Students often have difficulty in determining in lateral radiographs of the upper end of the femur which is the back and which is the front of the bone. The key is the bony projection formed by the trochanters: this is always posterior.

The hip region

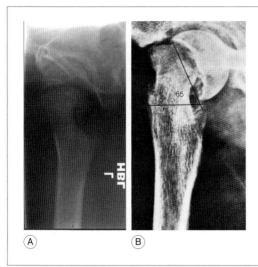

Fig. 17.39 Ⓐ Lateral radiograph of the left hip in the same child confirms that the epiphysis has slipped backwards on the femoral neck. Ⓑ Another patient. Slipped epiphysis of severe degree.

Diagnosis. Slipped upper femoral epiphysis should be suspected in every patient of 10–20 years of age who complains of pain in the hip or knee. The characteristic clinical features, together with the radiographic evidence of epiphysial displacement, are conclusive. The condition is nevertheless often missed, partly because pain may be predominantly in the knee, the hip therefore being not examined; or because lateral radiographs are not obtained (Fig. 17.38).

Complications. These include avascular necrosis of the epiphysis of the femoral head, cartilage necrosis, and late osteoarthritis.

Avascular necrosis (osteonecrosis) and consequent collapse of the epiphysis may occur if its blood supply is damaged. This complication is usually a consequence of attempted reduction of the slip by manipulation or of operation, but it may occur spontaneously, especially after a sudden acute slip.

Cartilage necrosis is a rare and unexplained thinning of the articular cartilage, with marked restriction of joint movement. It is commonest after operative treatment and may possibly represent an auto-immune reaction.

If severe displacement is allowed to remain uncorrected *osteoarthritis* is likely to develop in later life (Fig. 17.40).

It is necessary to emphasise that a careful watch must always be kept for slipping of the opposite femoral epiphysis, which may occur in up to 50% of patients and may justify prophylactic fixation in those thought to be at greater risk.

Treatment. The treatment depends upon the degree of displacement. This may be graded as *slight* or *severe*.

Slight displacement. When displacement is slight (less than 40° as measured on the lateral radiograph) (Fig. 17.39A) the position may be accepted and all that is necessary is to prevent further displacement. This is achieved by driving threaded wires or slender screws[1] along the neck of the femur into the

---

[1]A three-flanged nail, formerly sometimes used for fixation instead of threaded wires, is not recommended because it does not easily penetrate the hard epiphysis and may damage its blood supply.

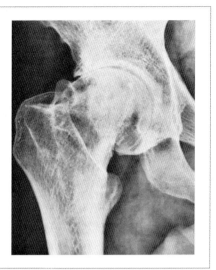

Fig. 17.40 Osteoarthritis developing twenty years after uncorrected slipped epiphysis.

epiphysis (Fig. 17.41). It should be remembered that even though the position that has been accepted may be imperfect, improvement can occur spontaneously in the succeeding years, through a process of remodelling.

Severe displacement. When displacement is severe (Fig. 17.39B) the position cannot easily be accepted because of the virtual certainty that painful osteoarthritis will develop in adult life. The position should therefore be improved. Three methods are available: manipulation, operative replacement of the epiphysis at the site of slipping, and compensatory osteotomy at a lower level.

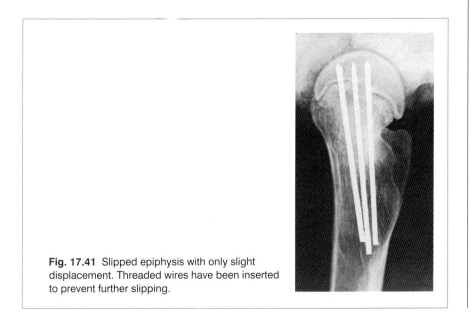

Fig. 17.41 Slipped epiphysis with only slight displacement. Threaded wires have been inserted to prevent further slipping.

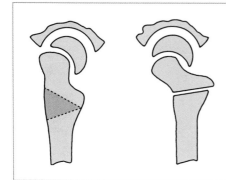

Fig. 17.42 Subtrochanteric osteotomy for slipped femoral epiphysis of severe degree. By removal of an appropriate wedge of bone (shown outlined in the left-hand diagram), the epiphysis is restored to its proper relationship with the acetabulum. The operation has the advantage that the blood supply of the epiphysis is not endangered.

Manipulation, with or without preliminary weight traction, is seldom successful; it is worth trying only in the rare cases of recent sudden displacement, especially if caused by injury. Manipulation – predominantly by medial rotation – should be carried out very gently lest the blood supply to the epiphysis be further damaged. After successful manipulative reduction further slipping should be prevented by inserting threaded wires or screws, as described above.

Operative replacement of the epiphysis, with fixation by wires or a screw, has sometimes been practised when symptoms have been present for less than 3 months, provided the growth plate is still open. At its best it can restore the hip virtually to normal. Nevertheless the operation has the serious hazard that it may destroy the blood supply to the femoral head, leading to avascular necrosis (osteonecrosis) of the femoral head and precipitating the onset of disabling osteoarthritis. In the opinion of many surgeons this major hazard negates any indication for the operation.

Compensatory osteotomy is an alternative method that is preferred by most surgeons. The osteotomy is done just below the trochanteric level (Fig. 17.42). An anteriorly based wedge of bone is removed so that the shaft of the femur is angled into flexion relative to the upper fragment. The operation thus compensates for the backward tilting of the epiphysis; correction should be sufficient to bring the epiphysis once more into the weight-transmitting segment of the acetabulum. The operation entails no risk of damage to the blood supply of the femoral head, so there is no risk of disastrous avascular necrosis (osteonecrosis); but it leaves the articular surface of the upper end of the femur deformed, and therefore does not altogether remove the risk of secondary osteoarthritis in later years.

EXTRA-ARTICULAR DISORDERS IN THE REGION OF THE HIP

COXA VARA

The general term *coxa vara* includes any condition in which the neck–shaft angle of the femur is less than the normal of about 125° (Fig. 17.43). The angle is sometimes reduced to 90° or less. The deformity is caused mechanically by the stress of body weight acting upon a femur that is defective or abnormally soft.

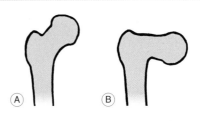

Fig. 17.43 Ⓐ Normal neck–shaft angle.
Ⓑ Coxa vara: the neck–shaft angle is reduced.

Causes. The most important causes of coxa vara are:

1. *Congenital*. Part of the femoral neck remains as unossified cartilage, which gradually bends during childhood (congenital coxa vara; infantile coxa vara). This type is uncommon.
2. *Slipped upper femoral epiphysis* (epiphysial coxa vara). This was described on page 371.
3. *Fracture*. Coxa vara is common after fractures in the trochanteric region with mal-union, and in ununited fractures of the neck of the femur.
4. *Softening of bone*, in general affections such as rickets, osteomalacia, or Paget's disease.

Effects. Coxa vara leads to true shortening of the limb. Approximation of the greater trochanter to the ilium slackens the abductor muscles of the hip and thus impairs their efficiency, leading in severe cases to a Trendelenburg 'dip', with consequent limp (p. 341).

Treatment. The treatment is mainly that of the underlying condition. Often a mild deformity is best accepted. In appropriate cases the neck–shaft angle can be corrected by osteotomy just below the greater trochanter.

SNAPPING HIP

Snapping hip is a harmless condition in which a distinct snap is heard and felt on certain movements of the joint. It does not denote any underlying injury or disease and it is seldom of practical significance. The snap is attributed to slipping of a tendinous thickening in the aponeurosis of the gluteus maximus over the bony prominence of the greater trochanter. It is heard easily when the patient flexes the hip actively, but it is not reproduced by passive movement with the muscles relaxed. Treatment is required only exceptionally, when disability is severe. The offending ridge of aponeurosis is simply divided transversely from its under surface.

EXTRINSIC DISORDERS SIMULATING DISEASE OF THE HIP

As has already been mentioned, it frequently happens that a patient complains of symptoms in the region of the hip or thigh when in fact they arise at a distance. The conditions that may confuse the diagnosis in this way fall into three main groups:

1. disorders of the spine or sacro-iliac joints
2. disorders of the abdomen or pelvis
3. occlusive vascular disease.

DISORDERS OF THE SPINE AND SACRO-ILIAC JOINTS

Prolapsed intervertebral disc

The pain of a prolapsed lumbar intervertebral disc is often referred to the gluteal region or lateral aspect of the thigh: indeed this is the commonest clinical feature in cases of intervertebral disc degeneration of slight or moderate degree. On examination other evidence of a spinal disorder will usually be found, whereas the hip itself is normal clinically and radiographically.

Sacro-iliac arthritis

The pain caused by arthritis of a sacro-iliac joint – whether it be tuberculous, pyogenic, or the early stages of ankylosing spondylitis – spreads diffusely over the gluteal area and may simulate an affection of the hip. Mistakes should be prevented by careful clinical examination and by routine radiography of the whole pelvis in cases of alleged hip complaints.

DISORDERS OF THE ABDOMEN AND PELVIS

Pelvic or lower abdominal inflammation

Inflammation involving the side wall of the pelvis may mimic a hip lesion very closely; indeed even experienced surgeons have been deceived. The condition responsible is usually a subacute suppurative lesion such as a deep peri-appendicular abscess or a pyosalpinx. The hip symptoms arise partly from irritation of the obturator nerve, causing referred pain in the thigh, and partly from irritative spasm of the hip muscles that have their origin within the abdomen or pelvis – namely the psoas, iliacus, pyriformis, and obturator internus. The muscle spasm may cause marked restriction of hip movements, with pain if movement is forced. Differentiation from an intrinsic lesion of the hip depends upon a careful history and a complete physical examination, including an investigation of the abdomen and pelvis.

OCCLUSIVE VASCULAR DISEASE

Thrombosis of lower aorta or main branches

Ischaemic pain in the muscles of the buttock or thigh, from occlusion of the lower abdominal aorta or its main branches, may occasionally simulate disease of the hip. Distinction should not be difficult: in occlusive vascular disease the pain is brought on by activity and is quickly relieved by rest; the femoral, popliteal and pedal pulses will be weak or absent and the hip will show a full range of painless movement.

18 | The thigh and knee

The knee depends for its stability upon its four main ligaments and upon the quadriceps muscle. The importance of the quadriceps cannot be overemphasised. So efficiently can a powerful quadriceps control the knee that it can maintain stability despite considerable laxity of the ligaments. In many injuries and diseases of the knee the quadriceps wastes strikingly, and to some extent the condition of the muscle is an index of the state of the knee: if it is wasted it is probable that there is a significant abnormality within the joint.

Apart from its vulnerability to injury, the knee is also particularly prone to almost every kind of arthritis. Moreover, it is the joint most commonly affected by osteochondritis dissecans and intra-articular loose body formation.

The region of the knee is the zone of most active bone growth in the lower limb (contrast the upper limb, where most growth occurs towards the shoulder and the wrist rather than towards the elbow). Perhaps partly for this reason the metaphyses near the knee are common sites of osteomyelitis and of primary malignant bone tumours.

The knee is, in fact, a region where nearly every kind of orthopaedic disorder may be represented.

In the diagnosis of knee complaints arthroscopy has secured for itself a role in investigation for any suspected intra-articular lesion although MRI has usurped this position. Arthroscopic techniques of surgery have become routine for such common disorders as meniscal tears and intra-articular loose bodies. Arthroscopic surgery has the advantages that formal opening of the knee is avoided and that recovery and convalescence are greatly accelerated. Stay in hospital is reduced, or increasingly the operation is performed as a 'day case procedure' without the need for admission.

In recent years total replacement arthroplasty of the knee has become established as the routine operation for the relief of disabling arthritis, whether rheumatoid or degenerative. The newer operation of unicompartmental arthroplasty is now producing results that allow it to be considered as an alternative to tibial osteotomy for the treatment of arthritis confined to a single tibio-femoral compartment.

SPECIAL POINTS IN THE INVESTIGATION OF THIGH AND KNEE COMPLAINTS

History

The history is of particular importance in the diagnosis of disorders of the knee. In a case of torn meniscus, for instance, the history is often the most important factor in the clinical diagnosis. When there has been a previous injury to the knee, the exact sequence of events at the time of the injury and afterwards must be ascertained. Enquiry is made into the mechanism of the injury; what the patient was doing at the time; whether he was able to carry on afterwards. Was he able to finish the game? If not, was he carried from the field or was he able to walk? How soon after the injury did the knee swell? Was he able to straighten the knee fully? If not, how did he eventually get it straight? Was he able to bend it? These and many other details must be elicited by careful questioning because they are so important in building up a picture of what exactly happened to the knee. Caution is necessary in accepting the patient's story of 'locking' at its face value. Many patients speak of 'locking' when the knee simply feels stiff and painful, or when it causes momentary jabs of pain on movement. Locking from a torn meniscus means simply that the knee cannot be straightened fully; it can usually be flexed freely. In locking from a loose body within the joint the knee may be jammed so that it will neither flex nor extend, but this is rather uncommon and the knee usually unlocks itself after an interval, or can be freed by judicious manoeuvring.

Exposure

For proper examination the whole length of the limb must be uncovered. It is impossible to examine a knee adequately when the thigh is half covered by tightly rolled trousers or underpants. The sound knee must also be exposed for comparison. For proper examination of the knee the patient must always be recumbent upon a couch.

Steps in clinical examination

A suggested routine for clinical examination of the thigh and knee is summarised in Table 18.1.

Determining the cause of a diffuse joint swelling

The knee exemplifies better than any other joint the different types of diffuse articular swelling. That the joint is in fact swollen should be obvious from inspection: comparison of the two knees will show that the concavities present at each side of the patella have been filled out on the affected side.

A diffuse swelling of the knee can arise only from three fundamental causes:

1. thickening of bone
2. fluid within the joint
3. thickening of the synovial membrane (in practice it is found that this is the only soft tissue about the knee that swells appreciably).

Determination of the particular cause or combination of causes in a given case depends entirely on careful palpation, as follows:

Thickening of bone. Thickening of bone is detected without difficulty by deep palpation if the affected side is compared with the normal. There may be a general enlargement, caused perhaps by a bone infection or by an expanding tumour or cyst; or there may be simply a local prominence, caused usually by osteophytes at the joint margin or by an exostosis.

Fluid within the joint. A fluid effusion is best detected by the fluctuation test. The palm of one hand is placed upon the thigh immediately above the patella – that is, over the suprapatellar pouch. The other hand is placed over the front of the joint, with the thumb and index finger just beyond the margins of the patella (Fig. 18.1A). Pressure of the upper hand upon the

Table 18.1 Routine clinical examination in suspected disorders of the thigh and knee

1. LOCAL EXAMINATION OF THE THIGH AND KNEE	
Inspection	**Power** (tested against resistance of bone
Soft-tissue contours	contours and alignment examiner)
Colour and texture of skin	Flexion
Scars or sinuses	Extension
Palpation	**Stability**
Skin temperature	Medial ligament
Bone contours	Lateral ligament
Soft-tissue contours	Anterior cruciate ligament: anterior draw
Local tenderness	test; Lachman test; pivot shift test
Measurements of thigh girth	Posterior cruciate ligament
Comparative measurements at precisely the	**Rotation tests** (McMurray)
same level in each limb give an indication of	(Of value mainly when a torn meniscus is
the relative bulk of the thigh muscles, and in	suspected)
particular of the quadriceps	**Stance and gait**
Movements (active and passive, against	
normal knee for comparison)	
Flexion	
Extension	
? Pain on movement	
? Crepitation on movement	
2. EXAMINATION OF POTENTIAL EXTRINSIC SOURCES OF THIGH OR KNEE SYMPTOMS	
This is important if a satisfactory explanation for the symptoms is not found on local examination. The investigation should include especially:	
1. the spine	
2. the hip	
3. GENERAL EXAMINATION	
General survey of other parts of the body. The local symptoms may be only one manifestation of a widespread disease	

suprapatellar pouch drives fluid from the pouch into the main joint cavity, where it bulges the capsule at each side of the patella and imparts an easily detectable hydraulic impulse to the finger and thumb of the lower hand (Fig. 18.1B). Conversely, by pressure of this finger and thumb the fluid can be driven back into the suprapatellar pouch, the hydraulic impulse being clearly received by the upper hand. In this way an unmistakable sense of fluctuation can be elicited between the two hands. With practice it is easy to detect even a small effusion in this way. The 'patellar tap' test (Fig. 18.1C), in which the patella is tapped backwards sharply so that it strikes the femur and rebounds, though still used, is less reliable. The test is negative in the presence of fluid in two circumstances: first, when there is insufficient fluid to raise the patella away from the femur; and secondly, when there is a tense effusion. If used at all, the 'patellar tap' test should be used only as a supplementary method.

Distinction between effusions of blood, serous fluid, and pus is made partly from the history, partly from the clinical examination. An effusion of blood (haemarthrosis) appears within an hour or two of an injury and rapidly becomes tense and therefore painful. An effusion of clear fluid develops slowly (12–24 hours) and is never as tense as an effusion of blood (haemarthrosis). An effusion of pus is associated with general illness and pyrexia.

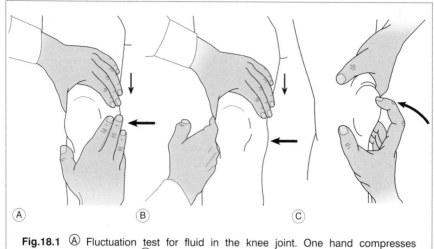

Fig.18.1 Ⓐ Fluctuation test for fluid in the knee joint. One hand compresses the suprapatellar pouch, Ⓑ while the thumb and finger of the other hand detects the fluid impulse on either side of the patella. Ⓒ In the patellar tap test the finger pushes the patella onto the front of the femoral condyle through the fluid resistance.

Thickening of synovial membrane. A thickened synovial membrane is always a prominent feature of chronic inflammatory arthritis. The thickening is often most obvious above the patella, where the reduplicated membrane forms the suprapatellar pouch. It has a characteristic boggy feel on palpation, rather as if a sheet of warm sponge-rubber had been placed between the skin and the underlying bone. It is worth emphasising that since it is highly vascular, a thickened synovial membrane is always associated with increased warmth of the overlying skin.

Movements

Accurate assessment of the range of movement is particularly important in the knee, because even a slight impairment of movement is significant. It is important to note also whether movement is painful and whether it is accompanied by crepitation.

Flexion. The normal range varies with the build of the patient. Thin patients can flex more than fat patients – usually enough to bring the heel in contact with the buttock. The range of the sound knee should always be taken as the normal for the individual.

Extension. There is a fairly wide variation in the normal range of extension: it is wrong to accept 0° as the starting-point of movement (0° = the anatomical position, with the knee straight). Many normal women can hyperextend their knees whereas some normal men cannot extend quite to the straight position. Variations are only of small magnitude but they may be significant. It is important to detect even a slight impairment of knee extension: therefore the range on the sound side must be taken as the yardstick of normal extension and a very careful comparison must be made between the two sides.

Tests for stability

The integrity of each of the four major ligaments is tested in turn.

Testing the medial and lateral ligaments. For this test the joint must be in a position just short of full extension, so that the posterior part of the joint capsule is relaxed: with the knee fully extended even marked laxity of the collateral ligaments can be masked by the intact posterior capsule, held taut. It must be remembered, however, that with the knee slightly flexed the medial and lateral ligaments are normally somewhat slack and allow a little side-to-side wobble. Technique: Support the limb by a hand gripping the ankle region and by the other hand behind the knee, flexing it slightly. Instruct the patient to relax the muscles. Using the more proximal hand as a fulcrum on the appropriate side of the knee, apply first an abduction force to test the medial ligament (Fig. 18.2A) and then an adduction force to test the lateral ligament. If the ligament is torn, the joint will open out more than in the normal knee when stress is applied.

Testing the anterior and posterior cruciate ligaments. The anterior cruciate ligament prevents anterior glide of the tibia on the femur; the posterior cruciate ligament prevents posterior glide. First the ligaments are tested with the knee flexed 90°. Technique: The patient's knee being flexed to a right angle and the foot placed firmly on the couch, sit lightly on the foot to prevent it from sliding (Fig. 18.2B). With the interlocked fingers of the two hands form a sling behind the upper end of the tibia, and clasp the sides of the leg between the thenar eminences. Place the tips of the thumbs one upon each femoral condyle. Ensure that the patient has relaxed the thigh muscles. Alternately pull and push the upper end of the tibia to determine the amount of antero-posterior movement. Normally there is an antero-posterior glide of up to half a centimetre; but since the normal is variable it is wise to use the patient's sound limb for comparison. Excessive glide in one or other direction indicates damage to the corresponding cruciate ligament.

In a second test the ligaments are examined with the knee flexed only 15° or 20° (Lachman test). One hand supports the thigh just above the knee, gripping the femoral condyles, while the other hand grasps the upper end of the tibia (Fig. 18.3). While the patient relaxes the muscles the extent of any anterior or posterior glide of the tibial condyles upon the femur is determined by push-and-pull movements of the tibia.

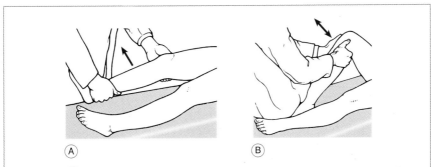

Fig. 18.2 Ⓐ Testing the medial ligament. The knee is held slightly flexed (see text). Ⓑ Testing the cruciate ligaments. The patient's foot is steadied by sitting upon it. Pulling the tibia forwards tenses the anterior ligament; pushing it backwards tenses the posterior ligament.

The thigh and knee

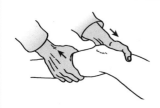

Fig. 18.3 In the Lachman test the amount of anterior or posterior glide of the tibia upon the femur is assessed with the knee flexed only about 20°.

Lateral pivot shift. The test for lateral pivot shift is supplementary to the tests described above for deficiency of the anterior cruciate ligament: it may be positive when the foregoing test is equivocal. The test depends on the fact that when the anterior cruciate ligament and the lateral ligament are deficient or lax the pivot between the lateral condyle of the femur and that of the tibia may be unstable. In that event the lateral tibial condylar surface may be displaced forwards in relation to the femoral condyle when the tibia is rotated medially with the knee straight. When the knee is then flexed the subluxation is spontaneously reduced with a visible or palpable 'jerk'. The test is thus an indication of antero-lateral instability.

Technique. The leg on the affected side is lifted by the examiner's corresponding hand (the right foot is lifted by the right hand; the left leg by the left hand) so that the knee drops into full extension with the muscles relaxed. The limb is supported under the arm, and with the other hand the examiner then presses against the outer aspect of the limb just below the knee, imparting a valgus strain (Fig. 18.4). At the same time the tibia is rotated medially upon the femur. The knee is now flexed slowly from the straight position. If the test is positive the lateral tibial condyle becomes spontaneously relocated on the femoral condyle when the knee reaches 30° or 35° of flexion. The relocation is evidenced by a visible or palpable jerk (hence the term 'jerk test' sometimes used for the manoeuvre).

Rotation test for pedunculated tag of meniscus

The object of this test, often known as McMurray's test and used only for suspected tears of the menisci, is to demonstrate a pedunculated tag of meniscus by causing it to be momentarily jammed between the joint surfaces: when the knee is then straightened a loud click may be heard and felt as the tag is disengaged.

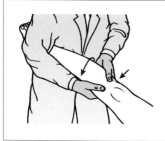

Fig. 18.4 Test for lateral pivot shift. The test depends upon first rotating the tibia medially to provoke subluxation of the lateral condyle of the tibia upon the lateral femoral condyle, and then correcting the subluxation by flexing the knee (see text).

The manoeuvre is carried out by repeatedly:

1. flexing the knee, first fully but in succeeding tests progressively less fully, then
2. rotating the tibia upon the femur, first laterally but in further tests medially, and finally
3. extending the knee while the rotation of the tibia is still maintained.

A loud click, distinct from the normal patellar click and usually associated with pain, suggests a tag tear (not a 'bucket-handle' tear) of a meniscus. Caution: Loud clicks can often be produced in normal knees. Most of them arise from movements of the patella, and they are not accompanied by pain. Discretion must be used in interpreting a click as an abnormal finding.

Extrinsic causes of pain in the thigh and knee

In most cases symptoms felt in the knee have their origin locally in or near the joint; but there are exceptions that may trap the unwary. Most importantly, pain in the knee may be the predominant feature of a disorder of the hip, such as arthritis or slipped upper femoral epiphysis. Less commonly sciatic pain, perhaps from a prolapsed intervertebral disc, has its greatest intensity at the level of the knee. In the investigation of pain in the knee we must therefore recognise the possibility that it may be referred from the spine or hip, and extend the examination to those regions if a satisfactory explanation for the trouble is not found on local examination.

Imaging

Radiographic examination. In a straightforward case antero-posterior and lateral films are sufficient. They should always include a reasonable length of the femur and of the tibia and fibula. Tangential projections of the femoral condyles with the knee flexed are sometimes helpful, especially when osteochondritis dissecans is suspected. Tangential ('sky-line') views of the patella may also be required.

When it is suspected that the knee symptoms might be referred from a lesion of the hip or spine appropriate radiographs of those regions should be obtained.

Radioisotope bone scanning. Occasionally this may be useful in the diagnosis of inflammatory or neoplastic lesions.

Magnetic resonance imaging. When adequate information cannot be obtained from plain radiography, magnetic resonance imaging may be helpful as a noninvasive alternative to arthroscopy.

Arthroscopy

Arthroscopy can be a useful adjunct to clinical and radiographic examination in the diagnosis of knee complaints (Fig. 18.5). Its use for diagnostic purposes has been largely replaced by MRI, but it is a well-established method of treating a number of intra-articular disorders by minimally invasive operation.

Arthroscopy is usually carried out with the patient anaesthetised, the joint cavity is filled with saline through a hollow needle, and a cannula and telescope are entered at the appropriate site – usually antero-laterally or antero-medially, depending upon whether the surgeon is concerned to inspect mainly the medial or the lateral compartment. By correctly manoeuvring and rotating the arthroscope, and if necessary by the use of alternative sites of entry, almost the whole extent of the interior of the joint can be brought into view with the possible

The thigh and knee

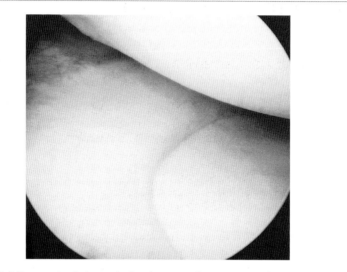

Fig. 18.5 Arthroscopic photograph showing normal appearance of medial meniscus. The medial femoral condyle is seen above, and the upper surface of the tibia is at the lower right. The concave edge of the meniscus is seen clearly lying upon the tibia.

exception of the postero-lateral recess. The information gained can be enhanced by probing the menisci and other intra-articular structures with an instrument introduced at a site away from the arthroscope.

DISORDERS OF THE THIGH

ACUTE OSTEOMYELITIS (General description of acute osteomyelitis, p. 85)

The femur is one of the bones most commonly affected by pyogenic osteomyelitis. The infection is carried to the femur either through the blood stream (haematogenous osteomyelitis), when it usually affects the lower metaphysis; or it is introduced through an external wound, especially in cases of compound fracture. The clinical features and treatment are the same as those of osteomyelitis elsewhere (p. 89).

CHRONIC OSTEOMYELITIS (General description of chronic osteomyelitis, p. 90)

Chronic pyogenic osteomyelitis is nearly always a sequel to acute infection that has been neglected or has responded poorly to treatment. As with the acute disease, the lower end of the femur is affected more often than the upper; but in many cases the infection spreads to involve a large part of the femoral shaft. Clinical features and treatment are like those of chronic osteomyelitis elsewhere (p. 91).

BONE TUMOURS IN THE THIGH

The femur is one of the commonest sites of the important bone tumours.

Benign tumours (General description of benign bone tumours, p. 106)

Of the four main types of benign bone tumour – osteoid osteoma, chondroma, osteochondroma, and giant-cell tumour – only the giant-cell tumour requires further consideration here, because of the special treatment requirements when it occurs close to the knee.

Giant-cell tumour (osteoclastoma)

The lower end of the femur is a particularly frequent site for this uncommon tumour. The upper end of the femur is affected much less often. The tumour usually arises in young adults. It begins in what was the metaphysial region, but since the epiphysis is fused there is no obstacle to its spread into the articular end of the bone (see Fig. 8.10A&B). The bone is gradually expanded, the cortex becoming very thin and pathological fracture may sometimes occur.

Though classed with the benign tumours, a giant-cell tumour tends to recur after inadequate removal and in rare cases it has the character of a sarcoma, metastasising through the blood stream.

Treatment. Thorough curettage of the tumour and filling of the resultant cavity with bone grafts or acrylic bone cement has been widely used but it is attended by a high incidence of recurrence. It may still be appropriate for small tumours but careful monitoring afterwards is essential so that any recurrence may be detected early. If the tumour is large many surgeons now prefer to excise the tumour-bearing lower end of the femur and to fit a custom-made metal prosthesis to replace the lower end of the femur and the knee joint.

Malignant tumours (General description of malignant bone tumours, p. 112)

The femur is a common site for all of the main types of malignant bone tumour occurring in younger patients. Three require mention – namely osteosarcoma, Ewing's sarcoma, and chondrosarcoma, though others such as lymphoma, malignant fibrous histiocytoma, and myeloma should be considered in the differential diagnosis of destructive femoral bone lesions. However, it should be remembered that metastatic tumours are much more common than any of the primary malignant tumours, particularly in patients over the age of 50.

Osteosarcoma (osteogenic sarcoma)

This is usually a tumour of childhood or early adult life: when it occurs in patients beyond middle age it is usually a complication of Paget's disease. Typically it arises in the metaphysis of a long bone, and the lower metaphysis of the femur is the favourite site. The tumour is highly malignant, with a mortality still in the region of 40% or more despite recent advances in treatment. Treatment is discussed on page 117.

Ewing's tumour

This also occurs mainly in children or adolescents. Unlike most bone tumours, it usually affects the shaft of the bone, which it expands in a fusiform manner. Over it, layer upon layer of new bone is laid down, giving a typical 'onion-peel'

The thigh and knee

appearance as seen in the radiographs. Although the tumour responds dramatically to chemotherapy, usually in combination with radiotherapy or surgical excision, the prognosis remains poor, with a mortality in the region of 50 per cent from blood-borne metastases. Treatment is discussed on page 121.

Chondrosarcoma

This tumour occurs more commonly in middle age and elderly patients suggesting that it represents a malignant change in a pre-existing chondroma. Clinically it presents with local pain and swelling and may reach a large size because of slow growth. Imaging shows an expanding lytic lesion with characteristic patchy calcification and cortical destruction. Treatment is entirely surgical since no chemotherapy is effective on the relatively avascular tumour.

Metastatic (secondary) tumours

The femur is commonly invaded by metastatic tumours, especially in its proximal half (Fig. 18.6).

Pathology. The tumours that metastasise most readily to bone are carcinomas of the lung, breast, prostate, kidney, and thyroid. The bone structure is usually destroyed by the tumour and pathological fracture is common (Fig. 18.6A).

Clinical features. Pain is the predominant symptom, but sometimes the tumour causes little disturbance until a pathological fracture occurs.

Treatment. The principles of treatment of metastatic tumours in bone were described on page 126. Most pathological fractures of the femur lend themselves well to internal fixation with a long modified intramedullary nail, though sometimes this requires the addition of acrylic bone cement to achieve stability (Fig. 18.6B). Where massive bone destruction has occurred in the proximal

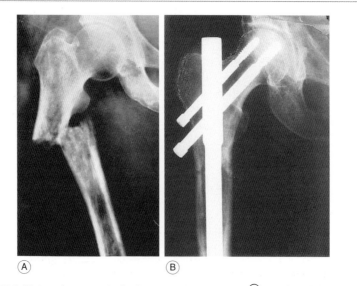

(A)   (B)

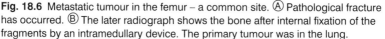

Fig. 18.6 Metastatic tumour in the femur – a common site. Ⓐ Pathological fracture has occurred. Ⓑ The later radiograph shows the bone after internal fixation of the fragments by an intramedullary device. The primary tumour was in the lung.

or distal femur, it may be necessary to replace this with a custom prosthesis. This facilitates nursing and greatly increases the quality of life because external splintage can be dispensed with and the patient mobilised.

ARTICULAR DISORDERS OF THE KNEE

PYOGENIC ARTHRITIS OF THE KNEE (General description of pyogenic arthritis, p. 96)

Pyogenic arthritis is commoner in the knee than in most other joints, partly because the knee is so exposed to injury and partly because of the close relationship of the joint cavity to the lower metaphysis of the femur, which is one of the commonest sites of acute osteomyelitis. The onset is acute or subacute, with pain, swelling, and loss of function. Radiographs do not show any abnormality in the early stages.

Treatment. Appropriate antibiotic therapy must be started immediately (see p. 98). Local treatment: The joint is rested in a plaster splint in a position of 20° of flexion. The purulent effusion is removed daily by aspiration so long as it re-forms or by arthrotomy. Rest is continued until the infection has been overcome; thereafter active movements are encouraged.

TUBERCULOUS ARTHRITIS OF THE KNEE (General description of tuberculous arthritis, p. 98)

After the hip, the knee is the limb joint most often affected by tuberculosis, usually in children or young adults. It is now an uncommon disease in Britain and other Western countries, though seen more often in developing countries and occasionally in immigrants to Britain. The knee is painful, diffusely swollen from thickening of the synovial membrane, and warm. Movements are restricted, the thigh muscles are wasted, and an abscess or sinus is sometimes apparent.

Radiographic features. The earliest change is diffuse rarefaction throughout the area of the knee (Fig. 18.7). Later, unless the disease is arrested, there is narrowing of the cartilage space and erosion of the underlying bone.

Treatment. Constitutional treatment, by antituberculous drugs, is the same as that for other tuberculous joints (p. 102). Local treatment is at first by rest in a splint or plaster, generally for two to three months in the first instance, depending on severity and progress. Subsequent management depends upon the response to treatment and the state of the joint at the end of this period of immobilisation. If the articular cartilage and bone are still intact, if the general health is good and the local signs have subsided, and if the erythrocyte sedimentation rate has steadily improved, it is likely that the disease has been aborted. In that event active joint movements are encouraged and walking is gradually resumed.

On the other hand, if the review at the end of the initial period of immobilisation shows that the disease is still active and that articular cartilage or bone has been destroyed, sound bony fusion should usually be the ultimate aim, though arthroplasty may sometimes be considered. Immobilisation is therefore continued until the disease becomes quiescent. Arthrodesis may then be undertaken, provided the growth epiphyses have closed. In children still growing it is better to defer arthrodesis lest growth be disturbed, and in the meantime to protect the knee in a walking caliper or splint.

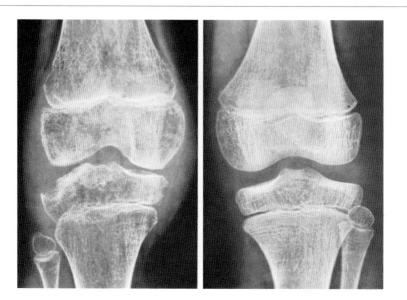

Fig. 18.7 Tuberculous arthritis of right knee in a child. The normal left knee is shown for comparison. Note the rarefaction, the diminution of cartilage space, and the small area of erosion near the lateral margin of the tibial joint surface. Destruction is only moderate, and a reasonably good result may be achieved with conservative treatment.

RHEUMATOID ARTHRITIS OF THE KNEE (General description of rheumatoid arthritis, p. 134)

The knees are among the joints most frequently affected by rheumatoid arthritis, and they often suffer severe permanent disability. Both knees are often affected simultaneously with several other joints.

The knees are painful, swollen from synovial thickening, and warm to the touch. Bow-leg, knock-knee, or flexion deformity may occur. Movement is impaired, and painful if forced.

Imaging. Radiographs do not show any abnormality at first. Later there is diffuse rarefaction of the bone in the area of the joint. In long-established cases destruction of articular cartilage leads to narrowing of the joint space (Fig. 18.8), and there may be clear-cut erosions of bone, characteristically at the articular margins. Radioisotope bone scanning shows increased uptake of isotope in the region of the joint.

Course and prognosis. The inflammation dies down after months or years, but the knee is seldom restored to normal. The joint surfaces are usually damaged and wear out sooner than those of a normal joint. Thus in the late stages osteoarthritis is liable to be superimposed upon the original rheumatoid condition.

Treatment. In the active stage the treatment is that for rheumatoid arthritis in general and requires coordinated care by a multi-disciplinary team (p. 137). Local treatment for the knees depends upon the severity of the inflammatory reaction. If it is severe, rest in bed or even temporary immobilisation with moulded plaster or polythene splints is advisable. When it is moderate or slight,

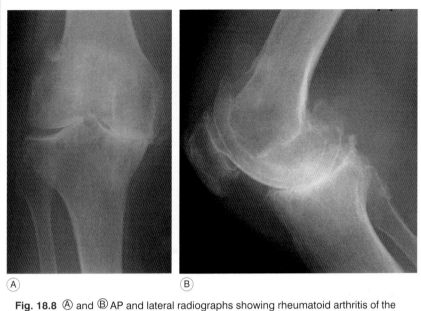

Fig. 18.8 Ⓐ and Ⓑ AP and lateral radiographs showing rheumatoid arthritis of the knee. The bone is porotic and there is complete loss of the medial joint space with irregularity of the articular surface indicating an underlying erosive process.

activity within the limits of pain is encouraged. Physical treatment is worth a trial. The most effective methods are exercises to preserve muscle power and joint movement, and local heat in the form of short-wave diathermy. Injections of hydrocortisone into the joint have sometimes given relief, but repeated injections are inadvisable because they may accelerate the destructive process.

Operative treatment. Three types of operation may be employed in treating more advanced stages of joint disease:

1. synovectomy
2. replacement arthroplasty
3. arthrodesis.

In deciding between them each case must be considered on its merits, and no hard-and-fast rules can be laid down.

Synovectomy. When there is persistent boggy thickening of the synovial membrane, but the articular cartilage is well preserved, the operation of synovectomy (excision of the synovial membrane) is worth considering. Comfort may be much improved and the advance of the disease is possibly slowed by the removal of the tissue producing the proinflammatory cytokines and enzymes responsible for cartilage destruction. This operation alone has no place in the later stages of the disease and is now used less frequently since the introduction of better drugs for the medical control of inflammatory disease.

Replacement arthroplasty. Replacement arthroplasty of the knee now gives as good results as have been achieved at the hip. Excellent and durable results are now being achieved in over 90 per cent of patients after ten years. In a favourable case pain is well relieved and good function is restored, with perhaps 90° or more of flexion movement. Replacement arthroplasty of the knee is particularly valuable for patients with severe disorganisation of the joint, and especially for elderly patients with involvement of several other joints.

Several techniques of knee arthroplasty are available: all of them rely upon replacement of the articular surfaces by a metal or plastic (polyethylene) prosthesis. Most of the earlier devices took the form of a hinge, but such devices are now seldom used because they do not mimic normal knee movement, and consequently there may be early implant loosening with bone destruction.

The present trend is to provide gliding articular surfaces rather than a pivoted hinge. Thus the femoral condyles may be replaced by a metal prosthesis cemented in place, and the tibial condyles by a matching polyethylene prosthesis, usually with a metal backing (total condylar replacement, Fig. 18.9A). When badly damaged, the patella may also be resurfaced with a matching polyethylene bearing. In unicompartmental arthritis, the medial or the lateral femoral condyle may be replaced alone (Fig. 18.9B). However, this is only suitable for osteoarthritis and in most cases of inflammatory arthritis, bicondylar replacement is preferred (Fig. 18.10). Many different types of total knee prosthesis are now available, including designs that incorporate artificial menisci, but medium-term results show no obvious advantages over the excellent results obtained with the original condylar replacements.

Arthrodesis. This is a reliable operation for the total abolition of pain and good stability, but it is appropriate only if the other joints of the lower limbs are healthy – a condition that is seldom met in rheumatoid disease. The joint is usually fused in about 20° or 25° of flexion, a position that is more convenient than the fully straight position, though a stiff knee is, of course, an awkward handicap.

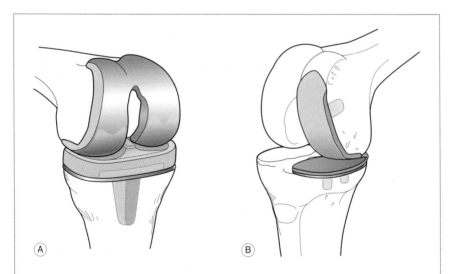

(A)   (B)

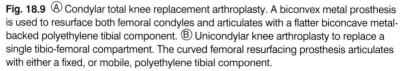

Fig. 18.9 Ⓐ Condylar total knee replacement arthroplasty. A biconvex metal prosthesis is used to resurface both femoral condyles and articulates with a flatter biconcave metal-backed polyethylene tibial component. Ⓑ Unicondylar knee arthroplasty to replace a single tibio-femoral compartment. The curved femoral resurfacing prosthesis articulates with either a fixed, or mobile, polyethylene tibial component.

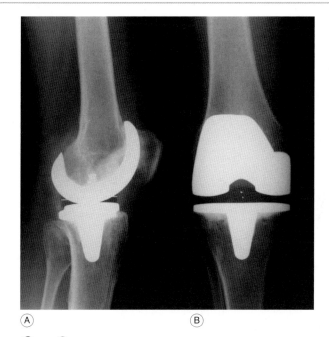

Fig. 18.10 Ⓐ and Ⓑ AP and lateral radiographs showing a total replacement arthroplasty of the knee. The metal prosthesis resurfacing both femoral condyles articulates with a polyethylene tibial prosthesis, which is not visible, but is supported by the metallic tibial stemmed implant.

OSTEOARTHRITIS OF THE KNEE (General description of osteoarthritis, p. 140)

The knee is affected by osteoarthritis more often than any other joint. The condition is particularly common in elderly, obese women.

Cause. It is caused by a degeneration of the articular cartilage of uncertain aetiology; but nearly always some factor is present that has caused the joint to wear out sooner than usual. Obesity is the commonest factor: for some reason it seems to impose a harmful stress upon the knee whereas it does not adversely affect the hip or ankle. Other important predisposing factors are: previous fracture causing irregularity of the joint surfaces; previous disease with damage to articular cartilage (especially old rheumatoid arthritis or infective arthritis); previous intra-articular mechanical damage, as from a torn meniscus or from osteochondritis dissecans; and mal-alignment of the tibia on the femur (as in long-established bow-leg or knock-knee deformity from any cause).

Pathology. The articular cartilage is worn away and the underlying bone becomes thickened and eburnated. There is hypertrophy of bone at the joint margins, with the formation of marginal osteophytes. The changes may affect predominantly the medial compartment of the femoro-tibial joint, or the patello-femoral joint; but usually the whole joint is affected.

The thigh and knee

Clinical features. The patient is commonly an elderly, heavy woman, in whom both knees may be affected. In another group, mostly in men, there is a history of previous mechanical derangement from a sports injury. There is slowly increasing aching pain in the joint, worse after unusual activity, and 'grating' may be felt or heard on movement. The symptoms are often exacerbated by a slight strain or twist. There is usually evidence of one of the predisposing factors mentioned above.

On examination the knee is slightly thickened from hypertrophy of bone at the joint margins, where a rim of osteophytes may be palpable. Effusion of fluid into the joint is unusual, except after much activity. Movement is moderately restricted and is accompanied by coarse crepitation. The quadriceps muscle is wasted. In severe cases there is a tendency to varus (bow-leg) deformity, less often a valgus (knock-knee) deformity, often with inability to straighten the knee fully.

Radiographic features. Narrowing of the cartilage space, which is the first sign of osteoarthritis in most joints, is often not discernible until a later stage in the case of the knee. An earlier sign in many cases is sharpening or 'spiking' of the joint margins, especially of the patella (Fig. 18.11) and tibia. Later, narrowing of the cartilage space is obvious, osteophytes form at the joint margins, and the subchondral bone may become sclerotic (Fig. 18.12). Opacities that appear to be loose bodies are often seen; most are not in fact loose but are attached to the synovial membrane.

Treatment. In the usual case of moderate severity, conservative treatment is often successful in relieving the symptoms, although the structural changes in the joint are clearly irreversible. The most effective method is by physiotherapy. Intensive active exercises are carried out to strengthen the wasted quadriceps muscle. Local heat therapy is often also given, but it is less important than the exercises. The knee is largely dependent upon the quadriceps for its stability, and if a powerful muscle can be developed symptoms may remain in abeyance despite a substantial degree of arthritis.

Intra-articular injections of hydrocortisone have been tried for pain relief, but the results are uncertain and any improvement is usually temporary. In general, steroid injections are not recommended because they have sometimes led to acceleration of the degenerative process. More recently injection of hyaluronan preparations has become popular, to provide viscosupplementation by increasing the viscosity of the synovial fluid, but the results have proved inconclusive.

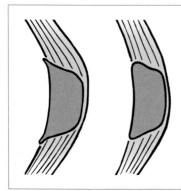

Fig. 18.11 Spiking of the articular margins of the patella, as seen in the lateral radiograph, is an early sign of osteoarthritis. The normal state (right) is shown for comparison.

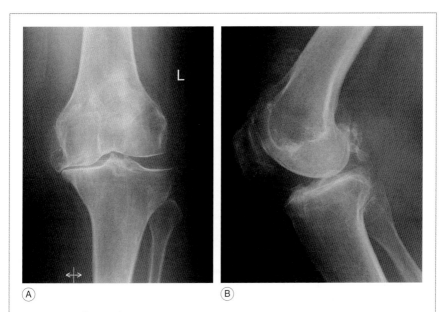

Fig. 18.12 Ⓐ and Ⓑ Radiographs of a knee with advanced osteoarthritis. There is marked narrowing of the medial joint space and the patello-femoral joint. However the bony cortex of tibia and femur remain clearly defined with subchondral sclerosis and numerous marginal osteophytes, some of which may have become loose bodies posteriorly.

Operative treatment. In advanced arthritis, with severe persistent pain, especially when associated with deformity and stiffness, operation may be advisable. Its nature will depend upon the circumstances of each case. The following are the operations most used:

1. arthroscopic washout
2. removal of loose bodies
3. upper tibial osteotomy
4. excision of patella
5. arthroplasty
6. arthrodesis.

Arthroscopic washout. Washout of the joint, often coupled with an arthroscopic debridement, has been used to treat early osteoarthritis in younger patients. However, its use in randomised controlled trials has indicated that its benefit may be doubtful and shortlasting.

Removal of loose bodies. When loose bodies cause recurrent locking of the joint they should be removed. This is a simple operation, usually carried out by an arthroscopic technique, that gives good results. Any evident irregularities or excrescences of the articular surfaces may be trimmed at the same time.

Upper tibial osteotomy. Tibial osteotomy aims to relieve pain and to correct deformity. It is especially valuable when wear of articular cartilage and bone has affected one half of the tibio-femoral joint more than the other. Commonly

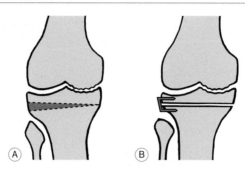

Fig. 18.13 Ⓐ Bow-leg deformity from uneven destruction of articular cartilage, that of the medial compartment being much thinner than that of the lateral. Body weight is now transmitted mainly through the diseased medial half of the joint. Interrupted line shows wedge of bone to be removed for correction of deformity. Ⓑ After corrective osteotomy and fixation with staples the line of weight transmission is shifted towards the more healthy lateral compartment.

the medial half of the joint is markedly narrowed whereas the lateral compartment remains relatively healthy. There will be obvious bow-leg deformity and pain is likely to be prominent in the degenerate medial compartment, which is forced by the mal-alignment to take most of the weight (Fig. 18.13A). Correction of the mal-alignment by removal of a wedge of bone based laterally (Fig. 18.13B) transfers the weight-bearing thrust towards the more healthy lateral compartment and is often effective in relieving pain. Likewise if the lateral compartment is worn more than the medial, with consequent genu valgum, a medially based wedge may be excised. The osteotomy is done about 1.5 cm below the upper articular surface of the tibia, and to permit early walking the fragments are usually fixed together at operation by metal staples (Fig. 18.13B).

Excision of patella. This is only appropriate in the unusual situation when the arthritic process is largely confined to the patello-femoral joint, the femoro-tibial joint being relatively healthy. With the introduction of successful techniques for patello-femoral arthroplasty this operation is now seldom performed.

Arthroplasty (see Fig. 18.10). This has now become established as the surgical treatment of choice for advanced osteoarthritis of the knee. It will correct deformity, relieve pain, and restore mobility in over 90% of patients, with results extending out for 10–15 years. Methods of replacement arthroplasty were outlined for the treatment of rheumatoid arthritis on page 392. Most commonly the same techniques of total replacement arthroplasty of both the tibio-femoral and patello-femoral joints are used in osteoarthritis. However, unicompartmental tibio-femoral arthroplasty is now being increasingly used as an alternative to upper tibial osteotomy in younger active patients to restore more movement when the arthritis is at an early stage and confined to one compartment. A curved metal prosthetic replacement is fixed to the affected femoral condyle and articulates with a polyethylene tibial component, either directly, or through a gliding polyethylene meniscal bearing to provide more physiological movement (Fig. 18.14). The results in appropriately selected cases are as good

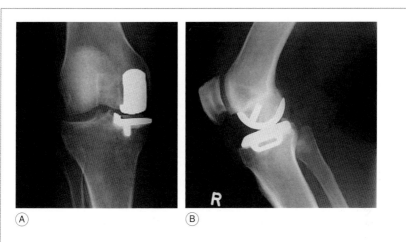

(A)   (B)

Fig. 18.14 Ⓐ and Ⓑ Radiographs of unicompartmental tibio-femoral arthroplasty with a metal resurfacing of one femoral condyle articulating with a polyethylene tibial prosthesis supported by a metal backing fixed to the bone.

as those from total joint replacement and still allow later revision to the full procedure if required at a later stage.

Arthrodesis. This is now seldom undertaken, but it may occasionally be appropriate in a severe case, or as a salvage procedure when other operations have failed and where the other knee and the hips are normal.

HAEMOPHILIC ARTHRITIS OF THE KNEE (General description of haemophilic arthritis, p. 145)

Haemophilic arthritis affects the knee more often than any other joint. It is uncommon because haemophilia itself is encountered only rather rarely.

Pathology. Initially there is simply a haemorrhage into the joint (haemarthrosis). With rest, this is slowly absorbed into the hypertrophic synovial membrane. But further bleeding usually occurs, and this leads eventually to degenerative changes in the articular cartilage and to fibrous thickening and contractures of the synovial membrane.

Clinical features. The findings on examination vary according to the phase and duration of the disease. After each fresh episode of bleeding the knee is swollen, partly from contained blood and partly from synovial thickening caused by interstitial extravasation of blood. The overlying skin is abnormally warm. Joint movements are restricted, and painful if forced.

In a quiescent phase between episodes of haemarthrosis there is some thickening of the joint from synovial fibrosis, movements are slightly or moderately impaired, and often there is moderate flexion deformity.

Investigations. The clotting time of the blood is increased.

Diagnosis. Because of the synovial thickening, increased warmth of the skin and restriction of knee movements, haemophilic arthritis is easily mistaken for chronic inflammatory arthritis. A history of previous bleeding incidents and the increased clotting time of the blood are the important distinguishing features. Biopsy should be avoided because it may cause further bleeding. A history of haemophilia in other male family members also provides a clue.

Treatment. In centres where the necessary haematological facilities are available the ideal treatment for acute haemarthrosis is to aspirate the knee under the temporary cover of antihaemophilic factor (factor VIII) as if it were an ordinary traumatic haemarthrosis. The leg should be elevated and ice packs should be applied to the knee, which should be rested in a polythene or plaster splint until the acute symptoms subside. With the increasing availability of recombinant factor VIII, many haemophilic patients retain their own supply at home and are able to initiate treatment by intravenous injection at the onset of symptoms of bleeding. This can be repeated for several days to manage the acute episode and reduce the need for hospital admission and delay the development of chronic joint changes. If antihaemophilic factor is not available the outlook for the future of the knee is much less favourable. Aspiration should usually be avoided. Instead, the knee should be bandaged and immobilised on a Thomas's splint or in a plaster backslab. After 2–4 weeks the residual blood is absorbed and cautious activity may be resumed under physiotherapy supervision.

The chronic degenerative arthritis that results from multiple repeated haemarthroses may have to be controlled by the permanent use of a polythene knee splint. Operative treatment to reduce this risk – such as arthroscopic synovectomy – is practicable, but only under the cover of adequate doses of antihaemophilic factor. When joint contractures or deformities develop, they may require tendon release or lengthening, or even corrective osteotomies. Advanced haemophiliac arthropathy (see Fig. 9.7, p. 147) may necessitate replacement arthroplasty of the joint to restore mobility. This is now possible under factor VIII cover, which needs to be continued for 2–3 weeks after surgery. The majority of patients get good results, but there is a greater risk of complications, particularly infection as many patients have acquired HIV from contaminated blood transfusions.

NEUROPATHIC ARTHRITIS OF THE KNEE (General description of neuropathic arthritis, p. 147)

Neuropathic arthritis (Charcot's osteoarthropathy) of the knee is now seen very seldom in Britain because of the rarity of tabes dorsalis, formerly the most prevalent underlying cause. Other occasional causes include denervation of the joint from a lesion of the cauda equina or from other neurological disease.

The pathological changes may be regarded as a much exaggerated form of osteoarthritis. The articular cartilage and parts of the underlying bone are worn away, but at the same time there is often considerable hypertrophy of bone at the joint margins. The ligaments become lax and the joint is unstable.

Clinically there is marked lateral laxity, often allowing severe bow-leg deformity. Pain is slight or absent.

Radiographs show marked destructive changes, usually with some new bone formation at the joint margins.

Treatment may be required if there is marked deformity or gross instability demanding some form of protective appliance (orthosis), such as a moulded plastic splint or a caliper. Arthrodesis is practicable but because of the absence of severe pain operation should usually be avoided.

ANTERIOR KNEE PAIN (Including chondromalacia of the patella)

Anterior knee pain is a generic term that almost certainly includes more than a single clinical entity. The non-specific nature of the label implies, correctly, that the pathogenesis of the pain is not always well understood. The clinical syndrome characteristically occurs in adolescents, especially girls, though it also affects athletes, particularly runners. The description that follows relates to one well-recognised type of lesion, namely chondromalacia of the patella. Similar symptoms may occur in the absence of demonstrable patellar changes, and their causation is often conjectural. Chondromalacia may represent part of a spectrum of conditions associated with patellar instability or malalignment. These also include the more severe disorders of recurrent or habitual dislocation (see p. 409).

Chondromalacia of the patella

In chondromalacia of the patella the cartilage of the articular surface of the patella – particularly the medial facet – is roughened and fibrillated for reasons that are unknown. It is surmised that friction between the damaged area and the corresponding femoral condyle is responsible for the pain. The condition is distinct from osteoarthritis but osteoarthritis may be superimposed upon it in later years.

Clinical features. The patient is often a girl aged 15–18 years. There is aching pain deep in the knee, behind the patella. Pain is exacerbated by climbing or descending stairs. There is often an effusion of fluid, and tenderness may be found on palpating the deep surface of the patella after displacing it to one side. There may also be a point of marked tenderness over the front of the medial femoral condyle. Movements may be accompanied by fine crepitation transmitted to the examiner's hand upon the patella, especially when the patient does a 'knees bend' exercise from the standing position.

Investigations. Radiographs are normal, though axial views are required to exclude lateral patellar tilt or subluxation. MRI scans may sometimes reveal defects or fissures in the articular cartilage of the patella, but this is not as reliable as direct visualisation by arthroscopy which will also demonstrate any associated synovial bands, if present.

Treatment. This should nearly always be non-operative. An elasticated bandage is applied and strenuous activities are curtailed. These precautions will usually reduce the symptoms to an acceptable level. Physiotherapy consisting of strapping the patella medially and strengthening the vastus medialis muscle can be of benefit. Operative treatment should be avoided unless significant patello-femoral malalignment is present, for although a variety of procedures has been devised the results are almost universally disappointing.

TEARS OF THE MENISCI

Injuries of the menisci (semilunar cartilages) are common in men under the age of 45. A tear is usually caused by a twisting force with the knee semiflexed or flexed. It is usually a football injury, but it is also common among men who work in a squatting position. Thus it was common among coal miners excavating shallow seams, before the advent of mechanisation. The medial meniscus is torn much more often than the lateral.

Pathology. In patients of athletic age there are three types of meniscus tear, but all begin as a longitudinal split (Fig. 18.15A) which must be distinguished from the iatrogenic transverse tear resulting from operative trauma (Fig. 18.15B). If the split extends throughout the length of the meniscus it becomes a bucket-handle tear, in which the fragments remain attached at both ends (Fig. 18.16A). This is much the commonest type. The 'bucket handle' (that is, the central fragment) is displaced towards the middle of the joint, so that the condyle of the femur rolls upon the tibia through the rent in the meniscus (Fig. 18.16A). Since the femoral condyle is so shaped that it requires most space when the knee is straight, the chief effect of a displaced 'bucket-handle' fragment is that it limits full extension (= 'locking').

If the initial longitudinal tear emerges at the concave border of the meniscus a pedunculated tag is formed. In posterior horn tear the fragment remains attached at its posterior horn (Fig. 18.16B); in anterior horn tear it remains attached at its anterior horn (Fig. 18.16C). The peripheral part of the meniscus is vascular and tears in the peripheral third can sometimes be sutured as they have some capacity for healing. The inner part is avascular and does not heal, tears in the inner third therefore need to be excised.

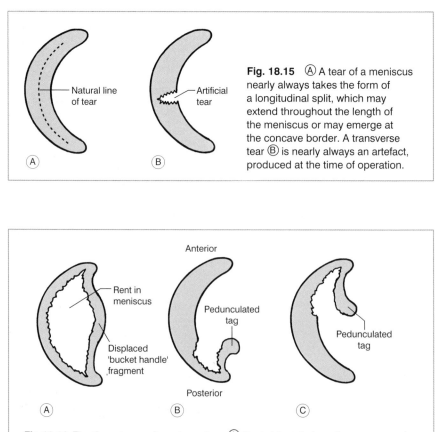

Fig. 18.15 Ⓐ A tear of a meniscus nearly always takes the form of a longitudinal split, which may extend throughout the length of the meniscus or may emerge at the concave border. A transverse tear Ⓑ is nearly always an artefact, produced at the time of operation.

Fig 18.16 The three types of meniscus tear. Ⓐ Bucket-handle tear, the commonest type. Ⓑ Posterior horn tear. Ⓒ Anterior horn tear.

As the inner parts of the meniscus are almost avascular, when they are torn there is not an effusion of blood into the joint. Instead there is an effusion of clear synovial fluid, secreted in response to the injury.

Clinical features of torn medial meniscus. The patient is usually male and 18–45 years old. The history is characteristic, especially with 'bucket-handle' tears. In consequence of a twisting injury the patient falls and has pain at the antero-medial aspect of the joint. He is unable to continue what he was doing, or does so only with difficulty. He is unable to straighten the knee fully. The next day he notices swelling of the whole knee. He rests the knee. After about 2 weeks the swelling lessens, the knee seems to go straight, and he resumes his activities. Within weeks or months the knee suddenly gives way again during a twisting movement; there are pain and subsequent swelling as before. Similar incidents occur repeatedly.

Locking. By 'locking' is meant inability to extend the knee fully. It is not a true jamming of the joint because there is a free range of flexion. Locking is a common feature of torn medial meniscus, but the limitation of extension is often so slight that it is not noticed by the patient. Persistent locking can occur only in 'bucket-handle' tears: tag tears cause momentary catching but not true locking in the accepted sense.

On examination in the recent stage the typical features are effusion of fluid, wasting of the quadriceps muscle, local tenderness at the level of the joint antero-medially, and (characteristically in 'bucket-handle' tears) limitation of the *last few degrees* of extension by a springy resistance, with sharp antero-medial pain if passive extension is forced.

In the 'silent' phase between attacks there are often no signs other than wasting of the quadriceps.

Clinical features of torn lateral meniscus. The features are broadly similar, but the clinical picture is often less clearly defined. The history may be vague. Pain is at the lateral rather than the medial side of the joint, Instead it is often poorly localised.

Imaging. Plain radiographs are usually normal, whether the tear be of the medial or of the lateral meniscus, but in untreated cases of long duration signs of early degenerative arthritis may be noted in the affected compartment. Arthrography will often demonstrate meniscal tears, but it is now seldom undertaken because MRI is even more reliable in demonstrating the various types of tear and is non-invasive (Fig. 18.17).

Arthroscopy. On arthroscopic examination a meniscal tear can be seen whatever its site, except sometimes at the posterior end of the lateral meniscus (Fig. 18.18).

Diagnosis. In the 'silent' phase clinical diagnosis often depends largely upon the history. The surgeon should be very cautious in diagnosing a torn meniscus unless there is a clear history of injury and unless there have been recurrent incidents, each followed by synovial effusion. If one is relying on clinical diagnosis alone a period of observation may be required before the diagnosis becomes reasonably certain. MRI, or arthroscopy if this is not available, should establish the nature of the lesion conclusively.

Late effects. Long-continued internal derangement from a torn meniscus predisposes to the later development of degenerative arthritis. Arthritis is also liable to develop many years after a meniscus has been removed.

Treatment. Once the diagnosis is established the standard treatment is to excise either the whole meniscus or, more appropriately in most cases, the

The thigh and knee

The thigh and knee

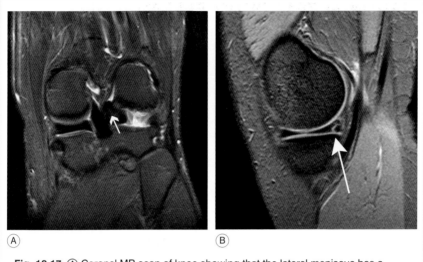

(A)   (B)

Fig. 18.17 (A) Coronal MR scan of knee showing that the lateral meniscus has a bucket handle tear with a large meniscal fragment displaced centrally into the joint (arrow). (B) Sagittal T2 weighted MR scan of the knee with a vertical tear of the posterior horn of the medial meniscus (arrow).

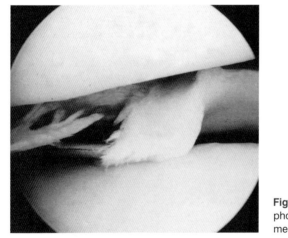

Fig. 18.18 Arthroscopic photograph showing tear of medial meniscus.

displaced 'bucket-handle' fragment alone. This operation is usually best carried out by the arthroscopic technique without formal opening of the joint – though of course the joint may be opened by incision if difficulty arises during the course of arthroscopic surgery. In selected cases of peripheral tear, repair by suture is sometimes undertaken using a semi-closed arthroscopic technique.

HORIZONTAL TEAR OF DEGENERATE MEDIAL MENISCUS

The meniscal tears described above are uncommon in patients over the age of 50, when the menisci begin to show degenerative changes. But a degenerate meniscus is liable to suffer a different type of lesion. The medial meniscus in particular may split horizontally at a point often near the middle of its convexity (Fig. 18.19). Such a split is usually of small dimensions, and since there is no separation of the fragments natural healing can occur.

Clinically there is troublesome and persistent pain at the medial aspect of the knee at the joint level. The pain may be noticed after a minor injury, but often an injury has not been remembered. In the early stages there is usually a small effusion of fluid into the joint.

Treatment should be expectant at first, by bandaging and quadriceps exercises. In most cases the symptoms resolve in the course of several months. In the occasional case in which they fail to do so, excision of the torn meniscal fragment by arthroscopic surgery should be advised.

CYSTS OF THE MENISCI

A cyst of a meniscus (semilunar cartilage) forms a tense, almost solid swelling at the level of the joint, usually on the lateral side.

Cause. Cysts arise spontaneously, but there is often a previous history of direct injury at the site of the cyst.

Pathology. The swelling is formed by a proliferation of fibrous tissue, which is honeycombed with small cystic cavities containing small quantities of clear gelatinous fluid.

Clinical features. The lateral meniscus is affected much more often than the medial. There is visible swelling, most obvious when the knee is held slightly flexed, at the level of the joint and usually anterior to the lateral (or medial) ligament (Fig. 18.20). The swelling tends to be painful at night and it is usually tender on firm pressure. The swelling is so tense that fluctuation can seldom be elicited – indeed it is sometimes mistaken for bone.

Imaging. Radiographs may show an indentation of the side of the tibial condyle where the cyst has been in contact with it. MRI scanning will confirm the origin of the cyst from the meniscus (Fig. 18.21) and exclude more serious soft-tissue tumours.

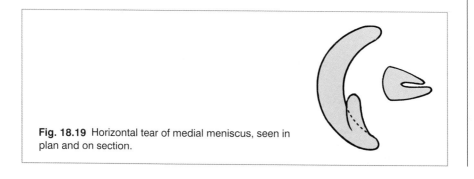

Fig. 18.19 Horizontal tear of medial meniscus, seen in plan and on section.

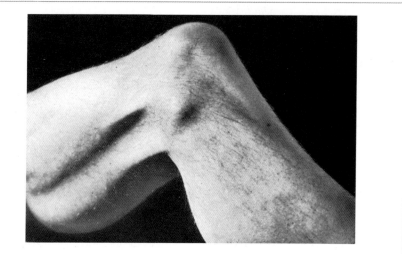

Fig. 18.20 Cyst of lateral meniscus.

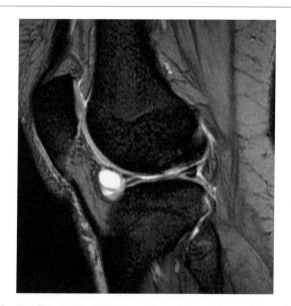

Fig. 18.21 Sagittal T2 weighted MR scan of knee. There is a cyst lying adjacent to the anterior horn of the lateral meniscus. The adjacent meniscus has a horizontal tear. Meniscal cysts are always associated with a meniscal tear.

Treatment. If the disability justifies operation the cyst should be excised together with the meniscus from which it arises. Very occasionally, it may be practicable to excise the cyst arthroscopically while leaving the meniscus intact.

DISCOID LATERAL MENISCUS

Rarely the lateral meniscus (semilunar cartilage) fails to assume its normal crescentic form during development, but persists in its embryonic form as a thick disc-like mass interposed between the lateral condyles of the femur and tibia.

A discoid meniscus may cause recurrent discomfort in the knee, with a tendency to giving way. Usually a loud 'clonk' can be demonstrated on flexion–extension movements. These symptoms often become prominent during childhood or adolescence. If the disability becomes troublesome the meniscus should be removed. There is a risk of the development of degenerative arthritis in later life.

OSTEOCHONDRITIS DISSECANS OF THE KNEE (General description of osteochondritis dissecans, p. 153)

Osteochondritis dissecans is characterised by local ischaemic necrosis of a segment of the articular surface of a bone and of the overlying articular cartilage, with eventual separation of the fragment to form an intra-articular loose body. The knee is affected much more often than any other joint.

Cause. This is unknown. Impairment of the blood supply to the affected segment of bone by thrombosis of an end artery has been suggested. Injury is possibly a predisposing factor. There is also a constitutional predisposition to the disease, because it may affect several members of a family or several joints in the same patient.

Pathology. The lesion nearly always affects the articular surface of the medial condyle of the femur (Fig. 18.22). The size of the affected segment varies – it is often about 2 cm in diameter. Within the area of the lesion the subchondral bone is avascular and the overlying cartilage softens. A clear line of demarcation

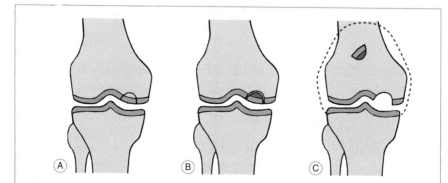

Fig. 18.22 The evolution of osteochondritis dissecans. Ⓐ A segment of the articular surface dies. Ⓑ A line of demarcation forms around it. Ⓒ The fragment breaks away and lies loose in the joint, leaving a cavity in the femoral condyle.

forms between the avascular segment and the surrounding normal bone and cartilage (Fig. 18.22A). After many months the fragment separates as a loose body (sometimes two or three), leaving a shallow cavity in the articular surface which is ultimately filled with fibrocartilage (Fig. 18.22B&C). The damage to the joint surface predisposes to the later development of osteoarthritis, especially when the fragment is large.

Clinical features. The patient is an adolescent or a young adult, who complains of discomfort or pain in the knee after exercise, a feeling of insecurity, and intermittent swelling. The condition is commoner in males and may affect both knees in 15–20% of patients. When a loose body has already separated within the joint the predominant symptom is recurrent sudden locking. On examination there is a fluid effusion. The quadriceps muscle is wasted. Movements are not usually impaired.

Imaging. Radiographs show a clear-cut defect of the bone at the articular surface of the medial femoral condyle (Fig. 18.23). At first the cavity is occupied by the separating fragment of bone; but later the cavity may be empty, and a loose body will then be seen elsewhere in the joint. The lesion is shown best in tangential postero-anterior projections with the knee semiflexed (Fig. 18.23B). The advent of MRI has provided more valuable information on the state of the overlying articular cartilage and whether this is healing or liable to separate (Fig. 18.24).

Arthroscopy. The osteochondritic lesion in the medial femoral condyle will be clearly evident in the later stages. Initially, however, the defect is concealed by articular cartilage that looks normal, though if it is probed an area of softening may be apparent.

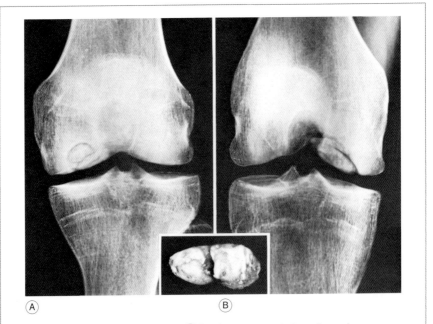

(A) (B)

Fig. 18.23 Osteochondritis dissecans. Ⓐ Routine antero-posterior radiograph. Ⓑ Tangential postero-anterior projection with knee semiflexed – the so-called intercondylar view. This shows clearly the large crescentic cavity in the medial femoral condyle, with the separating fragment in situ. Inset shows the loose fragment after removal.

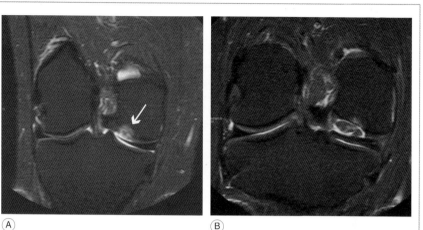

Fig. 18.24 Ⓐ Coronal MR scan of knee showing early osteochondritis dissecans. The arrow points to a defect of the cortex of the medial femoral condyle, which is the commonest site for this condition. Ⓑ Coronal MR scan of knee. In this case the area of osteochondritis has become separated from the underlying bone and can potentially become displaced forming an intra-articular loose body.

Treatment. In the developing stage treatment should be expectant: the knee is supported with a crepe bandage and strenuous activities are curtailed. Sometimes in these early cases the lesion will heal spontaneously, especially in young adolescents, and can be monitored by repeat MRI.

When the lesion shows a clear line of demarcation between the separating fragment and the surrounding normal bone – the loose piece should usually be removed, especially if it is small. This may be done arthroscopically. A shallow cavity is left in the femoral condyle, but this gradually fills with fibrocartilage and adequate function is usually restored.

Because of the risk of the later development of osteoarthritis if a large part of the femoral condyle has been excavated, some surgeons recommend that the loose fragment be replaced in position and fixed with a pin or pins. It has been shown that the fragment may unite again with its bed, but it is by no means certain yet that the incidence of late osteoarthritis will be reduced by this method of treatment. Attempts are now being made to use chondrocyte or osteochondral grafting of the defect for cases in which the separated fragment is large, but as yet the long-term results are uncertain.

LOOSE BODIES IN THE KNEE

The knee is the joint most commonly affected by the formation of loose bodies. There are four main causes:

1. osteochondritis dissecans (1–3 loose bodies)
2. osteoarthritis (1–10 loose bodies)
3. hip fracture of a joint surface (1–3 loose bodies)
4. synovial chondromatosis (up to 500 loose bodies).

Pathology. *Osteochondritis dissecans* was described on page 153. A loose body may be formed by spontaneous separation of a fragment of bone and cartilage from the articular surface of the medial femoral condyle. The loose body lies free in the joint, and a shallow cavity remains in the condyle.

Osteoarthritis was described on page 393. Some of the loose bodies that may be found in osteoarthritis are probably formed by detachment of marginal osteophytes. Most separated osteophytes, however, retain a synovial attachment and do not cause trouble: although they appear loose in radiographs they should not be regarded as such unless symptoms of locking indicate that they are moving freely within the joint. True loose bodies may possibly form from flakes of articular cartilage shed into the joint that gradually enlarge, nourished by synovial fluid.

Chip fracture of joint surface (osteochondral fracture) is an infrequent cause of intra-articular loose bodies. There is a clear history of the causative injury. A flake of bone with overlying articular cartilage is detached, always from a convex surface.

Synovial chondromatosis (osteochondromatosis) is a rare disease of the synovial membrane (p. 152). It is characterised by the formation of numerous small villous processes, which become pedunculated. Later their bulbous extremities become cartilaginous and they are detached to lie free in the joint. Finally, some or all of the numerous loose bodies become calcified.

Whatever the cause of a loose body, its repeated jamming between the joint surfaces will predispose to osteoarthritis after a long latent period, or will aggravate existing osteoarthritis.

Clinical features. The characteristic symptom of a loose body in the knee is recurrent locking of the joint from interposition of the loose piece between the joint surfaces. Suddenly, without warning, the knee becomes jammed during movement. Locking is accompanied by severe pain. After a variable interval the patient is usually able, by manoeuvring the limb, to disengage the loose body and free the joint. The next day the knee is found to be swollen with fluid. In many cases the patient is able to feel the mobile body through the soft tissues when it lies in a superficial part of the joint. It is common for such a body to lodge in the suprapatellar pouch.

On examination the findings are often slight, for a patient is seldom seen when the knee is locked. If he is seen soon afterwards a fluid effusion is present. Between attacks there may be no objective signs other than perhaps slight wasting of the quadriceps. Sometimes the loose body can be palpated, especially if it has migrated to the suprapatellar pouch. The features of an underlying condition such as osteoarthritis may be present.

Radiographic features. With few exceptions, loose bodies are shown radiographically. They often lie in the suprapatellar pouch (Fig. 18.25A). Care should be taken not to mistake the fabella (a seasmoid bone in the lateral head of the gastrocnemius) (Fig. 18.25B) for a loose body. The position of the fabella is constant: it lies slightly above the level of the joint well behind the femur and towards the lateral side, and it is always oval in shape with its long axis vertical.

Treatment. In general the treatment for an intra-articular loose body is to remove it, when possible by an arthroscopic technique. Removal should always be advised if the loose body is causing recurrent locking. If there are no symptoms of locking operation is not essential. In such cases the fragment, though appearing loose in the radiographs, is often attached to the synovial membrane and is kept out of harm's way. This applies particularly to detached osteophytes in cases of osteoarthritis.

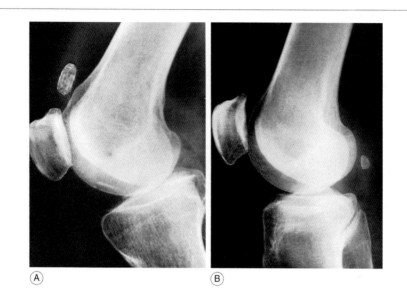

Ⓐ   Ⓑ

Fig. 18.25 Ⓐ Loose body in the knee. As in this case, loose bodies often lie in the suprapatellar pouch. Ⓑ The fabella, a sesamoid bone in the lateral head of the gastrocnemius, is present in many normal persons. It is sometimes mistaken for a loose body in the joint.

RECURRENT DISLOCATION OF THE PATELLA

The patello-femoral joint is one of the three joints that are most liable to recurrent displacement, the others being the shoulder and the ankle. In the case of the patello-femoral joint, unlike the other two, the instability is often caused by congenital factors rather than by an initial violent injury.

Pathological anatomy. In dislocations of the patella the displacement is always lateral, the patella slipping over the lateral condyle of the femur while the knee is flexed. Four factors, all of which may be inborn, predispose to recurrent dislocation:

1. general ligamentous laxity ('double-jointedness'), which may be an inherited defect of soft tissues
2. under-development of the lateral femoral condyle, with a shallow intercondylar groove
3. an abnormally high position of the patella (patella alta), which consequently does not lie so deeply as usual in the intercondylar groove and is often smaller than normal
4. genu valgum, which causes the line of pull of the quadriceps to lie too far to the lateral side.

This last factor is seldom an important one.

Clinical features. Recurrent dislocation of the patella is more common in girls than in boys. Often both knees are affected. Trouble usually begins during adolescence. Dislocation occurs while the patient is engaged in some activity that entails flexing the knees – not necessarily a violent exertion. Suddenly, while the knee is flexed or semiflexed, there is severe pain in the front of the knee, and the patient is unable to straighten it. Often the displacement of the patella is recognised and reduced on the spot, either by the patient herself or by an onlooker.

On examination in the dislocated state the knee is swollen, and the patella is seen and felt upon the lateral side of the lateral femoral condyle. After reduction the main signs are an effusion of fluid (usually blood-stained), and tenderness over the medial part of the quadriceps expansion, which is usually strained or torn. One of the minor anatomical anomalies mentioned above may be observed. In particular, generalised ligamentous laxity is often found, as evidenced by the patient's ability to hyperextend the knee (genu recurvatum) or other joints such as the wrists or the joints of the fingers and thumb; this double-jointedness may be present also in parents or other relatives. The patella is often found to lie higher than normal, and it may be unduly small.

Imaging. Radiographs are seldom obtained in the state of dislocation. After reduction the knee may appear normal radiographically, but commonly the patella is small and is seen at a slightly higher level than usual, often in both knees ('patella alta').

MRI scans may be more informative and may demonstrate damage to the articular surface of the patella and any defects or tears in the medial soft-tissue structures (Fig. 18.26).

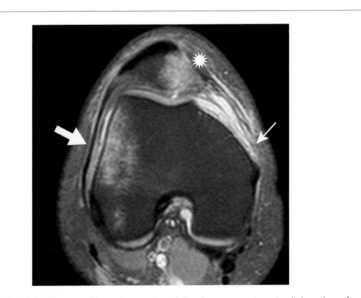

Fig. 18.26 Axial MR scan of knee in a patient following a recent acute dislocation of the patella. The large arrow indicates bone oedema where the patella has struck the condyle at the moment of dislocation. The star indicates the reciprocal bone oedema seen within the medial patellar facet. The small arrow indicates disruption of the medial patello-femoral ligament.

Course. Dislocation of the patella does not always become recurrent: some patients have no further trouble after an initial dislocation. But in most cases dislocations recur with ever-increasing ease and frequency, so that the patient may become seriously handicapped. Oft-repeated dislocations predispose to the later development of osteoarthritis.

Treatment. Treatment should be expectant at first. After a dislocation the patient should receive a course of physiotherapy designed to strengthen the quadriceps muscle, and especially the vastus medialis.

If the dislocations recur with such frequency that the patient is seriously disabled, operation should be advised. The method often recommended is to detach the bony insertion of the patellar tendon and transpose it to a new bed in the tibia, medial and distal to the original insertion (Fig. 18.27). In this way the patella is drawn lower into the deeper part of the intercondylar groove of the femur, and the line of pull of the quadriceps mechanism is transferred more to the medial side. This operation is often criticised on the grounds that it may be followed, after an interval of many years, by the development of degenerative arthritis. But such arthritis is an in-built complication of recurrent dislocation of the patella and cannot be ascribed solely to the operation. Other operations include release of tight soft tissues at the lateral side of the joint, reefing of the quadriceps expansion, and repair of the soft tissues on the medial side.

Habitual dislocation

It is important to distinguish between recurrent dislocation of the patella and habitual dislocation. Whereas in recurrent dislocation the knee may seem normal for weeks or months between dislocations, in habitual dislocation the patella dislocates laterally each time the knee is flexed beyond a certain range. This condition becomes apparent at an earlier age than recurrent dislocation – usually in early childhood. The underlying pathology is also distinct: there is an abnormality of the quadriceps muscle and in particular of the vastus lateralis, which may show a fibrous contracture; or there may be an abnormal fibrous band tethering the vastus lateralis to the ilio-tibial tract. It is this shortened vastus lateralis that pulls the patella laterally every time the knee is markedly flexed. In the absence of treatment the patella may eventually become permanently dislocated.

Treatment is by division of the tight muscle or band, by arthroscopy or open operation, so far as is necessary to allow full flexion of the knee without displacement of the patella.

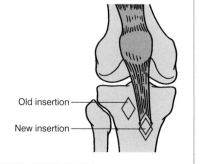

Fig. 18.27 Transposition of the insertion of the patellar tendon downwards and medially re-aligns the pull of the quadriceps and draws the patella down to lie in the intercondylar groove of the femur.

Old insertion

New insertion

EXTRA-ARTICULAR DISORDERS IN THE REGION OF THE KNEE

GENU VARUM AND GENU VALGUM

Genu varum (bow leg) and genu valgum (knock knee) occur commonly in childhood. In the vast majority of instances there is no underlying disease, and the deformity need not cause anxiety because it is gradually corrected spontaneously as the child grows.

Genu varum or genu valgum may also occur, either in children or in adults, as a consequence of injury or disease. The commonest causes are:

1. fracture of the lower part of the femur or of the upper part of the tibia with mal-union (for example, depressed fracture of the lateral tibial condyle causing genu valgum)
2. rheumatoid arthritis or osteoarthritis
3. rarefying diseases of the bones, such as rickets or osteomalacia
4. other bone-softening diseases such as Paget's disease (osteitis deformans) (see Fig. 6.5, p. 67)
5. in children, uneven growth of the epiphysial plates, such as may occur after injury or osteomyelitis or in dyschondroplasia (p. 65).

In assessing a case of genu varum or genu valgum the surgeon must always be careful to exclude such underlying organic disorders by full clinical examination, and if necessary by radiography, before diagnosing the benign childhood affections described in the following sections.

Benign genu varum of toddlers

The knee and leg are bowed outwards (Fig. 18.28A). A mild degree of this deformity is so common as to be almost normal in children aged 1 to 3 years. It does not require treatment unless it persists into later childhood. Care should be taken to exclude the possibility of rickets or other underlying bone disease.

Benign genu valgum of childhood

The knee is angled inwards, the tibia being abducted in relation to the femur. With the knees straight, the medial malleoli cannot be brought into contact (Fig. 18.28B). The 'knock-knee' deformity is common in children aged 3 to 5 years. In the absence of underlying bone disease it usually corrects itself spontaneously in the course of years.

Treatment. In early childhood treatment is unnecessary, but it is common practice (albeit of doubtful relevance) to fit a wedge, base medially and 3–5 millimetres deep, to the heel of the shoe. In theory this tends to shift the line of weight-bearing medially, which in turn favours correction of the deformity (see Fig. 19.20).

Severe genu valgum persisting after the age of 10 requires active treatment. In growing children two methods of correction are available. One is to retard the growth at the medial side of the epiphysial cartilage of the femur or tibia by bridging the epiphysis to the diaphysis with metal staples (epiphysiodesis). The other and more certain method is by supracondylar osteotomy of the

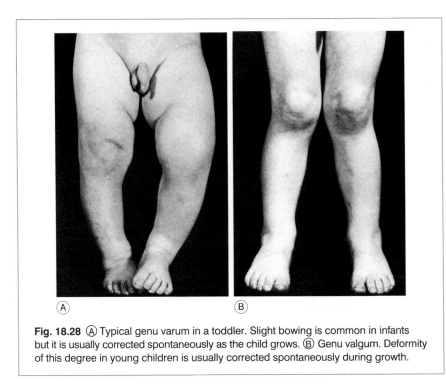

Fig. 18.28 Ⓐ Typical genu varum in a toddler. Slight bowing is common in infants but it is usually corrected spontaneously as the child grows. Ⓑ Genu valgum. Deformity of this degree in young children is usually corrected spontaneously during growth.

femur – or of the upper end of the tibia if the fault lies there – with excision of a suitable wedge from the medial side. After the cessation of epiphysial growth genu valgum can be corrected only by osteotomy.

RUPTURE OF THE QUADRICEPS APPARATUS

The quadriceps muscle gains insertion into the tibia through the medium of the patella (enclosed within the quadriceps expansion) and the patellar tendon. Complete rupture may occur at three points (Fig. 18.29):

1. at the point of attachment of the quadriceps tendon to the upper pole of the patella
2. through the patella and the surrounding quadriceps expansion (fractured patella)
3. at the attachment of the patellar tendon to the tibial tubercle.

In all cases the injury is caused by an unexpected flexion force, resisted automatically by a sudden contraction of the quadriceps.

Avulsion from patella

Avulsion of the quadriceps tendon from the upper pole of the patella occurs mainly in elderly men, in whom the quadriceps tendon is often degenerate. It is not a common injury. The clinical diagnosis is seldom in doubt, but can be confirmed by ultrasound or MR scanning (Fig. 18.30). The tendon should be re-attached to the bone by strong non-absorbable sutures passed through drill holes near the upper border of the patella.

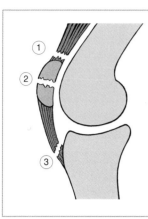

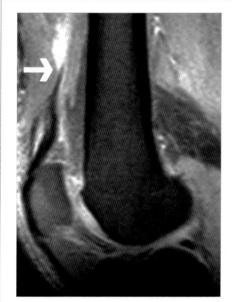

Fig. 18.29 The three points at which the quadriceps apparatus may rupture. 1. At insertion of quadriceps into patella. 2. Through the patella. 3. At insertion of patellar tendon into tibial tubercle.

Fig. 18.30 Sagittal T2 weighted MR scan of knee showing a degenerate tear of the quadriceps tendon (arrow).

Disruption through patella

This is the usual site of rupture, and it forms a common variety of fractured patella. The injury occurs mainly in adults of middle age. If the patella is cleanly broken into two pieces the fragments should be fixed together by a screw or cerclage wiring, with reinforcing sutures through the torn soft tissues on either side of the patella. If there are multiple patellar fragments, these should be excised and the quadriceps expansion repaired by sutures.

Avulsion at tibial tubercle

This is the least common injury, occurring mainly in children or young adults. A fragment of bone may be pulled off with the tendon. The torn tendon should be re-attached by sutures.

APOPHYSITIS OF THE TIBIAL TUBERCLE (Osgood–Schlatter's disease[1])

Apophysitis of the tibial tubercle is a childhood affection in which the tibial tubercle becomes enlarged and temporarily painful. Often known as Osgood–Schlatter's disease, it was formerly regarded as an example of osteochondritis juvenilis (p. 130), but it is now generally agreed that it is nothing more than a strain of the developing tibial tubercle, from the pull of the patellar tendon.

Clinical and radiographic features. The patient is a child or adolescent aged 10 to 16 years, usually a boy, and often active in athletic pursuits. The complaint is of pain in front of and below the knee, worse on strenuous activity. On examination the tibial tubercle is unduly prominent, and tender on palpation. Pain is increased when the quadriceps is tensed, as in raising the leg against resistance with the knee held straight. The symptoms and signs are confined to the region of the tibial tubercle, and the knee joint itself is normal.

Radiographs show enlargement and sometimes fragmentation of the tibial tubercle (Fig. 18.31).

Course. The disorder is usually self-limiting, and normal function is almost always restored by the time the apophysis of the tibial tubercle is fused to the main body of the bone.

Treatment. In most cases treatment is not required. If local pain and tenderness are severe and the symptoms persist into late adolescence, it may be necessary to rest the knee for a few weeks in an extension brace.

PREPATELLAR BURSITIS

The bursa that lies in front of the lower half of the patella and the upper part of the patellar tendon is prone to inflammation.

Types. There are two types of prepatellar bursitis:

1. irritative
2. infective or suppurative.

Irritative prepatellar bursitis

This is caused by repeated friction; it occurs especially in those who do much kneeling ('housemaid's knee'). There is fibrous thickening of the wall of the bursa, which is distended with fluid.

---

[1]Robert Osgood (1873–1956) was a famous American orthopaedic surgeon, but was working as a radiologist in Boston Children's Hospital when he described the condition in 1903. He worked with Robert Jones in England during the First World War and helped him found the British Orthopaedic Association.
Carl Schlatter (1864–1934) was a Swiss general surgeon who also reported the condition in 1903, he later became Professor of Surgery in Zurich in 1924.

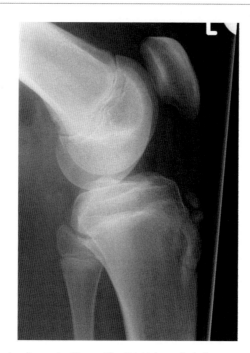

Fig. 18.31 Lateral radiograph of knee. The tibial tuberosity is fragmented. The normal appearance of the tibial tuberosity in adolescents is very variable. Diagnosis of Osgood–Schlatter's syndrome is principally clinical based on localised pain and tenderness. Many patients with radiographs similar to this are asymptomatic.

Clinical features. There is a softly fluctuant swelling in front of the lower part of the patella, which is clearly demarcated. It is manifestly confined to a plane in front of the joint, and the joint itself is unaffected.

Treatment. A trial may be made of aspiration under local anaesthesia, but the effusion tends to recur unless further friction can be avoided. The risk of recurrence may possibly be reduced if hydrocortisone is injected into the emptied sac. Operative excision of the bursa affords a more certain permanent cure.

Suppurative prepatellar bursitis

This is caused by infection of the bursa with pyogenic organisms, which reach the bursa directly through a puncture wound, or through the lymphatics from an infected lesion on the leg. The wall of the bursa is acutely inflamed and the sac is distended with pus.

Clinical features. There are pain and swelling in front of the knee. There may be mild constitutional disturbance, with pyrexia. The swelling is confined to the site of the prepatellar bursa. It is acutely tender on palpation, and the overlying skin is hot and reddened. The inguinal lymphatic glands are often enlarged and tender. The knee joint itself is unaffected, but the patient is unwilling to bend it fully because flexion increases the pain by tensing the skin over the bursa.

Treatment. Appropriate antibiotic therapy should be instituted and the bursal abscess should be drained by incision.

POPLITEAL CYSTS

Cystic swellings are not infrequently found in the popliteal fossa. Most are examples of irritative bursitis, usually of the semimembranosus bursa. A few are caused by herniation of the synovial cavity of the knee (Baker's cyst). Care must be taken to distinguish popliteal cysts from other, more serious swellings in this region, such as aneurysm of the popliteal artery and synovial sarcoma. This can be achieved by appropriate imaging using ultrasound or MRI scans.

Semimembranosus bursitis

The semimembranosus bursa lies between the medial head of the gastrocnemius and the semimembranosus. The bursa may become distended with fluid to form an elongated sac that bulges backwards between the muscle planes. Clinically, there is a soft cystic swelling at the back of the knee, close to the medial condyle of the femur.

Treatment is not always required. In children particularly, operation may usually be avoided because the cyst may disappear spontaneously. Nevertheless if the swelling becomes uncomfortably large, especially in an adult, the sac should be excised and then sent for routine histological examination to confirm the diagnosis.

Baker's cyst[1]

A Baker's cyst is simply a herniation of the synovial cavity of the knee, with the formation of a fluid-filled sac extending backwards and downwards (Fig. 18.32A). It is not a primary condition but is always secondary to a disorder of the knee with persistent synovial effusion, such as rheumatoid arthritis or osteoarthritis. In long-standing cases the hernial sac is much elongated, and may extend a considerable distance down the calf. Occasionally this may rupture and the resultant pain and local tenderness may be mistaken for a deep vein thrombosis.

Clinically there is a soft cystic bulge near the midline behind the knee or in the upper calf. The underlying abnormality of the knee, with synovial effusion, will usually be obvious.

Imaging. Where there is any uncertainty as to the diagnosis, it may be necessary to use ultrasound or MRI scanning to establish the nature and extent of the lesion (Fig. 18.32B).

Treatment. In most cases treatment should be directed towards the underlying condition of the knee rather than to the cyst itself. Nevertheless if the cyst is extensive it is sometimes advisable to excise it, with routine histological examination of the removed sac to confirm the diagnosis.

---

[1]William Morrant Baker (1839–1896) was a surgeon at St. Bartholomew's Hospital, London and first described synovial cysts connected to joints in 1877. He also invented the rubber tracheostomy tube.

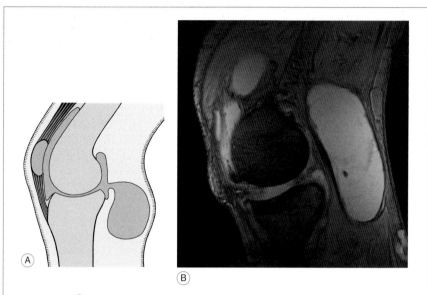

Fig. 18.32 Ⓐ To show how a Baker's cyst is formed as a herniation of the synovial membrane. Ⓑ Sagittal T2 weighted MR scan of knee showing the typical appearance of a large popliteal or Baker's cyst. The large high-signal lesion in the popliteal fossa is often associated with extensive degenerative changes in the knee joint, as seen here.

PELLEGRINI–STIEDA'S DISEASE[1]

Pellegrini–Stieda's disease is the name sometimes used to describe ossification in the subligamentous haematoma after partial avulsion of the medial ligament from the medial condyle of the femur. Clinically there is persistent discomfort at the medial side of the knee after an injury to the medial ligament. There are thickening and slight tenderness over the site of attachment of the ligament to the medial femoral condyle. Radiographs show a thin plaque of new bone close to the medial condyle.

Treatment is by active mobilising and muscle-strengthening exercises.

Calcified deposit in medial ligament

It is probable that some supposed cases of Pellegrini–Stieda's disease are in fact examples of calcified deposit within the medial ligament. A similar deposit may occur in the lateral ligament. These lesions are homologous with the calcified deposit that occurs more commonly in the supraspinatus tendon at the shoulder (p. 269). If the symptoms are acute the calcified material should be removed by aspiration or by operation. A steroid injection may also be of benefit in some patients.

[1]Augusto Pellegrini (1877–1958), who was Professor of Surgery in Florence and later Perugia, described post-traumatic ossification of knee ligaments in 1905. He was also a pioneer in the development of powered prostheses for the upper limb.
Alfred Stieda (1869–1945) was a German surgeon and Professor in Konigsberg who also reported the condition in 1905.

EXTRINSIC DISORDERS WITH REFERRED SYMPTOMS IN THE KNEE

From time to time patients are seen whose main complaint is of pain in the knee, but local examination reveals no satisfactory explanation for it. In such cases the possibility that the pain is referred from a disorder distant from the knee should always be considered. The commonest source of such referred pain is a disorder of the hip, particularly a slipped capital femoral epiphysis in children or osteoarthritis in the adult. Much less often a disorder of the spine is responsible, though referred pain to the leg from pressure of prolapsed disc material on lumbo-sacral nerve roots may sometimes cause confusion.

The thigh and knee

19 | The leg, ankle, and foot

In the orthopaedic out-patient clinic disorders of the foot are second in frequency only to disorders of the back. Their prevalence may have several causes. *Hereditary factors*: The foot is probably in a state of relatively rapid evolution consequent upon man's assumption of the upright posture, and perhaps for that reason it is prone to variations in structure and form which may impair its efficiency. *Postural stresses*: Overweight throws an increased burden on the feet, and they may be unable to withstand the stress without ill-effect, especially if the intrinsic muscles are poorly developed. *Footwear*: The wearing of shoes is a potent cause of foot disorders. Many types of shoe interfere seriously with the mechanics of the foot, and the ladies' shoe with high heel and pointed toe is particularly to blame.

SPECIAL POINTS IN THE INVESTIGATION OF LEG, ANKLE, AND FOOT COMPLAINTS

In nearly all cases symptoms in the leg, ankle, or foot can be explained by a local abnormality. Only rarely are they referred from a distant lesion. In this respect the lower limb differs markedly from the upper, for in many cases symptoms in the hand have no local cause but are referred from a proximal lesion.

History

The precise distribution of pain should be ascertained. The occupation and habits of the patient, including sporting activities, may be significant, as may also be a history of previous injury. Specific enquiry should be made into the effect upon the symptoms of standing and walking.

Exposure

It is essential that socks or stockings be removed and that the whole leg be exposed up to the knee. Both limbs must always be examined so that the two may be compared. The first part of the examination is conducted with the patient lying upon a couch. Later, the foot is examined while the patient stands.

Steps in clinical examination

A suggested plan for the routine clinical examination of the leg, ankle, and foot is summarised in Table 19.1.

Assessing the state of the peripheral circulation

An essential part of the examination of the foot that is often forgotten is to study the efficiency of the arterial circulation. A reasonably accurate assessment may

Table 19.1 Routine clinical examination in suspected disorders of the leg, ankle, and foot

---

1. LOCAL EXAMINATION OF THE LEG, ANKLE, AND FOOT

Inspection Bone contours and alignment Soft-tissue contours Colour and texture of skin Scars or sinuses	*At the toes*: Flexion Extension **Power** (tested against resistance of examiner) Each muscle group to be tested in turn. (Power of calf muscles is best tested with the patient recumbent and then standing) (Compare with other side)
Palpation Skin temperature Bone contours Soft-tissue contours Local tenderness	
State of peripheral circulation Dorsalis pedis pulse Posterior tibial pulse Popliteal pulse Femoral pulse ? Cyanosis of foot when dependent	**Stability** Integrity of ligaments—particularly the lateral ligament of the ankle **Appearance of foot on standing** Colour Shape of longitudinal arch Shape of forefoot Efficiency of toes Efficiency of calf muscles (? ability to raise heel from ground while standing on affected leg alone)
Movements (active and passive, compared with normal side) *At the ankle*: Plantarflexion Extension (dorsiflexion) *At the subtalar joint*: Inversion-adduction Eversion-abduction *At the midtarsal joint*: Inversion-adduction Eversion-abduction	**Gait** **Condition of footwear** Sites of greatest wear. (Compare with other side)

---

2. GENERAL EXAMINATION
General survey of other parts of the body. The local symptoms may be only one manifestation of a widespread disease

---

be made on clinical evidence alone, but if surgical treatment is contemplated and vascular insufficiency is suspected it is necessary to have more precise information which can be provided only by certain special investigations.

Clinical assessment. This is based on a study of the texture of the skin and nails, colour changes, skin temperature, the arterial pulses, auscultation, and exercise tolerance. *Texture of skin and nails*: The skin of an ischaemic foot loses its hair and becomes thin and inelastic. The nails are coarse, thickened and irregular. Ulceration of the tips of the toes may be noted. *Colour changes*. A brick-red rubor or cyanosis occurring when the foot is made dependent after a period of elevation (Buerger's test) denotes serious impairment of the arterial circulation. *Temperature*: A foot with impaired arterial supply is colder than normal, but little reliance can be placed on this test as applied clinically at the bedside. *Arterial pulses*: The pulses to be felt for are the dorsalis pedis, the posterior tibial, the popliteal and the femoral. The popliteal pulse is often difficult to feel even in normal individuals. Palpation should be made with the fingertips of both hands supporting the slightly flexed knee. Pulsation of the dorsalis pedis artery is best felt at the dorsum of the foot between the bases of the first and second metatarsals. The posterior tibial artery is felt about 2 cm behind and below the tip of the medial malleolus. Absence or impairment of arterial pulsation is an important sign of defective circulation. It should be remembered, however, that a normal pulse is easily masked by thickening or oedema of the soft tissues. *Capillary return*: In limb ischaemia capillary return is slowed after blanching of a digital pulp or nail by pressure. *Auscultation*: A bruit over one of the major limb vessels, caused by turbulence of blood flow, may denote partial obstruction or an arterio-venous communication.

Special investigations. These may be indicated when the clinical examination shows evidence of vascular impairment. They include ankle blood pressure recordings, Doppler ultrasound probe analysis, combined probe analysis and ultrasonography, pulse volume recording (plethysmography), and digital arteriography. For more detail on these and the treatment of limb ischaemia readers should consult a textbook of vascular surgery.

Movements at the ankle and tarsal joints

Since the joints are close together, movement at the tarsal joints is easily mistaken for movement at the ankle, and vice versa. Careful examination is required to determine the range at each individual joint.

Ankle movement. The ankle is strictly a hinge joint. The only movements are extension (dorsiflexion) and plantarflexion. The range should be judged from the excursion of the hindfoot rather than the forefoot, so that any contribution from the tarsal joints is disregarded. Similarly, in testing the passive range, the foot should be controlled from the heel (Fig. 19.1). The normal range of ankle movement varies in different subjects; so the normal ankle must be used as a control. An average range is about 25° of extension (dorsiflexion) and 35° of plantarflexion.

Subtalar and midtarsal movement. In normal use the subtalar and midtarsal joints work together as a single unit. The movements permitted are:

1. combined inversion and adduction (supination)
2. combined eversion and abduction (pronation).

In clinical examination the range of movement contributed by each component can be determined separately. To test *subtalar movement* support the lower leg by a hand gripping the ankle. With the other hand lightly grasp the calcaneus from below (Fig. 19.2). Instruct the patient alternately to invert and evert the foot, observing the range through which the heel rocks from side to side. Compare with the sound foot. The normal range is about 20° on each side of the neutral position.

To test *midtarsal movement* grasp the calcaneus firmly so that subtalar movement is eliminated. With the other hand lightly grasp the midfoot near the bases of the metatarsals (Fig. 19.3). Instruct the patient alternately to twist

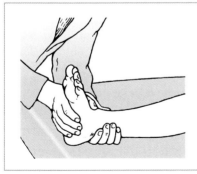

Fig. 19.1 Examining ankle movement. The examining hand grips the hindfoot rather than the forefoot, so that movements of the subtalar and midtarsal joints are eliminated.

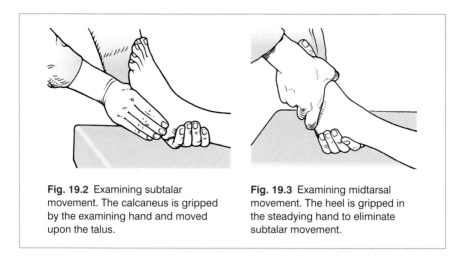

Fig. 19.2 Examining subtalar movement. The calcaneus is gripped by the examining hand and moved upon the talus.

Fig. 19.3 Examining midtarsal movement. The heel is gripped in the steadying hand to eliminate subtalar movement.

the foot inwards and outwards into inversion and eversion, and compare the range with that on the sound side. The normal is a rotation of about 15° on each side of the neutral position.

Toe movements. Determine the active and passive range at the metatarso-phalangeal and interphalangeal joints. It should be remembered that the normal range of dorsiflexion of the great toe at the metatarso-phalangeal joint is nearly 90° (Fig. 19.4). The range varies, but limitation to less than 60° of dorsiflexion is certainly abnormal. The range of downward flexion is about 15° but it varies between individuals. Movement at the lesser toes is variable: there should be not less than 30° of flexion at the metatarso-phalangeal joints and at the interphalangeal joints.

Examination of the feet under weight-bearing stress

Instruct the patient to stand evenly on both feet. Observe the general shape of the ankle, foot, and toes. Study the shape of the longitudinal arch. Is it of normal

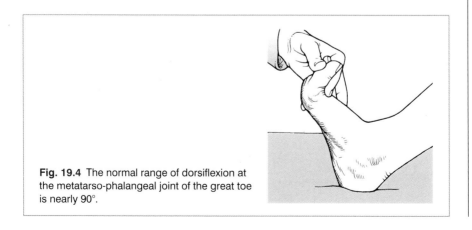

Fig. 19.4 The normal range of dorsiflexion at the metatarso-phalangeal joint of the great toe is nearly 90°.

shape? Is it flattened so that the navicular region is in contact with the ground (pes planus or valgus)? Or is it higher than normal (pes cavus)? It is important to view the heel from the back, so that any inward (varus) or outward (valgus) deviation may be noted. Next study the forefoot. Is it splayed and broader than normal? Assess the function of the toes. Normally they can be pressed upon the ground by the action of the intrinsic muscles so that the metatarsal heads are lifted up and relieved of weight-bearing pressure. Finally, examine the efficiency of the calf muscles. The crucial test is to ask the patient to stand on the affected leg and to raise the heel from the ground (see Fig. 19.5).

Examination of spine

Certain deformities of the foot – especially pes cavus with clawing of the toes – may be caused by a neurological abnormality in the thoraco-lumbar or lumbar region of the spine, associated with spina bifida or other developmental anomaly (see p. 171). Examination should therefore be made for a tell-tale dimple, pigmented area, or tuft of hair on the overlying skin.

Gait

Look especially for abnormal posture of the feet such as turning in (intoeing) or turning out, or drop foot (inability to dorsiflex the foot, necessitating high stepping gait). Observe whether weight is borne correctly on the sole of the foot or whether it is taken too much on the medial or lateral border. Observe also whether the heel is raised normally from the ground at the beginning of each step.

For a more refined analysis of gait special force plates may be incorporated in a walkway to record the pressure beneath each component part of the foot in all phases of the step. It is thus possible objectively to compare the pattern of

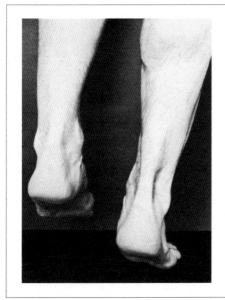

Fig. 19.5 The crucial test of intact calf function is to raise the heel from the ground while standing only on the affected leg. Inability to do this after an injury to the calcaneal tendon is diagnostic of complete rupture.

gait in a defective foot with the normal pattern; or to compare the gait pattern of a foot before and after operation. The patient's ability to negotiate stairs with normal rhythm should also be assessed.

Footwear

The examination of the foot is not complete until the patient's shoes have been inspected and compared on the two sides. Note the position of greatest wear. When the foot is normal the greatest wear in the sole occurs beneath the ball of the foot and slightly to the medial side. In the heel it is at the posterior border slightly to the lateral side. The state of the uppers is also important: excessive bulging on the medial side suggests a valgus foot and excessive bulging on the lateral side an inverted foot.

Radiographic examination

The ankle. Routine radiographs of the ankle comprise an antero-posterior and a lateral projection centred at the level of the joint. The films should include a reasonable length of the shafts of the tibia and fibula, and the whole of the talus.

When laxity of the lateral ligament is suspected a special inversion film is required. This is an antero-posterior projection taken while the heel is held in fullest inversion by an assistant. If the lateral ligament is torn or lax the talus will then be shown tilted in the ankle mortise (see Fig. 19.10, p. 433).

In cases of suspected ligamentous injury antero-posterior stability should also be tested. Rupture of the anterior talo-fibular component of the lateral ligament allows anterior subluxation of the talus in the mortise as shown in a lateral radiograph taken while the foot is pushed forward upon the tibia.

The foot. Routine radiographs should comprise an antero-posterior (strictly a supero-inferior) projection and a lateral projection, preferably taken while weight is borne on the feet. An oblique projection (non-weight-bearing) is used to show the mid-foot. Special techniques are available to show the calcaneus (axial view).

DISORDERS OF THE LEG

RUPTURE OF THE CALCANEAL TENDON

Surprising as it may seem, a ruptured calcaneal tendon (tendo Achillis) is often overlooked, the symptoms being wrongly ascribed to a strain or to a ruptured plantaris tendon.

Pathology. The rupture is nearly always complete. It occurs about 5 cm above the insertion of the tendon. If it is left untreated the tendon unites spontaneously, but with lengthening and loss of function.

Clinical features. While running or jumping, the patient feels a sudden agonising pain at the back of the ankle. He may believe that something has struck him. He is able to walk, but only with a bad limp. *On examination* of the back of the heel there is tenderness at the site of rupture. There is general thickening from effusion of blood and from oedema of the paratenon, but a gap can usually be felt in the course of the tendon. The power of plantarflexion at the ankle is greatly weakened, though some power remains through the action of the tibialis posterior, the peronei, and the toe flexors. A useful test, to be carried out with the patient prone, is to squeeze the bulk of the calf muscles from side to side. Normally this causes a slight plantarflexion movement of the foot, but not if the tendon is ruptured.

Diagnosis. The retention of some power of plantarflexion may deflect the unwary from the correct diagnosis. The crucial test is to ask the patient to lift the heel from the ground while standing only upon the affected leg (Fig. 19.5). This is impossible if the tendon is ruptured. In cases of doubt the gap in the tendon may be well demonstrated by ultrasound or MRI scanning (Fig. 19.6).

Treatment. Non-operative treatment may be used in selected cases, usually older and more sedentary patients who make less demands on their ankle function. The method is only applicable where passive ankle flexion can bring the torn ends of the tendon into apposition. The ankle is then immobilised in a below-knee plaster for 5 weeks, with the foot in slight equinus to relax the tendon and thus help to prevent lengthening.

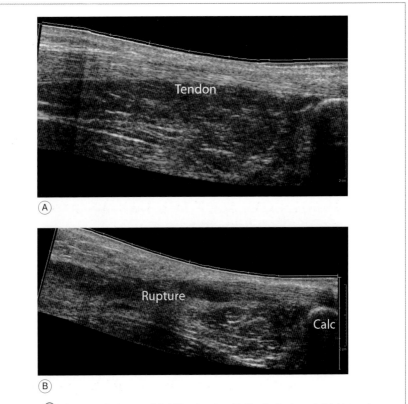

Fig. 19.6 Ⓐ Ultrasound of normal Achilles tendon. Patient's foot on right. Normal appearance of tendon seen above the word 'Tendon'. Ⓑ Compare with this ultrasound of a ruptured tendon.

In the majority of younger patients, particularly those who wish to continue athletic pursuits after healing, operative treatment is preferable. It entails repair of the tendon, using non-absorbable sutures of synthetic material, tension on the suture line being relaxed by immobilising the limb with right-angled knee flexion and moderate ankle plantarflexion for 2 weeks. For the next four weeks a below-knee plaster with the ankle at 90° is worn. Certain protocols allow earlier mobilisation of the ankle under close supervision of a physiotherapist.

Whether treatment is by plaster alone or by operation, it must be completed after removal of the plaster by increasingly vigorous exercises for the calf muscles, practised under the supervision of a physiotherapist until full strength is restored.

ACUTE OSTEOMYELITIS (General description of acute osteomyelitis, p. 85)

The tibia is one of the commonest sites of haematogenous osteomyelitis. Because of its liability to open (compound) fracture it is also the commonest site of osteomyelitis from direct contamination. The fibula is less often affected.

The pathological and clinical features and treatment conform to the general description on page 89.

CHRONIC OSTEOMYELITIS (General description of chronic osteomyelitis, p. 90)

Chronic osteomyelitis in the lower leg, as elsewhere, is nearly always a sequel of acute osteomyelitis. It may follow either the haematogenous type of infection or an infected open fracture.

Brodie's abscess. This rather uncommon lesion was described on page 92. It is a special form of chronic osteomyelitis which arises insidiously, without a recognised acute infection preceding it. The tibia is the commonest site (see Fig. 7.7, p. 93).

SYPHILITIC INFECTION OF THE TIBIA (General description of syphilitic osteitis, p. 95)

Although skeletal syphilis is now rare in Western countries, it still occurs in other parts of the world, and when it does occur the tibia is often the bone affected. The infection may take the form of a localised gumma or of diffuse osteoperiostitis (see Fig. 7.11A&B, p. 96). There is a gradually enlarging swelling, with moderate pain. It is important to bear the possibility of syphilis in mind, because the swelling is easily mistaken for a tumour.

TUMOURS OF BONE

Benign tumours (General description of benign bone tumours, p. 106)

Of the four main types of benign tumours of bone – osteoid osteoma, chondroma, osteochondroma, and giant-cell tumour – only chondroma and giant-cell tumour require further mention here.

Chondroma
In the tibia or fibula this is seldom found except in multiple form in the condition of dyschondroplasia (p. 65). The individual tumours in this condition resemble enchondromata. They arise from the growing epiphysial cartilage plate, and they interfere with the normal growth of the bone. An important effect is that the growth of the tibia and fibula may be unequal, with the consequence that the bones may become curved or the plane of the ankle joint may be tilted away from the horizontal (see Fig. 6.4A, p. 65).

Giant-cell tumour (osteoclastoma)
The upper end of the tibia or fibula, like the lower end of the femur, is a favourite site for this tumour. It usually arises in a young adult, expanding the bone and extending to within a short distance of the articular surface.

Treatment. If the tumour is in the fibula the whole of the affected end of the bone should be excised together with an adequate margin of healthy bone. If the tumour is in the upper end of the tibia, the problem of treatment is much more difficult. Curettage and packing with bone graft or acrylic cement is usually attempted unless the articular surface is already compromised. If this fails, or is impractical, as in the femur it may be necessary to excise the upper end of the tibia to ensure full eradication of the tumour. Function and continuity may be restored after excision by the use of a custom-made prosthesis to replace the knee joint and the upper half of the tibia, or the knee may be arthrodesed where this is not possible.

Malignant tumours (General description of malignant bone tumours, p. 112)
The tibia, like the femur, is a common site for primary malignant bone tumours, especially osteosarcoma and Ewing's tumour.

Osteosarcoma (osteogenic sarcoma)
This tumour usually affects the upper metaphysis of the tibia: the lower end of the tibia and the fibula are affected much less often. The tumour metastasises rapidly through the blood stream, especially to the lungs. Treatment was described on p. 117.

Ewing's tumour
This usually affects the shaft of a long bone, again in childhood or early adult life. The tibia is one of the commonest sites. Treatment was described on page 121.

INTERMITTENT CLAUDICATION
Intermittent claudication is a symptom of arterial insufficiency in the lower limb. In its typical form it is characterised by cramp-like pain in the calf, induced by walking and relieved by rest.

Cause. The usual underlying cause is arteriosclerosis with consequent partial or total obstruction of the main limb vessel. Thrombo-angiitis obliterans and arterial embolism are less common causes. Tobacco smoking is a major contributory factor.

Pathology. The basic disturbance is ischaemia of muscle, in consequence of which metabolites cannot be removed speedily enough when the muscle is exercised. The accumulation of metabolites is believed to be responsible for the pain, which subsides within a few minutes when the muscle is rested. The muscles usually affected are those of the calf, but in some instances other muscle groups are involved, according to the site of the arterial obstruction. The vascular lesion is usually a complete occlusion of the femoral or the popliteal artery. In claudication affecting the buttock the aortic bifurcation or the iliac artery may be occluded.

Clinical features. Intermittent claudication is much more common in men than in women. In the usual arteriosclerotic type the patient is past middle life, but in cases due to thrombo-angiitis obliterans or embolism the symptoms may develop in early adult life. The patient is usually a regular smoker.

With gradual arterial occlusion the onset is insidious and the symptoms are slowly progressive; but in cases precipitated by thrombosis or embolism the onset may be sudden. In a typical case the patient complains that after walking a certain distance – perhaps a hundred metres or so – he is forced to stop by severe cramp-like pain in the calf, or occasionally in another muscle group, such as the buttock. After a few minutes' rest the pain disappears and he is able to walk on again for a similar distance.

On examination there is objective evidence of impaired arterial circulation in the lower limb (p. 421). The posterior tibial, dorsalis pedis, and popliteal pulses are absent. There may be ischaemic changes in the skin of the foot. Evidence of widespread arterial or cardiac disease is nearly always found on general examination.

For further details on the **investigation, diagnosis** and **treatment** of this condition readers should refer to a textbook of vascular surgery.

DISORDERS OF THE ANKLE

PYOGENIC ARTHRITIS OF THE ANKLE (General description of pyogenic arthritis, p. 96)

Pyogenic arthritis of the ankle is uncommon. The organisms reach the joint through the blood stream or through a penetrating wound; local spread from a focus of osteomyelitis of the tibia or fibula is rare because the bony metaphyses are entirely extra-capsular (see Fig. 7.2, p. 87).

TUBERCULOUS ARTHRITIS OF THE ANKLE (General description of tuberculous arthritis, p. 98)

Tuberculosis is much less common in the ankle than it is in the hip and knee. In Britain it is now seen very seldom. When it is seen, it is often in an immigrant from a developing country.

The clinical features correspond to those of tuberculous arthritis of other superficial joints, with pain, swelling, increased warmth of the overlying skin, restriction of movement, and limp.

Treatment. Early conservative treatment (p. 102) may restore a mobile ankle, but if in a resistant case articular cartilage is badly eroded or destroyed arthrodesis may have to be undertaken.

The leg, ankle, and foot

RHEUMATOID ARTHRITIS OF THE ANKLE (General description of rheumatoid arthritis, p. 134)

One or both ankles are often affected by rheumatoid arthritis in common with other joints in the lower limb, particularly the foot. There may be marked destruction of the articular cartilage and subchondral bone with pain, stiffness, and deformity (Fig. 19.7).

Treatment. Medical treatment is along the lines suggested for the disease as a whole (p. 137). *Local treatment*: In the active phase rest in a plaster is sometimes required, but in most cases the patient should be encouraged to remain active as far as possible, with such help as may be gained from local support by a moulded polypropylene splint. Operation is advised mainly when destruction of articular cartilage has led to intractable pain with marked impairment of capacity for walking. Arthrodesis and replacement arthroplasty are the methods available. Arthrodesis is usually the operation of choice because it gives permanent relief of pain with good function. If the subtalar and midtarsal joints are also severely affected they should be included in the fusion. Replacement arthroplasty of the ankle is appropriate in some patients (Fig. 19.8). The operation is technically demanding because of the limited surgical access to the joint, while the long-term results are much less satisfactory than with the hip or knee because poor bone support may lead to early implant loosening.

OSTEOARTHRITIS OF THE ANKLE (General description of osteoarthritis, p. 140)

Degenerative destruction of the articular cartilage is less common in the ankle than in the knee or hip. There is nearly always a known predispos-

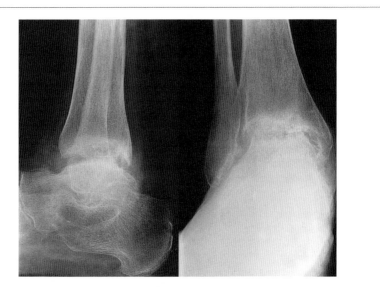

Fig. 19.7 Radiographs of the ankle with advanced rheumatoid arthritis showing loss of joint space and erosion of the articular surfaces of the tibia and talus.

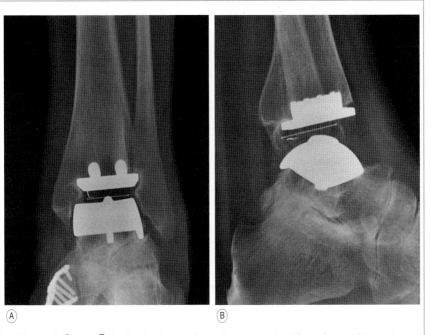

(A)   (B)

Fig. 19.8 Ⓐ and Ⓑ Radiographs of a Scandinavian total ankle replacement arthroplasty inserted for the treatment of advanced rheumatoid arthritis. Metal prostheses have been used to resurface the dome of the talus and the distal tibia and both articulate with a mobile polyethylene meniscal prosthesis placed between them (position shown by wire marker).

ing factor which causes the joint to wear out prematurely. The commonest is irregularity or mal-alignment of the joint surfaces after a fracture. Sometimes articular disease such as previous rheumatoid arthritis or osteochondromatosis is the primary factor.

Clinical features. The symptoms are pain which slowly increases over months and years, and limp. *On examination* the joint is a little thickened from hypertrophy of bone (osteophyte formation) at the joint margins. Movements are restricted slightly or severely according to the degree of arthritis.

Radiographs show the typical features of osteoarthritis – narrowing of the cartilage space, a tendency to sclerosis of the bone adjacent to the joint, and osteophyte formation at the joint margins (Fig. 19.9).

Treatment. In mild cases treatment is often unnecessary, because the patient may be willing to accept the disability when the nature of the trouble has been explained. When treatment is called for, conservative measures should be tried first if the disability is only moderate. Physiotherapy by short-wave diathermy, and active exercises are usually advised. Sometimes local splintage by a moulded polypropylene support will provide relief while allowing the patient to continue to walk. Such treatment, however, is only palliative, and if

The leg, ankle, and foot

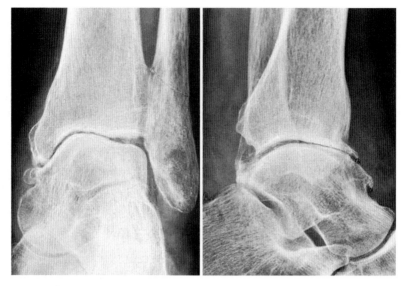

Fig. 19.9 Osteoarthritis of the ankle complicating fracture-subluxation 10 years before. Note the marked narrowing of the cartilage space and the prominent osteophytes.

the disability increases to the extent of becoming a serious handicap operation should be undertaken.

Surgical treatment should usually be by arthrodesis, which provides a painless stable joint for many years. A number of different methods are available to produce reliable bony fusion and with the introduction of arthroscopic techniques to remove the degenerate cartilage, combined with rigid internal fixation across the opposed bone surfaces, the post-operative rehabilitation is rapid. Unfortunately, after 10–15 years more than 50% of these patients develop further disability from hindfoot pain because of the accelerated onset of arthritis in the adjacent sub-talar and talo-navicular joints. In an attempt to overcome this problem in younger patients, replacement arthroplasty with resurfacing prostheses has been explored as a possible alternative (see Fig. 19.8). As with arthroplasty for rheumatoid arthritis, the long-term results are still uncertain because of bone resorption and implant loosening and it is not yet widely recommended.

NEUROPATHIC ARTHRITIS OF THE ANKLE (General description of neuropathic arthritis, p. 147)

Neuropathic arthritis is uncommon but nevertheless well recognised in the ankle. The underlying neurological disease is diabetic neuropathy, syringomyelia, cauda equina lesion, tabes dorsalis, or, where it is prevalent, leprosy.

Treatment. In many cases protection by a firm surgical boot, reinforced if necessary by a below-knee brace, is all that is required. Occasionally arthrodesis of the ankle may have to be considered. Appropriate treatment must be given for the underlying neurological disorder.

RECURRENT SUBLUXATION OF THE ANKLE

When the lateral ligament of the ankle is torn and fails to heal there may be persistent instability with recurrent attacks of giving way in which the talus tilts medially in the ankle mortise. Anterior displacement relative to the tibial articular surface may also occur. The causative injury is always a severe inversion force.

Clinical features. The patient complains that the ankle 'goes over' at frequent intervals, often causing him to fall. Each incident is accompanied by pain at the lateral side of the ankle. There is always a history of previous severe injury, followed by much swelling and extensive bruising at the lateral side of the joint.

On examination there is often some oedema about the ankle. There is tenderness over the site of the lateral ligament. The normal ankle movements – dorsiflexion and plantarflexion – are unchanged, but abnormal mobility is present as shown by the fact that the heel can be inverted passively beyond the normal range permitted at the subtalar joint. Moreover, when the heel is fully inverted a dimple or depression of the skin may be visible in front of the lateral malleolus, where the soft tissues have been 'sucked' into the gap created between tibia and talus.

Radiographic features. Routine radiographs do not show any abnormality. Antero-posterior films must be taken while the heel is held fully inverted. If the lateral ligament is torn or lax the talus will then be shown tilted away from the tibio-fibular mortise at the lateral side through 20 or 30° or more (Fig. 19.10). Anterior displacement of the talus relative to the tibial articular surface may sometimes also be demonstrated in lateral radiographs taken while the foot is pushed forwards.

Diagnosis. Chronic strain of the lateral ligament may cause similar symptoms, but in that condition radiographs will not show the talus tilted significantly on forced inversion. (It should be noted that the talus may tilt up to

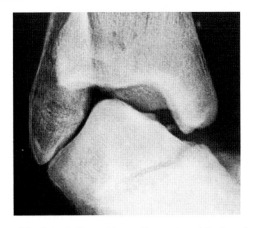

Fig. 19.10 Tilting of the talus in the ankle mortise under adduction stress; an indication of torn lateral ligament.

10° or even 15° in a normal ankle. Tilting beyond that amount is demonstrated only when the ligament is torn.)

Treatment. If the disability is slight it may be sufficient to strengthen the evertor muscles (mainly the peronei) by exercises, to enable them to control the ankle more efficiently. Stability may also be enhanced by broadening and 'floating out' the heel of the shoe. If the disability is severe operation is required. A new lateral ligament may be constructed either from the peroneus brevis tendon or from the peroneus tertius. Trials are also proceeding with the use of artificial ligaments, either as substitutes or as a means of promoting the growth of new ligamentous tissue.

DISORDERS OF THE FOOT

CONGENITAL CLUB FOOT (Talipes equino-varus)

The rather vague term 'club foot' has come to be synonymous in the minds of most surgeons with the commonest and most important congenital deformity of the foot—talipes equino-varus (Fig. 19.11). The less common, and usually less serious, form of club foot, talipes calcaneo-valgus, will be considered later under that title.

Cause. This is still under debate. In most cases a defect of fetal development is responsible, with imbalance between the invertor-plantarflexor muscles and the evertor-dorsiflexor muscles. A neuromuscular defect is possibly relevant. Minor degrees of the deformity may possibly be explained by prolonged mal-position of the foetal foot in the uterus, but this cannot be accepted as the usual cause.

Pathology. The crucial component of the deformity is subluxation of the talo-navicular joint, so that the navicular bone lies partly on the medial aspect of the head of the talus instead of on its distal aspect (Fig. 19.12). The soft tissues at the medial side of the foot are under-developed and shorter than

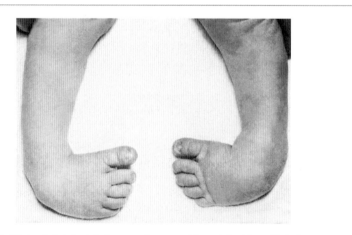

Fig. 19.11 Bilateral club foot (talipes equino-varus) in an infant boy. Note the poor development of the calf muscles.

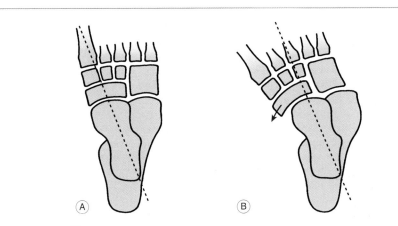

Fig. 19.12 Ⓐ Normal alignment of the forefoot upon the long axis of the talus. Ⓑ Subluxation of the navicular bone medially on the head of the talus – the crucial component in the pathology of talipes equino-varus. Interrupted line shows forward projection of the long axis of the talus passing lateral to the first metatarsal – a useful radiological sign. In the normal state the line passes through or medial to the first metatarsal Ⓐ.

normal. The foot is adducted and inverted at the subtalar, midtarsal, and anterior tarsal joints, and is held in equinus (plantarflexion) at the ankle. In most cases under-development of the calf and peroneal muscles is a striking feature. Thus if only one foot is affected there is a marked discrepancy in the girth of the calf between the two sides.

In the absence of early effective treatment the developing tarsal bones assume an abnormal shape as growth occurs, perpetuating the deformity.

Clinical features. The deformity is much commoner in boys than in girls. (Contrast developmental dysplasia (congenital dislocation) of the hip, which is much commoner in girls.) One or both feet may be affected. When the infant is born it is noticed that the foot is turned inwards so that the sole is directed medially (Fig. 19.11). The deformity, to be more precise, consists of three elements:

1. inversion (twisting inwards) of the foot
2. adduction (inward deviation) of the forefoot relative to the hindfoot
3. equinus (plantarflexion).

The foot cannot be pushed passively through the normal range of eversion and dorsiflexion. There may be obvious under-development of the muscles of the lower leg, especially noticeable when only one foot is affected.

Diagnosis. New-born infants should be examined routinely for evidence of club foot. It is not sufficient, for purposes of diagnosis, that the foot be found to rest in the position described, for often the feet of normal infants tend to lie naturally in a somewhat inverted position. The criterion for the diagnosis of club foot is that the deformity cannot readily be corrected and over-corrected to bring the foot into eversion and dorsiflexion. It should be remembered that in normal infants under 1 year old it is possible to evert and dorsiflex the foot far enough to bring the little toe into contact with the shin.

Radiographic features. In the antero-posterior radiograph of a normal foot a line projecting the long axis of the talus forwards passes medial to the first metatarsal bone or coincides with it (Fig. 19.12A). In uncorrected or incompletely corrected club foot the line passes lateral to the metatarsal (Fig. 19.12B).

Prognosis. The prognosis depends largely upon the age at which primary treatment is begun, and upon the efficiency with which it is carried out. The longer the delay before treatment, the smaller is the prospect of complete cure. Yet even with prompt treatment the outcome is uncertain. In a proportion of cases, despite the greatest care from the time of birth, there is a tendency to relapse when treatment is discontinued. These are usually the cases that show marked hypoplasia of the muscles of the lower leg, especially of the peroneal group. Even in the most severe cases, however, it should always be possible to ensure a plantigrade foot, if not a normal foot, by operative means.

Treatment in a fresh case. Although it is seemingly a simple deformity, talipes equino-varus presents difficult problems in treatment. The most widely accepted practice is to rely upon conservative treatment by correction and splintage during the first year of life (often using the so-called Ponseti technique[1]) and often well beyond that; if casting and splintage fail to correct the position then operative correction is carried out.

Primary conservative treatment. Ideally treatment should be begun immediately after birth – certainly not more than 1 week later. The principles of treatment are:

1. to correct and over-correct the deformity by firm manual pressure, repeated at appropriate intervals (usually weekly at first)
2. to hold the foot in the over-corrected position to counteract the natural tendency for the deformity to recur.

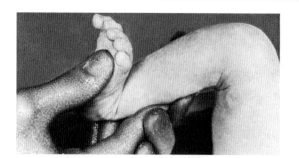

Fig. 19.13 Correcting a club-foot deformity by manual pressure without anaesthesia. Note that pressure is applied under the midfoot, not under the forefoot.

[1]Ignacio Ponseti (1914–) Spanish born orthopaedic surgeon emigrated to Iowa in USA in 1941 and developed his innovative conservative treatment for clubfoot, which he still teaches and is widely used throughout the world.

Correction of deformity. The deformity is corrected by firm manual pressure without anaesthesia (Fig. 19.13). The Ponseti technique involves first correcting the cavus deformity, then the adduction and heel varus, and finally the equinus deformity. Depending on the severity of the deformity, it may be possible to correct it fully by two or three manipulations, or as many as five or six manipulations at weekly intervals may be required.

Maintenance of correction. Three methods are available for holding the foot in the corrected position between manipulations:

1. a plaster of Paris cast
2. metal splints as advocated by Denis Browne
3. adhesive strapping.

Retention in a plaster is much to be preferred, because it holds the foot in the over-corrected position more efficiently and for a longer period than do metal splints or strapping – even though the technique of applying a plaster correctly is not easy to learn. The plaster must extend to the upper thigh, with the knee flexed 90° (Fig. 19.14); otherwise the infant is able to draw the foot up inside the plaster, with consequent loss of correction. The plaster must be changed every week at first, but the interval may be extended to two and then three weeks as the child grows larger.

Operative treatment. Opinions vary on the correct duration of conservative treatment and on the timing of corrective operations in infants. If treatment by manipulation and retention fails, operation should usually be undertaken before the age of 9 months: some would say much earlier. If at the end of three or four months the feet are not normal clinically and radiologically, operation should be advised. The idea behind early operation is to set the tarsal bones in normal relationship to one another and to remove deforming forces, thus allowing the bones to develop in their normal shape from an early age. All taut ligaments at the medial side of the ankle and foot are divided and any tendon that is too tight to allow full correction is lengthened – including the calcaneal tendon. Finally the tarsal bones, thus released, are restored to their normal

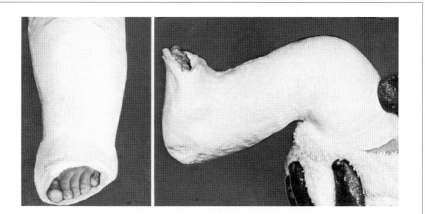

Fig. 19.14 Plaster for maintaining correction in congenital club foot. It is essential to include the thigh, with the knee flexed to a right angle.

relationships, particular attention being paid to the talus and the navicular bone. After operation a plaster is worn for 2 or 3 months.

Treatment in neglected or relapsed cases. Repeated manipulation and retention in plaster can produce worthwhile improvement in children of up to two years of age. If significant deformity is still present after the age of two, operative treatment is required. It should be appreciated that in these late cases no method of treatment – whether conservative or operative – is capable of restoring the foot to normal. The most that can be done is to restore a plantigrade foot.[1]

Types of operation. In children aged 2 to 12 years there is the option to employ any of seven operations, depending upon the circumstances of each case:

1. division of the short soft tissues at the medial side of the foot, the foot thereafter being forced into a plantigrade position and immobilised in plaster for three months
2. transfer of the tendon of the tibialis anterior to the outer side of the foot
3. transfer of the tibialis posterior tendon through the interosseous membrane to the outer side of the foot, to supplement the action of the evertor muscles
4. lengthening of a short calcaneal tendon
5. arthrodesis of the calcaneo-cuboid joint, with excision of a wafer of bone to shorten the lateral border of the foot
6. when inversion of the heel is a prominent feature, Dwyer osteotomy of the calcaneus with insertion of a bone wedge in the medial side to correct the line of weight-bearing
7. application of a circular (Ilizarov) external fixation frame which allows gradual correction of the deformity.

In children over the age of 12 resort must be had to operation upon the bones: a wedge of bone of appropriate size (with base dorso-laterally) is removed from the tarsus so that when the resulting gap is closed the foot is plantigrade. This operation is not recommended for children under 12 because the active bone growth of the foot is likely to be impaired.

CONGENITAL TALIPES CALCANEO-VALGUS

This is the opposite deformity to talipes equino-varus. The foot is everted and dorsiflexed. It is usually a less serious deformity than talipes equino-varus and with few exceptions, in which there is displacement at the talo-navicular joint (see congenital vertical talus, below), it responds readily to treatment.

Cause. The cause is unknown. In some cases it may simply be a postural deformity, from folding of the foot against the shin for a long time in intra-uterine life.

Clinical features. One foot or both feet may be affected. The foot rests in a position of eversion and dorsiflexion, so that its dorsum lies almost in contact with the shin (Fig. 19.15). Tightness of the dorso-lateral soft tissues prevents the foot from being brought down easily into inversion and equinus, though with steady pressure a fair degree of correction can usually be obtained.

Treatment. In most cases the deformity will respond to repeated manual stretching by the parents, who should be carefully instructed how to coax the foot into the over-corrected position of inversion and equinus by steady

---

[1]Plantigrade = sole walking; with the sole on the ground.

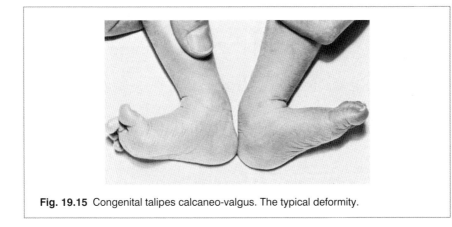

Fig. 19.15 Congenital talipes calcaneo-valgus. The typical deformity.

pressure upon the dorsum of the foot. The manipulations should be begun immediately after birth and should be carried out several times a day.

If calcaneo-valgus deformity still persists when the child is a month old more intensive supervision is required. The surgeon should gently over-correct the deformity as far as possible by manipulation without anaesthesia, thereafter applying a plaster with the foot in the over-corrected position. The plaster is changed weekly until a full range of inversion and equinus is gained. At that stage the plaster may be discarded without fear of relapse.

Congenital vertical talus

In a small proportion of cases of talipes calcaneo-valgus there is an underlying skeletal deformity at the talo-navicular joint. The navicular bone is displaced onto the dorsal aspect of the head of the talus, which is thus pushed downwards so that the long axis of the talus becomes almost vertical. The condition may sometimes be associated with muscular imbalance consequent upon neurological deficit, as for instance in spina bifida. In most of these cases operative correction will be required.

ACCESSORY BONES IN THE FOOT

Many accessory bones have been described in the foot, but most are of little or no practical importance. The commonest is the **os trigonum**, which lies immediately behind the talus, on the upper surface of the tuberosity of the calcaneus (Fig. 19.16). It does not cause symptoms. It may be confused with a fracture of the talus.

The only tarsal accessory bone that is frequently responsible for symptoms is the **os tibiale externum**[1] (accessory navicular bone) (Fig. 19.17). This lies medial to the navicular bone, and forms a well-marked prominence at the inner border of the foot which may become painful and tender from the pressure of the shoe. If the symptoms justify operation the accessory bone should be removed.

[1]The term os tibiale externum may seem confusing in so far as the ossicle is on the inner side of the foot. The title however relates to the embryonic position of the foot, in which the ossicle forms on the outer side.

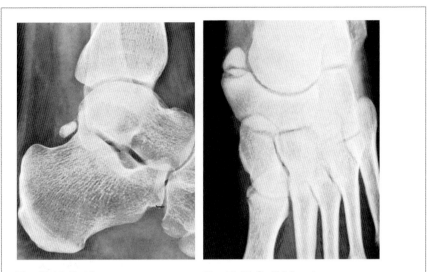

Fig. 19.16 Os trigonum.   **Fig. 19.17** Os tibiale externum.

PES CAVUS

In pes cavus or 'hollow foot' the longitudinal arch of the foot is accentuated.

Cause. In many cases the deformity has a congenital basis. It is sometimes familial. In other cases there is an underlying neurological disorder causing muscle imbalance. For instance, it is often associated with a minor degree of spinal dysraphism (p. 171), or it may follow poliomyelitis.

Pathology. The metatarsal heads are lowered in relation to the hind part of the foot, with consequent exaggeration of the longitudinal arch. The soft tissues in the sole are abnormally short, and eventually the bones themselves alter shape, perpetuating the deformity. There is always associated clawing of the toes, which are hyperextended at the metatarso-phalangeal joints and flexed at the proximal and distal interphalangeal joints (Fig. 19.18). This clawing seems to result from defective action of the intrinsic muscles – lumbricals and interossei. The effect is that the toes are almost functionless, and unable to take their normal share in weight-bearing. Consequently excessive weight falls upon the metatarsal heads on walking or standing, and hard callosities form in the underlying skin. The mal-alignment of the tarsal joints predisposes to the later development of osteoarthritis.

Clinical features. The deformity often becomes evident in childhood. It may affect one foot or both feet. In some cases the symptoms are negligible. When symptoms do arise they may take three forms:

1. painful callosities beneath the metatarsal heads
2. tenderness over the deformed toes from pressure against the shoe
3. pain in the tarsal region from osteoarthritis of the tarsal joints.

On examination the deformity is characteristic and easily recognised (Fig. 19.18). The longitudinal arch is high; the forefoot is thick and splayed; the toes are clawed; the metatarsal heads are prominent in the sole. Callosities beneath

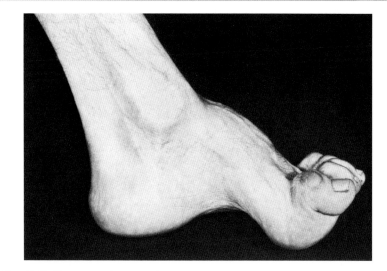

Fig. 19.18 Pes cavus. Typical deformity with high arch, clawed toes, and prominence of the metatarsal heads in the sole. In such a case the spine should always be examined for evidence of dysraphism.

the metatarsal heads indicate that they take excessive weight. The toes cannot be straightened at will by the patient, nor can they be pressed firmly upon the ground to take a share in weight-bearing. There may also be tender callosities where the tops of the toes have rubbed against the shoes.

The base of the spine should be examined for a congenital anomaly such as spina bifida, which may be suggested by the presence of a dimple, a tuft of hair, or an area of pigmentation. If suspicion of spinal dysraphism exists radiographs of the spine should be obtained.

Treatment. In many cases treatment is not required. Mild symptoms can often be relieved by regular chiropody and by the provision of a resilient pad beneath the metatarsal heads to distribute the weight more widely. It is often helpful to prescribe surgical shoes, made to fit the altered shape of the feet.

If the symptoms are severe operation may be required. The nature of the operation should depend upon the cause of the main symptoms.

Operations on the toes. When local pressure upon the toes or beneath the metatarsal heads is the main complaint, adequate relief can often be afforded simply by straightening the clawed toes. This may be done by arthrodesing all the interphalangeal joints or, if the toes are still mobile, by transplanting the long flexor tendon into the extensor expansion to supplement the action of the intrinsic muscles.

Operations on the soft tissues of the sole. In appropriate cases arthrodesis of the toes may be supplemented by the Steindler muscle-slide operation, in which the taut ligamentous tissues in the sole of the foot are detached from the calcaneus and allowed to slide forwards as the height of the arch is reduced by strong manual force. After operation the correction is maintained by immobilising the foot in plaster for 2 months.

Operations on the tarsal joints. When osteoarthritis of the tarsal joints is the main cause of the symptoms arthrodesis of the affected joints – usually the subtalar, calcaneo-cuboid, and talo-navicular joints (the so-called triple arthrodesis) – is required. At the same time the deformity is corrected by excising a wedge of bone, base upwards, from the metatarsus. When necessary, this operation may be combined with operations to straighten the toes.

PES PLANUS (Flat foot; valgus foot)

In this common condition the longitudinal arch of the foot is reduced so that, on standing, its medial border is close to, or in contact with, the ground (Fig. 19.19). It is usually associated with some degree of twisting outwards of the foot on its longitudinal axis (eversion or valgus deformity).

Cause. In many cases it probably has a congenital basis, but it may be caused by selective muscle weakness or paralysis.

Pathology. All infants have flat feet for a year or two after they begin to stand. When the deformity persists into adult life it becomes a permanent structural defect, the tarsal bones being so shaped that when articulated they tend to form a straight line rather than an arch.

Clinical features. In children, flat feet are usually symptomless, but the parents commonly complain that the uppers of the shoes persistently bulge inwards and that the heels wear down quickly at the inner sides.

In adults, too, flat feet are often free from symptoms, but they are more liable than are normal feet to suffer foot strain (p. 444), and when pain is complained of it is usually from that cause.

In later life pain may also arise from osteoarthritis of the tarsal joints consequent upon their mal-alignment.

Treatment. In children under 3 years old treatment is not required. In children over 3 the accepted method of treatment is to tilt the shoe slightly to the

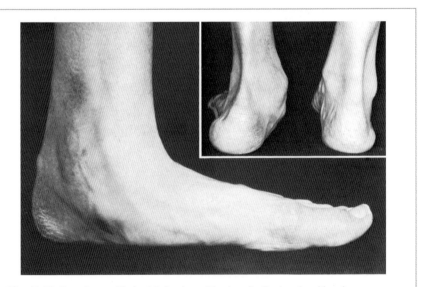

Fig. 19.19 Pes planus. Marked flattening of the longitudinal arch, with valgus deformity seen well from behind (inset).

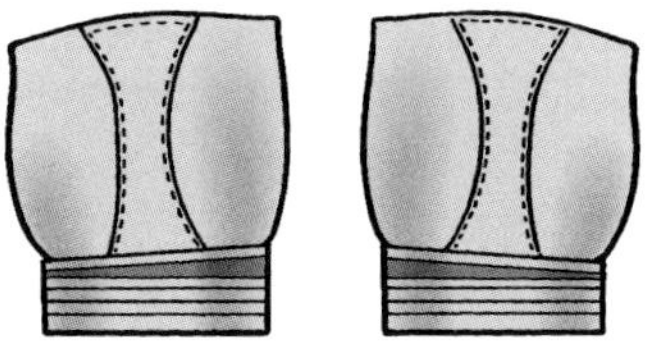

Fig. 19.20 Shoes drawn from behind, to illustrate medial heel wedges.

lateral side by inserting a wedge, base medially, between the layers of the heel (not the sole) (Fig. 19.20). This may help to overcome the valgus twist and to reduce the bulging-over of the uppers at the medial side, but it must be accepted that in most cases it is little more than a placebo. In older children it is better to insert a valgus insole (arch support) into the shoe, and this may be supplemented by a course of supervised exercises to strengthen the intrinsic muscles of the foot.

In cases of severe valgus deformity – which is usually the consequence of selective muscle imbalance, as after poliomyelitis – operation to restore the correct relationship between talus and calcaneus, and to fuse the two bones together (talocalcaneal arthrodesis), may be considered. In children this operation may be done by placing bone grafts extra-articularly in the sinus tarsi, from the lateral side.

In adults treatment is not needed unless symptoms are present, when the advisability of fitting an arch support should be considered. Supports are seldom of benefit when the foot is completely flat, but they often afford relief when the longitudinal arch is diminished but not lost.

If the symptoms in a case of long-established flat foot are ascribed to superimposed osteoarthritis of the tarsal joints, treatment should be directed against the arthritis (see below).

Peroneal spastic flat foot (spasmodic painful flat foot) and tarsal coalition

Whereas in most cases flat foot is painless, in a small number the flattening may be associated with pain and intermittent spasm of the peroneal muscles, provoked by weight-bearing. Peroneal spastic flat foot is important because it is often associated with congenital tarsal coalitions which, if not treated by early surgical excision, may lead to secondary arthritic changes in the tarsal joints.

Pathology. Tarsal coalitions represent an inherited failure of bony development and are present in 1–2% of the population. The characteristic feature is the existence of a cartilaginous or bony bar bridging two adjacent tarsal bones. The two commonest types are:

1. calcaneo-navicular coalition
2. talo-calcaneal coalition.

Clinical features. Symptoms usually begin in early adolescence, when the patient presents with a painful, rigid, valgus hindfoot. The symptoms are aggravated by prolonged standing or walking. Examination shows marked restriction of subtalar movement. Attempted eversion of the heel passively often provokes spasm of the peroneal muscles.

Diagnosis. Special oblique or axial radiographs may be required to show the abnormal bony bar, though this can be demonstrated more clearly on a CT scan. Later, secondary osteoarthritic changes may be seen in the tarsal joints.

Treatment. If coalition is diagnosed early, excision of the abnormal bar may relieve pain and restore some mobility. In the later stages, if degenerative arthritis causes severe disability arthrodesis of the affected joints may be required.

FOOT STRAIN

The term 'foot strain' implies a subacute or chronic strain of the tarsal ligaments, not an acute injury from sudden violence.

It may be caused in a normal foot by excessive standing or walking by a person unaccustomed to it: but it occurs mostly in those with a long-established foot deformity such as pes planus (flat foot) or pes cavus, when the ligaments of the foot may be inadequately protected by muscles.

The main symptoms are prolonged aching in the feet, worse on standing or walking, often with aching also in the calves.

It is important to eliminate other causes of foot problems such as ischaemia, neurological deficit and, in boys, particularly muscular dystrophy.

Treatment should be by reducing the time spent in standing and walking, by the fitting of an arch support if indicated, by supervised foot and toe exercises, and sometimes by electrical stimulation to strengthen the muscles of the leg and foot.

OSTEOARTHRITIS OF THE TARSAL JOINTS

Osteoarthritis may affect any of the tarsal joints, but in practice it is seen most often in the subtalar and midtarsal joints. It seldom arises primarily: there is nearly always a predisposing cause such as previous fracture or disease involving the joint surfaces (especially fractures of the calcaneus), or mal-alignment of the tarsal bones (as in severe flat foot or severe pes cavus).

Clinical features. The main symptom is pain, which gradually increases over months or years and finally leads to a limp and impaired capacity for walking. Pain is localised fairly accurately to the particular joint or joints affected. A history will usually be obtained of previous injury, disease, or deformity of the foot. *On examination* movement of the affected joint is impaired, and painful if forced.

Radiographs confirm the diagnosis and may give an indication of the primary underlying cause.

Treatment. In mild cases treatment is not required, especially if the patient's activities can be curtailed. When the disability is troublesome more active measures are needed. Conservative treatment is only palliative, but it is usually worth a trial. It should take the form of short-wave diathermy, muscle exercises, and support from an elastic bandage or moulded polypropylene heel seat. A trial may also be made of local injection of hydrocortisone into the affected joint; but repeated injections are not advised.

If conservative treatment fails to give adequate relief operation must be considered. The only effective method is by arthrodesis of the affected joint or joints.

OTHER FORMS OF ARTHRITIS OF THE TARSAL JOINTS

Like all true synovial joints, the tarsal joints are liable to any of the recognised forms of arthritis, including pyogenic arthritis, rheumatoid arthritis, tuberculous arthritis, gouty arthritis, and neuropathic arthritis. Of these, the only one that is at all common is rheumatoid arthritis, which affects particularly thesubtalar joint.

OSTEOCHONDRITIS OF THE NAVICULAR BONE
(Köhler's disease[1])

The general subject of osteochondritis was discussed in Chapter 8 (p. 130). The growing navicular bone is one of its best-recognised sites. The developing nucleus of the bone is temporarily softened and usually becomes compressed by the mechanical forces entailed in walking. A disturbance of blood supply is possibly a causative factor, but the pathogenesis is not fully understood.

Pathology. The pathology is believed to be like that of osteochondritis of other growing bony nuclei (see Table 8.2, p. 131). The bone, presumably necrotic from ischaemia, loses its normal trabecular structure and may become fragmented as it is gradually absorbed and replaced by new living bone. After about two years the normal bone structure is restored and the bone may regain almost its normal size and shape. If slight deformation of the bone does remain, the growing foot seems to adapt itself to the altered shape and little or nodisability persists.

Clinical features. Köhler's disease is confined to children aged about 3 to 5 years. The child complains of pain in the midtarsal part of the foot and is noticed to limp. *On examination* there may be slight swelling in the midtarsal region, with tenderness on firm palpation over the navicular bone and sometimes a slight increase in warmth. There may be some restriction of midtarsal movements with pain on forcing, but these signs are slight and sometimes absent.

Radiographic features. Radiographs are diagnostic. The ossifying nucleus of the navicular bone appears squashed antero-posteriorly (Fig. 19.21A); it is

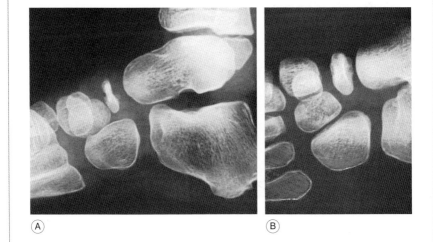

(A)   (B)

Fig. 19.21 Köhler's osteochondritis of the navicular bone. (A) Early stage. Bony nucleus dense and flattened antero-posteriorly. (B) Two years later. Bone texture restored; slight residual flattening.

[1] Alban Köhler (1874–1947) German pioneer in radiology worked in Wiesbaden and described the condition in 1908.

denser than normal, and may have a fragmented appearance. Serial radiographs during the 2-year span of the disease show the gradual evolution of the bone changes. After a stage of maximal density and deformation a few months after the onset there is gradual improvement until normal bone texture is restored (Fig. 19.21B).

Treatment. Despite the slow evolution of the bone changes prolonged treatment is not required. Good results follow symptomatic treatment. Usually all that is necessary is to rest the foot for 6–8 weeks in a walking plaster.

PAINFUL HEEL

The causes of painful heel are conveniently classified according to the site of the pain (Fig. 19.22).

Pain within the heel Disease of the calcaneus (osteomyelitis; tumour; Paget's disease) Arthritis of the subtalar joint	**Pain behind the heel** Rupture of the calcaneal tendon (p. 425) Calcaneal paratendinitis Post-calcaneal bursitis Calcaneal apophysitis
Pain beneath the heel Tender heel pad Plantar fasciitis	

DISEASE OF THE CALCANEUS

The calcaneus is subject, although rarely, to all types of infection of bone, the commonest being pyogenic infection (osteomyelitis). Occasionally it is the seat of a benign or malignant tumour. It may also be affected by other disorders of bone, such as Paget's disease.

Arthritis of the subtalar joint

The commonest type of arthritis in the subtalar joint is osteoarthritis secondary to fracture of the calcaneus (p. 444). The joint is occasionally subject to other forms of arthritis, such as pyogenic arthritis, rheumatoid arthritis, tuberculous arthritis, and gout.

Calcaneal paratendinitis (calcaneal tenosynovitis)

The calcaneal tendon is surrounded by loose connective tissue, or paratenon, which allows gliding movements. Rarely, this becomes inflamed from excessive friction. The condition should be termed paratendinitis rather than tenosynovitis, because there is no true synovial sheath.

Clinical features. The patient is usually an active athletic young adult. There is pain in the region of the calcaneal tendon, made worse by activities such as running or dancing. *On examination* there is tenderness on palpation between finger and thumb deep to the tendon (Fig. 19.22), and there is slight local thickening in this region. The tendon itself is of normal size and consistency.

The leg, ankle, and foot

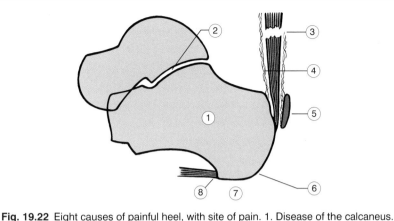

Fig. 19.22 Eight causes of painful heel, with site of pain. 1. Disease of the calcaneus. 2. Arthritis of the subtalar joint. 3. Ruptured calcaneal tendon. 4. Calcaneal paratendinitis. 5. Post-calcaneal bursitis. 6. Calcaneal apophysitis. 7. Tender heel pad. 8. Plantar fasciitis.

Treatment. Local physiotherapy may be helpful, particularly by the application of ultrasound therapy to the affected area, or from eccentric calf muscle training. In many cases relief is afforded by local injection of hydrocortisone deep to the tendon. (The tendon itself must not on any account be injected lest it be weakened, with serious risk of rupture.) In a resistant case operation may be required: it consists in excising the loose connective tissue surrounding and deep to the tendon.

Post-calcaneal bursitis

This is the commonest cause of pain behind the heel. It is often a cause of troublesome disability in young women.

Pathology. An adventitious bursa forms at the back of the heel, between the tuberosity of the calcaneus and the skin. Repeated friction against the back of the shoe leads to chronic inflammation and thickening of the walls of the bursa, and the sac may be distended with fluid. Prominence of the underlying bone aggravates the bursitis.

Clinical features. There is troublesome tenderness where the swelling is in contact with the shoe (Fig. 19.22). The symptoms are aggravated by walking, and they tend to be worse in winter than in summer; hence the term 'winter heel'. *On examination* there is an obvious gristly prominence at the back of the heel; the overlying skin is thickened and may be red.

Treatment. In mild or recent cases the symptoms can be controlled by protecting the back of the heel with a double layer of elastic adhesive strapping and by wearing shoes with soft backs. If these measures fail the bursa should be excised: its recurrence must be prevented by excising the prominent upper posterior corner of the calcaneal tuberosity, immediately above the attachment of the calcaneal tendon.

Calcaneal apophysitis (Sever's disease[1])

This harmless condition occurs only in children, during the period of active growth of the calcaneal apophysis. It was formerly believed to be an example of osteochondritis (p. 130), but it is now generally agreed that it is nothing more than a chronic strain at the attachment of the posterior apophysis of the calcaneus to the main body of the bone, possibly from the pull of the calcaneal tendon. It may thus be regarded as analogous to Osgood–Schlatter's disease of the tibial tubercle (p. 415), and totally unrelated to osteochondritis.

Clinical features. The child, usually between 8 and 13 years old, complains of pain behind the heel, and a slight limp may be noticed. *On examination* there is tenderness over the lower posterior part of the tuberosity of the calcaneus (Fig. 19.22). *Radiographs* usually fail to show any alteration from the normal. Importance has sometimes been attached to an appearance of fragmentation of the calcaneal apophysis, but this is a normal state, often seen in children without pain in the heel.

Treatment. In most cases treatment is not required, because the symptoms will gradually subside spontaneously. If the pain is troublesome, rest for a few weeks in a below-knee walking plaster will afford adequate relief.

Tender heel pad

This is a distinct clinical condition characterised by pain beneath the hind part of the heel on standing or walking.

Pathology. The site of the tenderness is the tough fibro-fatty tissue beneath the prominent weight-bearing part of the calcaneus. In some cases the lesion is probably no more than a simple contusion; but in most cases injury seems to play no part and it must be assumed that there is mild inflammation, of uncertain origin.

Clinical features. Pain beneath the heel on standing or walking is the only symptom. *On examination* there is well-marked local tenderness on firm palpation over the heel pad (Fig. 19.22).

Treatment. There is a tendency to slow spontaneous improvement. Recovery may be hastened by the injection of hydrocortisone locally at the site of greatest tenderness, and by providing a sponge-rubber heel cushion on an insole. Ultrasound therapy to the tender area is also worth a trial if pain persists. Anti-inflammatory medication should also be prescribed.

Plantar fasciitis

In this condition, which is believed to be inflammatory, there is pain beneath the anterior part of the calcaneus. It may be part of a more widespread inflammatory condition such as Reiter's disease.

Pathology. The lesion affects the soft tissues at the site of attachment of the plantar aponeurosis to the inferior aspect of the tuberosity of the calcaneus (Fig. 19.22).

Clinical features. The complaint is of pain beneath the heel on standing or walking; the pain extends medially and into the sole. The disability is sometimes severe. When the condition is part of a widespread inflammatory disorder both heels may be affected. *On examination* there is marked

---

[1] James Sever (1878–1964) American orthopaedic surgeon who was Chief at Boston Children's Hospital for 40 years and described the condition in 1912. He also wrote articles on neonatal brachial plexus injuries.

tenderness over the site of attachment of the plantar fascia to the calcaneus. The site of tenderness is further forward than it is in tender heel pad, just described. *Radiographs* usually do not show any abnormality. A sharp spur projecting forwards from the tuberosity of the calcaneus is sometimes found, but its significance is doubtful because such spurs may be present in patients without heel symptoms.

Treatment. Conservative treatment usually suffices if pursued energetically, though recovery may be slow. A course of non-steroidal anti-inflammatory drugs is usually prescribed. The heel should be protected by a resilient cushion on an insole. If these measures fail, local injection of hydrocortisone into the tender area may be tried. If the fasciitis is part of a widespread inflammatory disorder (notably Reiter's syndrome) treatment appropriate to the underlying condition should be instituted.

PAIN IN THE FOREFOOT (METATARSALGIA)

Pain in the forefoot is one of the commonest orthopaedic complaints. There are three main causes, of which the first is the most frequent:

1. anterior flat foot (dropped transverse arch)
2. stress fracture of a metatarsal bone (march fracture)
3. plantar digital neuritis (Morton's metatarsalgia).

Anterior flat foot (dropped transverse arch)

Permanent flattening of the transverse arch of the foot, with excessive weight-bearing pressure beneath the metatarsal heads, is the commonest cause of metatarsalgia. In most cases the primary cause is inefficiency of the intrinsic muscles of the foot.

Pathology. Even in normal feet the transverse arch is only a potential arch, not a constant one. But in the normal state the metatarsal heads can be raised from the ground at will by the action of the toes, held straight at the interphalangeal joints by the intrinsic muscles and flexed strongly at the metatarsophalangeal joints by the intrinsic muscles in conjunction with the long and short flexors (Fig. 19.23A). Thus the weight is shared between the metatarsal heads and the toes. If the intrinsic muscles are inefficient the toes are unable to fulfil their important weight-sharing function and all the pressure falls upon the metatarsal heads (Fig. 19.23B). The excessive pressure leads to the formation of callosities.

Clinical features. The main complaint is of pain beneath the forefoot. There may be secondary symptoms from pressure of the shoes upon deformed toes. *On examination* the forefoot is often splayed, appearing broader than normal. There are callosities beneath some or all of the metatarsal heads. The toes are often curled. The patient is unable to raise the metatarsal heads from the ground by pressing downwards with the toes – an indication that the intrinsic muscles are inefficient.

Treatment. In patients under 50 worthwhile improvement can usually be gained by a prolonged course of physiotherapy, designed to strengthen the intrinsic muscles by special exercises. In older patients this treatment is seldom effective, and instead a trial may be made of soft moulded orthotic insoles to

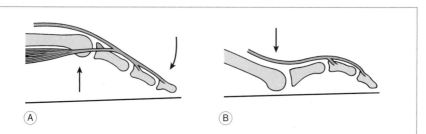

Fig. 19.23 Ⓐ Diagram to show the normal action of the toes in raising the metatarsal heads from the ground, whereby they share the weight with the metatarsal heads. This action is controlled mainly by the intrinsic muscles, which, by producing flexion at the metatarso-phalangeal joints and extension at the interphalangeal joints, cause the toes to press upon the ground, lifting the metatarsal heads. Ⓑ If the intrinsic muscles are inefficient all the weight must be borne by the metatarsal heads.

distribute the weight-bearing pressure over a wide area of the metatarsus. If there is a prominent callosity it may be pared away, with temporary relief.

If disability is severe, pain from local prominence of an individual metatarsal head in the sole may be relieved by osteotomy of the neck of the metatarsal and dorsal displacement of the head.

Stress fracture of a metatarsal bone (march fracture; fatigue fracture)

Stress or fatigue fractures are unusual in that there is no history of violence. The possibility of fracture may therefore be overlooked. A stress fracture of a metatarsal is not a common cause of pain in the forefoot but the possibility of its occurrence should be remembered.

Cause. The fracture is ascribed to long-continued or oft-repeated stress, hence the name as it is common in new military recruits subjected to excessive route marching; it has been likened to the fatigue fractures that sometimes occur in metals.

Pathology. The fracture usually affects the shaft of the second or third metatarsal bone, near its neck. It is no more than a hair-line crack, and there is no displacement of the fragments. In the process of healing a large mass of callus may form around the bone at the site of fracture. (This has occasionally been mistaken for a tumour.)

Clinical features. The complaint is of severe pain in the forefoot on walking. The onset is rapid but the patient is usually unable to ascribe it to an obvious cause. Enquiry may reveal, however, that he has recently done an unusual amount of walking or marching before the onset. *On examination* there is swelling at the dorsum of the forefoot, with marked and well-localised tenderness over the affected metatarsal bone.

Radiographs at first show only a faint hair-line crack which is easily overlooked (Fig. 19.24A), but after two or three weeks the callus surrounding the fracture is clearly visible and usually abundant (Fig. 19.24B).

Treatment. The fracture heals spontaneously; so treatment is purely symptomatic. Indeed in some cases treatment is not needed; but if pain is severe immobilisation in a below-knee walking plaster for three or four weeks is advised.

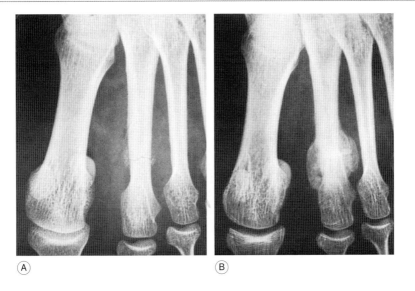

Fig. 19.24 Stress fracture of second metatarsal. (A) shows the initial radiograph, taken a week after the onset of pain. The fracture is seen as a fine crack across the bone. (B) shows the condition three weeks later, in the stage of healing. Abundant callus has formed about the site of fracture.

Plantar digital neuritis (Morton's metatarsalgia[1]; interdigital neuroma)

This condition, which is primarily an affection of a digital nerve, is characterised typically by metatarsal pain combined with a radiating pain in the third and fourth toes.

Pathology. The underlying lesion is a fibrous thickening or 'neuroma' of the digital nerve of the 3–4 cleft just proximal to its point of division into terminal branches. It takes the form of a fusiform swelling, usually about a centimetre long, surrounding the nerve as it lies in the space between the heads of the third and fourth metatarsals (Fig. 19.25). Occasionally the nerve to the 2–3 cleft is the one affected. The cause of the fibrous thickening is uncertain.

Clinical features. The patient is often a woman of middle age. She complains of pain in the forefoot on standing or walking. A characteristic feature is that the pain, arising in the metatarsal region, radiates forwards into the contiguous sides of the third and fourth toes, or to the fourth toe alone. Rarely, the cleft between the second and third toes is affected. The pain, like nerve pain in general, is piercing and disabling. Patients often state that they can relieve the pain by taking the shoe off and squeezing or manipulating the forefoot.

[1]Thomas Morton (1835–1903) American Civil War surgeon and founder of Philadelphia Orthopedic Hospital described the condition in 1876.

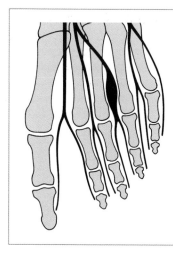

Fig. 19.25 Fibrous thickening of an interdigital nerve, a characteristic feature of plantar digital neuritis (Morton's metatarsalgia). The 'neuroma' is usually in the 3–4 cleft.

On examination the forefoot is often splayed, as in anterior flat foot. Sometimes a painful click can be elicited by compressing the metatarsal heads together from side to side, and upward pressure on the sole between the third and fourth metatarsal heads is painful.

Imaging. Plain radiographs are normal, but the abnormality of the nerve can be visualised with ultrasound or MRI scanning (Fig. 19.26) confirming the diagnosis.

Treatment. The patient should try first the effect of wearing a sponge-rubber metatarsal pad to support the anterior arch. If this fails to relieve the symptoms operative excision of the thickened segment of the nerve is recommended, though the patient must be warned that this leaves some residual numbness in the toe.

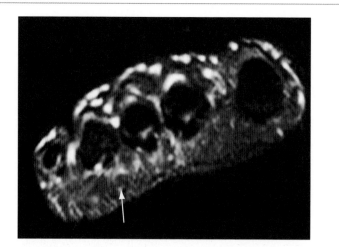

Fig. 19.26 Morton's neuroma shown on an axial T1 weighted MR scan of forefoot. The great toe is on the right of the image and the arrow indicates the small soft-tissue nodule in the interspace between the 3rd and 4th metatarsal heads.

PLANTAR WART (Verruca pedis; verruca plantaris)

Plantar warts may occur in any part of the sole of the foot, including the under surface of the heel. They are like warts elsewhere, except that they do not project beyond the skin surface. They are distinct from plantar callosities, which are simply localised thickenings of the skin at points of excessive pressure.

Cause. A virus infection is responsible.

Pathology. A wart is a simple papilloma, growing outwards from the basal layers of the skin. It is prevented by the pressure of weight-bearing from projecting much beyond the skin surface, but the surrounding skin is thickened, so the wart may have a total depth of up to half a centimetre. It slowly enlarges, but seldom reaches a diameter of as much as a centimetre.

Clinical features. The chief complaint is of severe localised pain on walking. *On examination* the skin surrounding the wart is thickened and therefore raised. The wart, a little darker in colour and with a mosaic surface, is seen in the centre of the raised area (Fig. 19.27). Its edge is clearly demarcated from the surrounding skin: this can be discerned easily if the skin is stretched away from the wart, when a tiny cleft becomes apparent between wart and skin. There is always marked local tenderness on pressure over the wart.

Diagnosis. The main difficulty is to distinguish warts from callosities. Warts occur anywhere on the sole, callosities only over points of pressure. Warts are also much more tender than callosities. But the most reliable distinguishing feature is that a wart has a mosaic surface and a clearly defined margin with a potential cleft between it and the skin (Fig. 19.28A), whereas a callosity blends imperceptibly with the surrounding normal skin (Fig. 19.28B).

Treatment. The local application of appropriate caustics is often successful. If this treatment fails the wart should be curetted out and the base lightly cauterised.

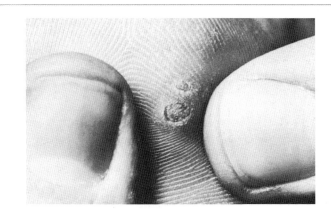

Fig. 19.27 Plantar wart. Note the clearly circumscribed outline and the slight cleft when the skin is stretched away from the wart.

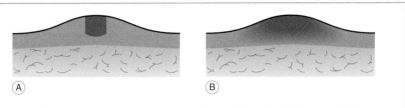

Fig. 19.28 Ⓐ Diagrammatic section of a plantar wart. It is clearly demarcated from the surrounding skin. Ⓑ Diagrammatic section of a callosity. It blends imperceptibly with the surrounding normal skin.

CALLOSITIES

A callosity is simply a localised thickening of the skin in response to abnormal pressure. It is nearly always secondary to a pre-existing disorder of the foot.

Plantar callosities are callosities on the sole of the foot. They occur under a prominent bone. They are commonest beneath the metatarsal heads when deficient intrinsic muscles prevent the toes from taking their proper share in weight-bearing (anterior flat foot, p. 449). They are also common beneath the base of the fifth metatarsal in patients who for any reason walk with the foot inverted.

Callosities on the toes often take the form of localised thickenings, when they are termed *corns*. They are caused by pressure against the shoe, and they are especially common when the dorsum of a toe is made unduly prominent by a fixed flexion deformity, as in hammer toe (see Fig. 19.33A, p. 459).

Treatment. The treatment is mainly that of the underlying condition. Palliative measures include paring of excess epidermis (preferably by a chiropodist, though simple instruments are available for use by the patient), and sponge-rubber padding to distribute the weight-bearing pressure over a wider area.

GANGLION

Ganglia are common on the dorsum of the foot and around the ankle. They are similar in all respects to the ganglia that occur at the back of the wrist and hand. They consist of thin-walled sacs filled with glairy viscous fluid, and the fibrous wall is usually connected deeply with a ligament, tendon sheath, or joint capsule. Clinically, a ganglion appears as a fluctuant subcutaneous swelling, which may be either soft or tense. If it causes trouble it should be excised.

DISORDERS OF THE TOES

HALLUX VALGUS

In hallux valgus the great toe is deviated laterally at the metatarso-phalangeal joint. It is common in women past middle age, and is not infrequent even in young women.

The leg, ankle, and foot

Cause. In some cases, particularly in children and adolescents, hereditary factors are responsible. But in most the deformity is caused by the toes being persistently forced laterally by enclosure in narrow pointed shoes. The wearing of high heels favours the development of hallux valgus because the forefoot is forced into the narrow pointed part of the shoe.

Pathology. Outward deviation of the great toe is the most obvious feature of the deformity, but a further, almost constant feature is that the first metatarsal is deviated medially, so that the gap between the heads of the first and second metatarsals is unduly wide (metatarsus primus varus). Indeed this may often be the primary defect. After several years two secondary changes occur. One is the formation of a thick-walled bursa (bunion) over the medial prominence of the metatarsal head; this may become inflamed, occasionally with suppuration. The second, a later development, is osteoarthritis of the metatarso-phalangeal joint consequent upon its mal-alignment (see Fig. 19.30B).

Clinical features. The patient is nearly always a woman, who is often at or past middle age when she seeks advice but may sometimes be a young woman or even an adolescent girl. The early symptoms arise from tenderness over the bunion from pressure against the shoe. There is also difficulty in getting comfortable footwear. Later, additional symptoms arise from osteoarthritis of the metatarso-phalangeal joint, and from flattening of the transverse arch (anterior flat foot, p. 449), which is a common associated deformity.

On examination the deformity is obvious at a glance (Figs 19.29A and 19.30A). The skin over the prominent joint is hard, reddened, and tender. Often a thick-walled bursa can be felt, and occasionally it is distended with fluid (Fig. 19.30B). In relatively early cases metatarso-phalangeal joint movements are free and painless, but in severe cases of many years'

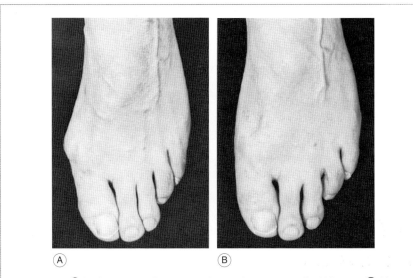

Ⓐ Ⓑ

Fig. 19.29 Ⓐ Hallux valgus of moderate degree in a woman of middle age. Ⓑ After correction by displacement osteotomy of the neck of the first metatarsal. Normal appearance restored.

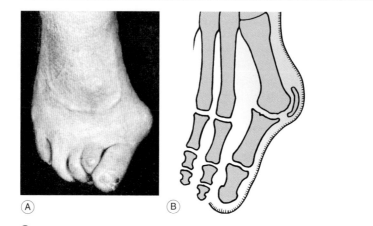

Fig. 19.30 Ⓐ Severe hallux valgus. The great toe is over-riding the deformed second toe. Ⓑ Diagram showing the prominent metatarsal head with overlying bunion, and osteoarthritis from long-standing mal-alignment of the joint.

duration the secondary osteoarthritis makes movement limited and painful. In late cases the forefoot is often flat and splayed, and the toes may be severely curled (Fig. 19.30A).

Treatment. In mild cases treatment is not required, but footwear must be selected with care to obtain adequate width. It may also be worthwhile to protect the bunion with pads of felt, and to wear a wedge of plastic foam between the great toe and the second toe to reduce the deformity.

If disability is troublesome operation is advisable. There is much variation of opinion among different surgeons on the choice of treatment. Mention will be made here of only four of the many methods that are available.

Trimming of 'exostosis'. When the deviation of the toe is slight, but troublesome symptoms arise from localised prominence or 'exostosis' of the first metatarsal head at the medial side of the foot, it may sometimes be sufficient simply to excise the bursa and chisel away the medial prominence of the metatarsal head without disturbing the joint itself. There is, however, a tendency for the symptoms to recur after this operation, and in general the results are so disappointing that the operation is now seldom recommended.

Displacement osteotomy of the neck of the first metatarsal bone. This is illustrated in Fig. 19.31. After division of the neck of the metatarsal the head fragment is displaced markedly laterally (Fig. 19.31B). The outward shift of the metatarsal head eliminates the prominence of the 'exostosis' without the need for its removal. The soft tissues between the heads of the first and second metatarsals are also relaxed, allowing permanent reduction of the subluxation at the first metatarso-phalangeal joint. After operation the toe may be immobilised in plaster for 6 weeks or fixed with a screw to ensure union at the site of osteotomy without loss of position.

By a process of remodelling, the alignment of the first metatarsal is gradually altered after operation so that it lies closer to the second metatarsal (Fig. 19.31B).

In this operation the joint itself is left undisturbed, indeed unopened. The operation gives good results in patients with relatively slight deformity (Fig. 19.29B): it does not shorten the toe appreciably or impair active movement,

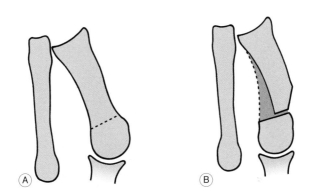

Fig. 19.31 Displacement osteotomy of the neck of the first metatarsal. Ⓐ Before operation. Note the wide gap between the first and second metatarsals. Ⓑ After division of the first metatarsal through its neck the head fragment is displaced markedly laterally, so that its medial prominence (the 'exostosis') disappears. The metatarso-phalangeal subluxation is automatically reduced. Remodelling (interrupted line) alters the shape of the metatarsal and the intermetatarsal gap is narrowed.

and it is therefore particularly suitable for young patients who wish to lead an energetic life.

Excision arthroplasty of the first metatarso-phalangeal joint by Keller's[1] method is widely used in elderly patients. The object is to create a flail, freely movable false joint between the first metatarsal and the proximal phalanx, with correction of the mal-alignment. This is done by excising the proximal half of the proximal phalanx so that a gap is left between the two bones: at the same time the bursa is excised and the medial prominence of the metatarsal head is smoothed off with a chisel (Fig. 19.32A).

The space created by excision of the base of the phalanx fills with rubbery fibrous tissue, and a false joint forms which allows a reasonable range of movement (Fig. 19.32B).

This operation leaves the great toe markedly shorter than normal and rather floppy, with poor active control over toe movements. The patient should be warned about this in advance. Nevertheless the main symptoms are relieved and the result is usually satisfactory in elderly patients who do not wish to walk long distances or to indulge in athletic pursuits.

Arthrodesis of the metatarso-phalangeal joint of the hallux in a position of slight extension allows full and permanent correction of the valgus deformity, even if it is very severe – but at the cost of loss of mobility.

When severe hallux valgus in an elderly patient is associated with flattening of the transverse arch and marked clawing of the toes (see Fig. 19.30A), operation of any type may be disappointing and it may be wiser to rely upon well-made surgical shoes.

[1]William Keller (1874–1959) Distinguished American Army surgeon who served as a general surgeon throughout his long military career, while developing his operation for bunions in 1904.

The leg, ankle, and foot

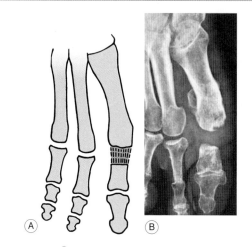

Fig. 19.32 Hallux valgus. Ⓐ Excision arthroplasty (Keller's operation): removal of the proximal half of the proximal phalanx. The resulting gap fills with flexible fibrous tissue. The bursa and the underlying prominence of the metatarsal head have also been removed. Ⓑ Radiograph 10 years after Keller's operation for hallux valgus.

HAMMER TOE

The term hammer toe denotes a fixed flexion deformity of an interphalangeal joint.

Cause. Presumably an imbalance of the delicate arrangement of flexor and extensor tendons is responsible; but the precise explanation of its occurrence is unknown. Hammer deformity, especially of the second toe, is often associated with severe hallux valgus (see Fig. 19.30A).

Pathology. The proximal interphalangeal joint of the second toe is that most commonly affected. The affected joint is sharply angled into flexion. Secondary contracture of the plantar aspect of the joint capsule fixes the deformity, and a callosity usually forms over the dorsum of the flexed joint, from pressure against the shoe (Fig. 19.33A).

Clinical features. Typically the deformity affects only one toe – usually the second. In the characteristic deformity the proximal interphalangeal joint is in fixed flexion, and the distal interphalangeal joint, though still mobile, rests in compensatory hyperextension (Fig. 19.33A). The symptoms, if any, are caused by the overlying callosity or 'corn' or pain from bearing weight on the end of the toenail.

Treatment. If symptoms are slight the deformity may be accepted, or conservative treatment by protective felt pads may be sufficient. In severe cases operation gives gratifying results. The joint surfaces are excised and the joint is arthrodesed or pseudarthrosed in the corrected position (Fig. 19.33B).

UNDER-RIDING TOE (Congenital curled toe)

Children are often brought for advice because one of the smaller toes, often the fourth, is curled inwards and lies beneath the adjacent toe. The condition does

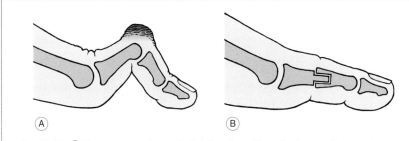

Fig. 19.33 Ⓐ Hammer toe: the typical deformity, with callosity over the prominent proximal joint. Ⓑ Peg arthrodesis, for correction of hammer toe.

not cause any symptoms during childhood, and it should be left alone until adolescence or early adult life, when the toe can easily be straightened if it begins to cause symptoms. Similar principles apply to the management of over-riding toe.

RHEUMATOID ARTHRITIS OF THE TOE JOINTS

Deformity of the forefoot is a common cause of pain and disability in rheumatoid arthritis, but may be underdiagnosed because of the more visible problems in the patient's other lower limb joints. Characteristically the metatarso-phalangeal joints are most affected, with destruction of articular cartilage, dorsal subluxation of the phalanges and clawing of the toes. Painful skin callosities then develop on the sole beneath the prominent metatarsal heads and on the dorsum of the flexed toes from the pressure of footwear.

In the early stages *radiographs* show only joint narrowing and marginal erosions. In the later stages there may be subluxation or dislocation of the metatarso-phalangeal joints with marked destruction of bone (Fig. 19.34).

Treatment. Minor deformity may be managed by the provision of moulded insoles and broad-fitting shoes with soft uppers. In advanced disease with fixed painful deformities forefoot reconstruction is advisable and should normally precede surgery for the hindfoot or knee joints to reduce the risk of ulceration and infection. There are a number of different operative procedures to restore the forefoot alignment by excision of the bases of the proximal phalanges and trimming of the metatarsal heads (excision arthroplasty). Following wound healing, patients may require the provision of orthotic insoles and surgical shoes to allow them to walk in comfort.

OSTEOARTHRITIS OF THE TOE JOINTS

In practice, osteoarthritis in the toes is seen commonly only in the metatarso-phalangeal joint of the great toe. This has been termed *hallux rigidus*. Occasionally the metatarso-phalangeal joint of one of the smaller toes is affected, usually as a late result of Freiberg's disease of a metatarsal head (p. 462).

Hallux rigidus

This is osteoarthritis of the metatarso-phalangeal joint of the great toe. Like osteoarthritis elsewhere, it is caused by wear and tear, but previous injury or disease of the joint is an important predisposing factor.

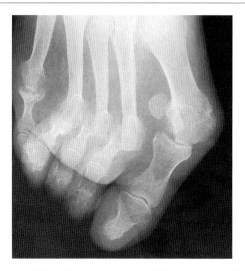

Fig. 19.34 Severe toe deformities from long-established rheumatoid arthritis. Note the subluxation of the metatarso-phalangeal joint of the great toe, and dislocation of several of the lesser toes at the metatarso-phalangeal joints. Some of the metatarsal heads show erosion of bone.

Pathology. The changes are like those of osteoarthritis in other joints. The articular cartilage is gradually worn away from both surfaces of the joint until eventually the subchondral bone is exposed. The exposed bone becomes hard and glossy (eburnation). The marginal bone hypertrophies to form osteophytes, which often cause obvious thickening, especially at the dorsum of the toe.

Clinical features. The complaint is of pain in the base of the great toe on walking. *On examination* the metatarso-phalangeal joint is palpably thickened from osteophyte formation. If an osteophyte is especially prominent on the dorsal or medial aspect of the joint a thick-walled bursa (bunion) may form over it; occasionally the bursa is distended with fluid. Flexion and extension of the toe at the metatarso-phalangeal joint are restricted – usually markedly so by the time the patient seeks advice (Fig. 19.35A). Forced dorsiflexion of the painful joint on walking is the main source of the disability. (It should be remembered that the normal range of dorsiflexion at the metatarso-phalangeal joint of the great toe is nearly 90°.)

Radiographs confirm the presence of osteoarthritis. The cartilage space is narrowed, the subchondral bone tends to be sclerotic, and there is osteophytic spurring of the joint margins (Fig. 19.35B).

Treatment. In mild cases treatment is not required. When treatment is called for, conservative measures are usually worth a trial first. A metatarsal bar should be fitted beneath the sole of the shoe at the metatarso-phalangeal level. This acts as a rocker in walking, and so reduces the dorsiflexion required of the toes when weight is brought onto the forefoot from the heel.

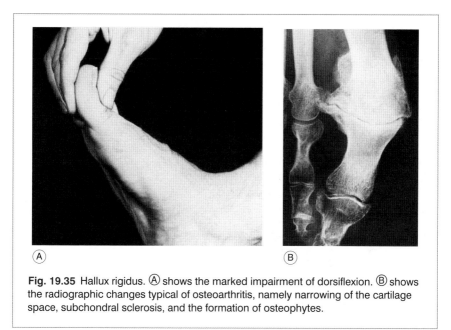

Fig. 19.35 Hallux rigidus. Ⓐ shows the marked impairment of dorsiflexion. Ⓑ shows the radiographic changes typical of osteoarthritis, namely narrowing of the cartilage space, subchondral sclerosis, and the formation of osteophytes.

When the disability is severe operation should be advised. One method is to create a flail joint by excision of the base of the proximal phalanx (Keller's arthroplasty), as for hallux valgus. Many surgeons find, however, that arthrodesis of the metatarso-phalangeal joint (see Fig. 4.1B) in a position of slight extension gives better results, with complete relief of pain.

Osteoarthritis of other toe joints

Osteoarthritis of the other metatarso-phalangeal joints is uncommon except as a sequel to Freiberg's disease of a metatarsal head (see below).

GOUTY ARTHRITIS OF THE GREAT TOE JOINTS (General description of gouty arthritis, p. 143)

The joints of the great toe are those most often affected in gout, especially in the first attack.

Clinical features. The patient is usually over 40, and more commonly a man than a woman. There is a sudden onset of severe pain in the great toe, often during the night.

On examination the toe is swollen, red, and extremely tender. Joint movements are impossible because of pain. There is sometimes slight pyrexia. The patient will usually recall previous similar attacks lasting a few days, with freedom from pain in the intervals. *Radiographs* are normal in the early stages. *Investigations*: There is sometimes a mild leucocytosis. The plasma urate level is usually raised.

Chronic gout. In this form deposits of sodium biurate in and around the joints of the great toe lead to persistent nodular thickening. *Radiographs* show rounded areas of transradiance in the bone ends; these represent deposits of sodium biurate (which is transradiant) in the subchondral bone.

Diagnosis. Acute gout is easily mistaken for acute infective arthritis. Features suggestive of gout are: a raised plasma urate level; a history of previous attacks, with symptom-free intervals; and the presence of tophi in the ears or elsewhere.

Course. Gout usually occurs in recurrent attacks. In the early years, an acute attack subsides within a few days, leaving the joint clinically normal. In chronic gout the joint is gradually disorganised, causing permanent disability.

Treatment. Acute attacks respond to selected non-steroidal anti-inflammatory drugs such as indometacin or naproxen, begun in high dosage which is reduced after two or three days, or to colchicine. Meanwhile the foot should be rested, and the toe should be protected from pressure by a bulky wool dressing. The treatment of recurrent and chronic gout was detailed on page 145.

FREIBERG'S DISEASE OF A METATARSAL HEAD[1]
(Metatarsal osteochondritis)

Freiberg's disease of a metatarsal head is regarded by some as an example of osteochondritis juvenilis (p. 130) and by others as osteochondritis dissecans (p. 153). It may therefore be advisable to use the non-committal eponymous title for the present. The essential feature of Freiberg's disease is partial necrosis and fragmentation of a metatarsal head, which may become deformed under the pressure of weight-bearing. It is an uncommon condition.

Pathology. The epiphysis of one of the metatarsal heads – nearly always the second or third – is the part affected. The bony nucleus becomes necrotic and granular. Part of the articular surface separates, usually remaining attached only by a hinge of articular cartilage. While it is in this crumbly state the metatarsal head is crushed by the pressure against it of the base of the proximal phalanx of the toe. The articular surface of the metatarsal head thus loses its normal dome-shaped contour and becomes flat (Fig. 19.36). After about 2 years the texture of the bone returns to normal, but flattening of the articular surface remains. Later, the distortion of the joint surface often leads to osteoarthritis.

Clinical features. At the time of onset the patient is 14 to 17 years old. There is pain in the affected metatarso-phalangeal joint, worse on standing or walking. *On examination* there is slight thickening in the region of the head of the metatarsal, which is tender on pressure. Movements of the metatarso-phalangeal joint are slightly restricted and painful. *Radiographs* reveal the nature of the trouble, though at first the changes are very slight and may be overlooked. Later the head of the metatarsal appears fragmented, with patches of increased density. Finally, the articular surface is flattened, so that the end of the bone appears square-cut instead of round (Fig. 19.36).

---

[1]Albert H. Freiberg (1868–1940) American orthopaedic surgeon worked throughout his career in Cincinnati, Ohio. He described the condition, which he described as an infarction from local trauma, in 1914.

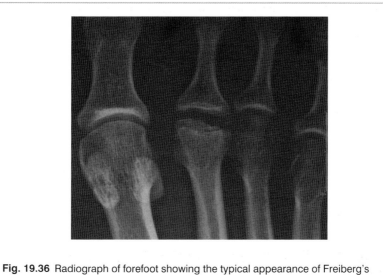

Fig. 19.36 Radiograph of forefoot showing the typical appearance of Freiberg's disease in the second metatarsal. There is an abnormal appearance of the metatarsal head, which is flattened and sclerotic due to osteochondritis.

Treatment. When the diagnosis can be made in the early stage – before marked radiographic changes are apparent – operation offers a hope of preventing permanent distortion of the joint surface. Through a window cut in the dorsal surface of the metatarsal neck the necrotic bone of the head is curetted out and replaced by cancellous chip bone grafts, packed firmly enough to restore the normal dome-shaped contour of the articular surface. Thereafter the toe is supported in a plaster cuff for 6 weeks.

When deformity of the metatarsal head is already well established at the time of diagnosis attempted restoration of the articular surface is of no avail. Expectant treatment is then recommended. If pain is troublesome rest in a walking plaster for 2 months may afford relief; but if disabling osteoarthritis develops later the head of the metatarsal should be excised.

INGROWING TOE NAIL (Embedded toe nail)

Ingrowing toe nail is common only in the great toe.

Cause. Some persons have toes that are prone to develop ingrowing toe nail. But the main causative factors are incorrect cutting of the nail, pressure on the nail-wall (lateral skin fold) by the shoe or by the adjacent second toe, and accumulation of dirt and sweat.

When the nail is cut its sides should be left long enough to project beyond the terminal pulp (Fig. 19.37A): if it is cut too short a sharp corner of nail lies in contact with the lateral skin fold (Fig. 19.37B), and this corner may tend to embed itself in the skin, especially if there is local pressure at the side of the toe. In the presence of dirt and sweat, infection is then liable to arise.

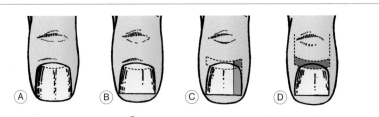

Fig. 19.37 (A) Nail cut correctly. (B) Nail cut too short: corners dig into pulp. (C) Operation for ingrowing toe nail. A strip of nail is avulsed and its re-growth is prevented by excision of a segment of the germinal matrix. (D) Operation for permanent ablation of the whole nail. After avulsion of the nail, only the germinal matrix need be excised to prevent re-growth. The raw area is covered by advancing the proximal skin flap.

Clinical features. The lesion may be at the medial or (more commonly) the lateral border of the nail, or both. There is pain at the affected anterior corner of the nail. *On examination* the skin fold is inflamed, and there may be local suppuration where the corner of the nail digs into the skin.

Treatment. In mild cases conservative treatment may suffice. Pledgets of gauze soaked in alcohol (surgical spirit) are tucked beneath the corner of the nail twice a day, and the nail is allowed to grow until its edges project beyond the skin folds (Fig. 19.37A).

In long-standing cases operation is advisable. If only one side of the nail is involved it is sufficient to avulse a strip of nail at the affected side and then to prevent re-growth of this part. Since the nail is formed only from the germinal matrix – the proximal curved segment of the nail bed that corresponds to the lunula – and not from the nail bed as a whole, it is necessary to remove only an appropriate piece of the germinal matrix to prevent regrowth (Fig. 19.37C).

In the worst cases, with infection at both sides of the nail, permanent ablation of the entire nail by excision of the whole of the germinal matrix is more satisfactory (Fig. 19.37D). The small raw area that remains can be covered simply by advancing a dorsal skin flap, based proximally and with its free edge at the nail fold.

SUBUNGUAL EXOSTOSIS

A subungual exostosis is a bony outgrowth from the dorsal surface of the distal phalanx of a toe – usually the great toe. It projects upwards and forwards between the tip of the nail and the terminal pulp. The nail is raised and deformed, and the skin of the pulp overlying the outgrowth is thickened and hard. There is sharp pain when pressure is applied over the nail or terminal pulp. *Radiographs* show the exostosis, which is seen best in the lateral projection.

Treatment. The exostosis should be excised through a terminal incision just beyond the tip of the nail.

ONYCHOGRYPOSIS

Translated from the Greek, this means 'hooked nail'. The term is descriptive. The nail – usually of the great toe – is enormously thickened, discoloured and curved, eventually resembling a miniature ox-horn (Fig. 19.38). The condition is due to a chronic fungal infection of the nail.

Treatment. Simple removal of the nail is an adequate temporary measure; but the new nail will become similarly deformed. The chance of this is reduced with appropriate oral antifungal therapy. For permanent cure the nail bed must be ablated by excision of the germinal matrix, as described in the section on ingrowing toe nail (p. 464).

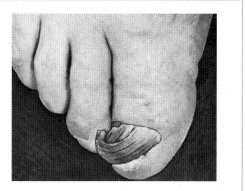

Fig. 19.38 Onychogryposis.

Index

Note: Page numbers in *italics* refer to figures.

Index

Index

Index